ADVANCES IN

Pediatrics

Editor-in-Chief
Carol D. Berkowitz, MD, FAAP, FACEP

Chief, Division of General Pediatrics,
Department of Pediatrics Aurora,
Harbor-UCLA Medical Center,
Distinguished Professor of Pediatrics,
David Geffen School of Medicine at UCLA,
Torrance, California

ELSEVIER

PHILADELPHIA LONDON TORONTO MONTREAL SYDNEY TOKYO

ADVANCES IN
Pediatrics

VOLUMES 1 THROUGH 64 (OUT OF PRINT)

VOLUME 65

Director, Continuity Publishing: Taylor Ball
Editor: Kerry Holland
Developmental Editor: Donald Mumford

Editorial Office:
Elsevier
1600 John F. Kennedy Blvd,
Suite 1800
Philadelphia, PA 19103-2899

International Standard Serial Number: 0065-3101
International Standard Book Number: 13: 978-0-323-75629-7

ADVANCES IN
Pediatrics

CONTRIBUTORS

ANA M. ALVAREZ, MD, FAAP, FPIDS, Associate Professor, Pediatric Infectious Diseases and Immunology, University of Florida College of Medicine Jacksonville, University of Florida Center for HIV/AIDS Research, Education and Service (UF CARES), Wolfson Children's Hospital, Jacksonville, Florida, USA

NELLY AMARIGLIO, PhD, Clinical Psychologist, Department of General Pediatrics, Children's Hospital of Los Angeles, Los Angeles, California, USA

SHAARA ARGO, MD, University of South Florida, Tampa, Florida, USA

CAROL D. BERKOWITZ, MD, FAAP, FACEP, Chief, Division of General Pediatrics, Department of Pediatrics, Harbor-UCLA Medical Center, Distinguished Professor of Pediatrics, UCLA David Geffen School of Medicine, Torrance, California, USA

KIRSTEN BIBBINS-DOMINGO, MD, PhD, Department of Epidemiology and Biostatistics, University of California, San Francisco, San Francisco, California, USA

MARIA DEMMA I. CABRAL, MD, FAAP, Assistant Professor, Department of Pediatric and Adolescent Medicine, Western Michigan University Homer Stryker M.D. School of Medicine, Kalamazoo, Michigan, USA

HEATHER CAMPBELL, MD, Neonatal-Perinatal Medicine Fellow, The University of North Carolina at Chapel Hill, Chapel Hill, North Carolina, USA

AILEEN CANNON, MD, Assistant Professor of Pediatrics, University of South Florida, Morsani College of Medicine, Tampa, Florida, USA

ELIZABETH DAWSON-HAHN, MD, MPH, FAAP, Acting Assistant Professor of Pediatrics, Division of General Pediatrics, University of Washington, Seattle, Washington, USA

KALYANI DERASARI, MD, Assistant Professor of Pediatrics, University of South Florida, Morsani College of Medicine, Tampa, Florida, USA

LISA DINH, MD, University of South Florida, Tampa, Florida, USA

CARLA FRANCISCO, MD, Assistant Clinical Professor, Pediatric Neurology and Multiple Sclerosis Clinic, University of California, San Francisco, Pediatric Brain Center, San Francisco, California, USA

RODNEY FRIEND, MD, Assistant Professor of Pediatrics, University of South Florida, Morsani College of Medicine, Tampa, Florida, USA

GISELLE Y. GUERRERO, MD, Sleep Medicine Fellow, University of South Florida, Tampa, Florida, USA

MELISSA HARADA, MD, Developmental-Behavioral Pediatric Fellow, Department of Pediatrics, UCLA David Geffen School of Medicine, Los Angeles, California, USA

KAM LUN HON, MD, FAAP, Professor, Department of Pediatrics, The Chinese University of Hong Kong, Shatin, Hong Kong

EMILY M. HSIEH, MD, Center for Cell and Gene Therapy, Baylor College of Medicine, Houston Methodist Hospital and Texas Children's Hospital, Texas Children's Cancer and Hematology Centers/Baylor College of Medicine, Houston, Texas, USA

ROBERT S. KAHN, MD, MPH, University of Cincinnati College of Medicine, Cincinnati Children's Hospital Medical Center, Cincinnati, Ohio, USA

RUSSELL S. KIRBY, PhD, MS, FACE, Distinguished University Professor and Marrell Endowed Chair, Strategic Area Faculty Lead for Population Health Science, College of Public Health, University of South Florida, Tampa, Florida, USA

IRENE KOOLWIJK, MD, MPH, Assistant Professor, Department of Pediatrics, UCLA David Geffen School of Medicine, Los Angeles, California, USA

ABIGAIL L.H. KROENING, MD, FAAP, Assistant Professor of Pediatrics, Division of Developmental and Behavioral Pediatrics, Golisano Children's Hospital, University of Rochester, Rochester, New York, USA

ANDA K. KUO, MD, Department of Pediatrics, University of California, San Francisco, San Francisco, California, USA

MEGAN M. LANGILLE, MD, Assistant Professor, Pediatrics, University of California, Los Angeles, Harbor-UCLA Medical Center, Torrance, California, USA

LATASHIA-LIKA LELEA, MD, MPH, MSc, Obstetrics and Gynecology Resident, University of Central Florida College of Medicine, UCF/HCA Consortium – Gainesville, North Florida Regional Medical Center, Gainesville, Florida, USA

ALEXANDER A.C. LEUNG, MD, MPH, FRCPC, MRCP (UK), FACP, Assistant Professor of Medicine, Departments of Medicine, Community Health Sciences, and Oncology, The University of Calgary, Calgary, Alberta, Canada

ALEXANDER K.C. LEUNG, MBBS, FRCPC, FRCP (UK & Irel), FRCPCH, FAAP, Clinical Professor of Pediatrics, The University of Calgary, Pediatric Consultant, The Alberta Children's Hospital, Calgary, Alberta, Canada

JACLYN LEWIS-CROSWELL, PsyD, Licensed Clinical Psychologist, Tampa General Hospital, Tampa, Florida, USA

ABIMBOLA MICHAEL-ASALU, MBBS, MPH, Department of Community and Family Health, College of Public Health, University of South Florida, Tampa, Florida, USA

TANYA L. KOWALCZYK MULLINS, MD, MS, Associate Professor of Pediatrics, Division of Adolescent and Transition Medicine, Cincinnati Children's Hospital Medical Center, Department of Pediatrics, University of Cincinnati College of Medicine, Cincinnati, Ohio, USA

SAGARIKA NALLU, MD, Assistant Professor, Director of Pediatric Sleep Medicine, Chief of Pediatric Neurology, Department of Pediatrics, University of South Florida, Morsani College of Medicine, Tampa, Florida, USA

REBECCA M. PLANT, MD, Assistant Professor of Pediatrics, Associate Program Director of Residency Program, University of South Florida, Tampa, Florida, USA

JOSEPH A. PUCCIO, MD, Associate Professor of Pediatrics, University of South Florida, Morsani College of Medicine, Tampa, Florida, USA

MOBEEN H. RATHORE, MD, CPE, FAAP, FPIDS, FSHEA, FIDSA, FACPE, Professor, Pediatric Infectious Diseases and Immunology, University of Florida College of Medicine Jacksonville, University of Florida Center for HIV/AIDS Research, Education and Service (UF CARES), Wolfson Children's Hospital, Jacksonville, Florida, USA

MARY K. ROJEK, PhD, Chair, Sex and Gender Health Collaborative, American Medical Women's Association, Schaumburg, Illinois, USA

RAYNE H. ROUCE, MD, Center for Cell and Gene Therapy, Baylor College of Medicine, Houston Methodist Hospital and Texas Children's Hospital, Texas Children's Cancer and Hematology Centers/Baylor College of Medicine, Houston, Texas, USA

ALICE RUTATANGWA, DO, MS, Pediatric Multiple Sclerosis/Neuroimmunology Clinical Fellow, Pediatric Neurology and Multiple Sclerosis Clinic, University of California, San Francisco, Pediatric Brain Center, San Francisco, California, USA

MONICA SHAH, MD, University of South Florida, Tampa, Florida, USA

PAMELA S. SINGER, MD, MS, Assistant Professor of Pediatric Nephrology, Cohen Children's Medical Center, Donald and Barbara Zucker School of Medicine at Hofstra/Northwell, New Hyde Park, New York, USA

DAVID H.M. STEFFIN, MD, Center for Cell and Gene Therapy, Baylor College of Medicine, Houston Methodist Hospital and Texas Children's Hospital, Texas Children's Cancer and Hematology Centers/Baylor College of Medicine, Houston, Texas, USA

DIANE M. STRAUB, MD, MPH, Professor of Pediatrics, Division of Adolescent Medicine, University of South Florida, Tampa, Florida, USA

NICOLE M. SUMMERS, PhD, MS, Department of Population Science and Policy, Southern Illinois University, Springfield, Illinois, USA

GENEVIEVE TAYLOR, MD, Neonatal-Perinatal Medicine Fellow, The University of North Carolina at Chapel Hill, Chapel Hill, North Carolina, USA

ALAN TOMINES, MD, Clinical Associate Professor, Department of Pediatrics, UCLA David Geffen School of Medicine, Medical Director of Information Systems, Enterprise Information Services, Cedars-Sinai Medical Center, Adjunct Professor, Department of Health Policy and Management, UCLA Fielding School of Public Health, Los Angeles, California, USA; Clinical Associate Professor, Harbor-UCLA Medical Center, Torrance, California, USA

SAMEER VOHRA, MD, JD, MA, Department of Population Science and Policy, School of Medicine, Southern Illinois University, Springfield, Illinois, USA

JANICE L. WERBINSKI, MD, FACOG, NCMP, Clinical Associate Professor Emerita, Department of Obstetrics and Gynecology, Western Michigan University Homer Stryker M.D. School of Medicine, Kalamazoo, Michigan, USA; Executive Director, Sex and Gender Health Collaborative, American Medical Women's Association, Schaumburg, Illinois, USA

HOPE WILLS, MA, RD, CSP, IBCLC, Clinical Dietitian IV, Department of Clinical Nutrition Services, Children's Hospital of Los Angeles, Los Angeles, California, USA

LARA M. WITTINE, MD, FCCP, Assistant Professor, University of South Florida, Morsani College of Medicine, Tampa, Florida, USA

CONTENTS

VOLUME 66 • 2019

Tall Stature in Children

Alexander K.C. Leung, Alexander A.C. Leung, and Kam Lun Hon

Updates on Hypertension and New Guidelines

Pamela S. Singer

Cerebral Palsy: Diagnosis, Epidemiology, Genetics, and Clinical Update

Abimbola Michael-Asalu, Genevieve Taylor, Heather Campbell, Latashia-Lika Lelea, and Russell S. Kirby

Resurgence of Syphilis

Joseph A. Puccio, Aileen Cannon, Kalyani Derasari, and Rodney Friend

Nonoccupational Postexposure Prophylaxis and Preexposure Prophylaxis for Human Immunodeficiency Virus Prevention in Adolescents and Young Adults

Diane M. Straub and Tanya L. Kowalczyk Mullins

Clostridium difficile Infection in Children

Ana M. Alvarez and Mobeen H. Rathore

Advances in Pediatrics 66 (2019) xix–xx
ADVANCES IN PEDIATRICS

Introduction

Carol D. Berkowitz, MD, FAAP, FACEP

The pace of change of medical practice has escalated exponentially in recent years. The classic adage that it takes 17 years between medical discoveries and the implementation of recommendations is no longer acceptable. Even knowing which drug to recommend is challenging. The number of FDA-approved drugs increased from 2000 in 1940 to 12,000 by 2010. Clinical medicine is changing so rapidly, clinicians recently out of residency may find that the guidelines they were taught are no longer contemporary. And one must be not only aware of what's new but also of what is no longer recommended. Reversals in medical practice occur regularly, impacting standard of care and decision-making. It is reported that 40% of the articles published in *New England Journal* between 2002 and 2012, recommended reversal in clinical practice protocols. Patients and parents, with ready access to the Internet, may be more aware of these changing recommendations than many practitioners. Additionally, there is greater emphasis on precision medicine and individualizing patient care. It is increasingly challenging for the practicing physician to remain up-to-date in what's new and recommended and what's no longer endorsed. As in the past, *Advances in Pediatrics* will review some of the newest emerging areas including precision population health, sex and gender differences, gene therapy and telehealth. Other chapters focus on common pediatric problems such as feeding and sleep disorders, tall stature and hypertension as well as the unique health care needs of immigrant and refugee children. Neurological conditions including cerebral palsy and multiple sclerosis are also reviewed and clinical updates provided. Infectious disease remain on the forefront with the resurgence of syphilis, *Clostrium difficile* and prophylactic management for HIV. Staying current is always a challenge for the practicing physician, especially in this age of complex medical conditions and complex

https://doi.org/10.1016/j.yapd.2019.05.001

health-care systems which may not have embraced a personalized approach to the individual patient.

Carol D. Berkowitz, MD, FAAP, FACEP
Division of General Pediatrics
Department of Pediatrics
Harbor-UCLA Medical Center
David Geffen School of Medicine at UCLA
1000 West Carson Street
Torrance, CA 90509, USA

E-mail address: cberkowitz52@gmail.com

Advances in Pediatrics 66 (2019) 1–13

ADVANCES IN PEDIATRICS

The Promise of Precision Population Health

Reducing Health Disparities Through a Community Partnership Framework

Anda K. Kuo, MD[a,*], Nicole M. Summers, PhD, MS[b], Sameer Vohra, MD, JD, MA[c], Robert S. Kahn, MD, MPH[d], Kirsten Bibbins-Domingo, MD, PhD[e]

[a]Department of Pediatrics, University of California, San Francisco, 1001 Potrero Avenue, MS6E, San Francisco, CA 94110, USA; [b]Department of Population Science and Policy, Southern Illinois University, 201 East Madison, Springfield, IL 62794, USA; [c]Department of Population Science and Policy, School of Medicine, Southern Illinois University, 201 East Madison, PO Box 19664, Springfield, IL 62794-9664, USA; [d]University of Cincinnati College of Medicine, Cincinnati Children's Hospital Medical Center, 3333 Burnet Avenue, Cincinnati, OH 45229, USA; [e]Department of Epidemiology and Biostatistics, University of California, San Francisco, 550 16th Street, San Francisco, CA 94158, USA

Keywords

- Precision medicine • Population health • Precision population health
- Precision public health • Community partnerships • Community engagement
- Community-based participatory research • Health disparities

Key points

- Precision medicine approaches provide opportunities to understand health and disease across populations and to target interventions that will simultaneously improve health and reduce health disparities.

Continued

Health care in the United States is characterized by extremes, with novel scientific breakthroughs and state-of-the-art, specialty care juxtaposed by some of the worst health outcomes [1]. The United States ranks lowest in maternal mortality, infant mortality, and life expectancy compared with other high-income nations and also has the highest total spending on

None of the authors have any commercial or financial conflicts of interest.

*Corresponding author. *E-mail address:* anda.kuo@ucsf.edu

https://doi.org/10.1016/j.yapd.2019.03.002

Continued

- Inclusion of community members as experts is foundational to the promise of precision population health, allowing an accurate understanding of the root causes of poor health and the identification of effective interventions.
- The authors provide a framework that illustrates the iterative interplay between the key elements of precision population health and community-based participatory research to achieve health equity.
- Institutions have a critical role in precision population health by providing the infrastructure to support and sustain community engagement and by carefully monitoring and balancing ethical implications.

health as a percentage of the gross domestic product. Health outcomes are not evenly distributed across US populations, because there are large differences by race and zip code. As a stark example, a baby born in 1 neighborhood can be expected to die as much as 25 years earlier than a baby born just a few miles away [2]. In addition, infant mortalities are twice as high for black mothers compared with white mothers with socioeconomic status accounting for only part of the difference [3].

In the United States, child health disparities are widening largely due to factors outside the scope of traditional medical care. As a result, health care, health care delivery, and research practices are developing novel mechanisms to improve health outcomes. For example, pediatric practices are piloting ways to screen and integrate care for the social determinants of health [4,5], and health systems are moving toward value-based care and population-based metrics [6]. However, there is no clear algorithm for tackling the historically and systemically embedded roots of health inequities. Improving the health of a population with an equity lens is complex, requiring health and academic institutions to create and transform different approaches to fulfilling their mission; these approaches must inevitably include multisector collaboration, integrated data systems, and policy changes [7].

Precision medicine has been touted by many as an approach that can improve health by tailoring prevention and treatments to individuals [8]. Tailoring is not new, but the advent of "big data," with large-scale biological databases, the ability to characterize patients across multiple biological domains, and the computational efficiency to consider multiple biological characteristics in a way to influence clinical decision making and practice, is the promise articulated by those espousing precision medicine [8]. Precision medicine has been criticized by some who argue that genomic and other "omic" variation leveraged in precision medicine are unlikely to address the major sources for poor health and variability in health outcomes observed in the United States [9]. Another criticism is that a focus on precision medicine will funnel resources away from addressing important social determinants of health that make larger contributions to poor health outcomes observed in the United States [10]. Without dismissing these critiques, others have argued that the precision approaches to understanding health and disease can also be applied to broader public and population health endeavors. These arguments have focused on broader concepts of precision health (rather than just precision medicine) and even have included notions of precision public health or precision population health (PPH). Those who have advocated for these views note that assuring diversity in efforts at biological characterization is essential for good science; integrating social, environmental, and behavioral determinants with the biological determinants of health will increase the ability to tailor prevention and treatments; and computational and technological advances can be applied effectively to public health problems as well [11]. Here, the authors embrace these notions under the framework of PPH and explore those principles of community engagement that will be necessary for assuring that current precision advances can be effectively applied to achieving improved health for the population.

In fact, the premise and promise of PPH suggest an inherent research practice based on community engagement whereby those in a population are active participants in setting research priorities, collecting and submitting individual data as "citizen scientists," determining relevant data to analyze, and offering explanatory models for findings [11]. However, descriptions of PPH do not clearly integrate well-established research frameworks that include community, such as community-based participatory research (CBPR). Instead, if mentioned in PPH efforts, community involvement is raised in the context of the importance of including diverse populations and disseminating interventions [12]. True community partnership using approaches such as CBPR will allow for the creation of targeted, precise interventions that understand the culture and relationships required for sustained health improvement.

In this article, the authors establish the context of precision medicine in improving population health, the history of community-based participatory research, and the application of CBPR to reducing health disparities and provide a framework for integrating the important and promising practices of PPH and community-based participatory research to achieve health equity.

PRECISION MEDICINE AND POPULATION HEALTH

Advancements in biomedical science, such as the mapping and sequencing of the human genome and proteomics, have led to an explosion of information and a new understanding of rare and more common diseases at an individual level [13]. For example, the subtyping of pediatric cancers has allowed for nuanced treatment protocols and improved outcomes [14]. Similarly, hundreds of genetic mutations are linked to autism, potentially explaining the wide spectrum of the disorder and offering the possibility of targeted treatments [15]. Although the concept of precision medicine has been in use for decades, including practices such as blood typing and newborn screening, the term "precision medicine" evolved in the past decade to describe "an emerging approach for disease treatment and prevention that takes into account individual variability in genes, environment, and lifestyle for each person" [16].

Widening health disparities are in stark contrast to the rapid evolution of precision medicine sciences. Despite the opportunity for better outcomes via more precise health care, fundamental health indicators like infant mortality and life expectancy are vastly different between populations [17]. There is increasing recognition of the health impact of the "conditions in which people are born, grow, live, work and age" or the *social determinants of health* [18]. With medical care estimated to account for only 10% to 20% of the modifiable contributors to good health [19], health systems are developing innovative approaches to address the social determinants of health and improve health outcomes of populations.

The application of precision medicine to improve populations has been in existence for decades. Newborn screening, for example, allows for the early identification, diagnosis, and treatment of a growing number of genetic disorders and is a public health program that is mandated throughout the United States. More recently, the application of precision medicine to the social determinants of health is emerging as a potential method to reduce health disparities [20]. For example, using data on asthma admission rates, researchers have been able to link asthma "hot spots" to specific public housing properties, identifying exacerbating environmental conditions, such as extensive mold and cockroach infestations. The medical treatment, in this case, was not access to health care or a specific pharmacologic intervention; rather, the "prescription" was better housing conditions. There is incredible power in the ability to analyze data to accurately and efficiently connect the "dots" and reveal the full landscape of multiple, individual experiences.

PPH has 4 general components: the collection of data for disease surveillance and detection, the prediction of risk, the targeting of interventions, and an understanding of the disease. Disease surveillance and detection require the accurate collection and review of data and can be applied to a gamut of conditions, including infectious diseases and environmental hazards. Technology, such as mobile phone and GPS data, enhances surveillance by better tracking affected individuals [21]. Enhanced surveillance and detection of conditions also allow for the possibility of more accurately predicting health risks in subpopulations and individuals. Enhanced surveillance and detection allows for the identification of subpopulations at risk for conditions, including infectious disease outbreaks [21], higher asthma admissions [22], premature birth [21], and "social" conditions, such as justice involvement [23]. The refined detection of conditions and prediction of risk do little to improve health if not paired with the application of effective, targeted interventions. These interventions are appropriately broad in scope given the range of risks being identified and include the early treatment of inborn errors of metabolism identified from newborn screening to the concentration of social programming to community "hot spots" for juvenile justice involvement. These 3 attributes of precision public health: surveillance and detection, predicting risk, and targeted interventions, also allow one to understand disease in new and different ways and to provide a better grasp of how to diagnose and treat diseases as varied as diabetes, influenza, and preterm birth [24].

An accurate and applicable understanding of disease also requires that PPH efforts collaborate with community stakeholders and that these collaborations acknowledge the deeply entrenched and systematically reinforced mistrust that communities, particularly those most impacted by health inequities, have of academic and health institutions. Fortunately, the field of research has developed approaches to involve community stakeholders that can serve as powerful guides for the practice of precision medicine in improving the health of populations.

COMMUNITY RESEARCH PARTNERSHIPS AND REDUCING HEALTH DISPARITIES

There are several approaches that support a spectrum of community involvement in research, including community-engaged research and participatory action research. The authors recognize that not all PPH efforts can support the ideal of equal partnership in the cocreation of research across the research process. However, the authors also think it is critical to highlight the far end of the partnership spectrum as the optimal approach to reducing health disparities [25]. Community-based participatory research (CBPR) is a collaborative research approach whereby academic and community stakeholders are equal partners across the spectrum of the research process [26–28]. In the past 20 years, CBPR emerged as a research framework combining "action" and "participatory" research processes with the goal of improving the lives of those targeted by the research. The "action" approach involves a cyclic process, incorporating action, reflection, problem solving, and decision making between partnerships [29]. "Participatory research" [30] emphasizes the lived experience, particularly of oppressed social groups, and recognizes issues of power and privilege. Specifically, CBPR combines the importance of coparticipation, with self-awareness of issues like power and privilege. There are 4 general expectations of CBPR projects: (a) capacity building, (b) colearning, (c) shared benefits among partners, and (d) reduction of disparities [26,27,31].

Principles in CBPR have been elaborated on by past research and vary in their application to each study [32]. *Capacity building* is aimed at creating the infrastructure needed to plan for future steps (eg, staffing, networking, and training). *Colearning* is defined as the process of exchanging knowledge (eg, data interpretation) and skills (eg, data analysis) between institutions and community members. *Shared benefits* are when the institution and partners involved both profit from the research, including the results that can be reaped. Results should further research agendas and translate into action for the community. Finally, and a particularly important principle, is that CBPR should aim to reduce disparities. In other words, researchers should aim to partner with communities to reduce the differences various neighborhoods, ethnic populations, and socioeconomic statuses experience in health outcomes.

CBPR provides the potential to include diverse community voices and build infrastructure with key community partners for sustainability. However, in communities most impacted by inequities, CBPR research faces challenges of careful navigation in power and privilege [26,27]. First, to reduce health inequities, it is essential to consider the power dynamic and assumptions introduced into the investigation. Researchers may have a "perceived power base" because they serve as experts [26]. Physicians, regardless of whether they are researchers, may also function as a perceived power base if they are seen as experts. Second, physicians should be aware of the assumptions they may bring to understanding the causes of poor health outcomes and the drivers of individual behavior, especially given the growing percentage of medical students who come from the highest levels of family household income [33]. Third, in small communities, investigators have to be cognizant of the ramifications from misrepresenting their expertise, because community members may rely on their word in the absence of local resources. Last, future investigators should also consider that power and bias issues brought from university or hospital affiliations may extend to other stakeholders. Selecting community stakeholders that are nonresidents, from highly educated fields, or part of the ethnic majority may all pose challenges in gaining an honest community perspective [34], and stakeholders may not be community residents. With heightened awareness of their own biases, academics, physicians, and other stakeholders have the opportunity to combine community expertise with their own skill sets and create relevant change to reduce disparities.

PRECISION POPULATION HEALTH AND COMMUNITY-PARTNERED RESEARCH

The intentional integration of community expertise into the practice of PPH offers a potent, complementary approach to reducing health disparities by creating tailored interventions with the community as partners. Although precision medicine uses databases to empower one to identify populations at risk for and affected by disease, approaches such as CBPR provide the mechanism to understand the nuances of associated risk factors, root causes, and effective interventions. Indeed, without using approaches such as CBPR, PPH efforts risk making false assumptions about research priorities, the data to examine, the interpretation of results, and effective interventions.

The authors' belief is that true partnerships with community should be an essential core competency of PPH at every step. They propose a PPH framework (Fig. 1) with the central goal of reducing disparities while understanding disease. To achieve this goal, the PPH framework embeds CBPR within the PPH disciplines [24] through an iterative, progressive set of stages that evolves via lessons learned and layers of relationship and trust building. To provide context, the authors discuss the PPH framework using the common childhood condition of asthma.

SURVEILLANCE AND DETECTION

Surveillance and detection require infrastructure for researchers and community members to gather the most useful data relevant to the desired health

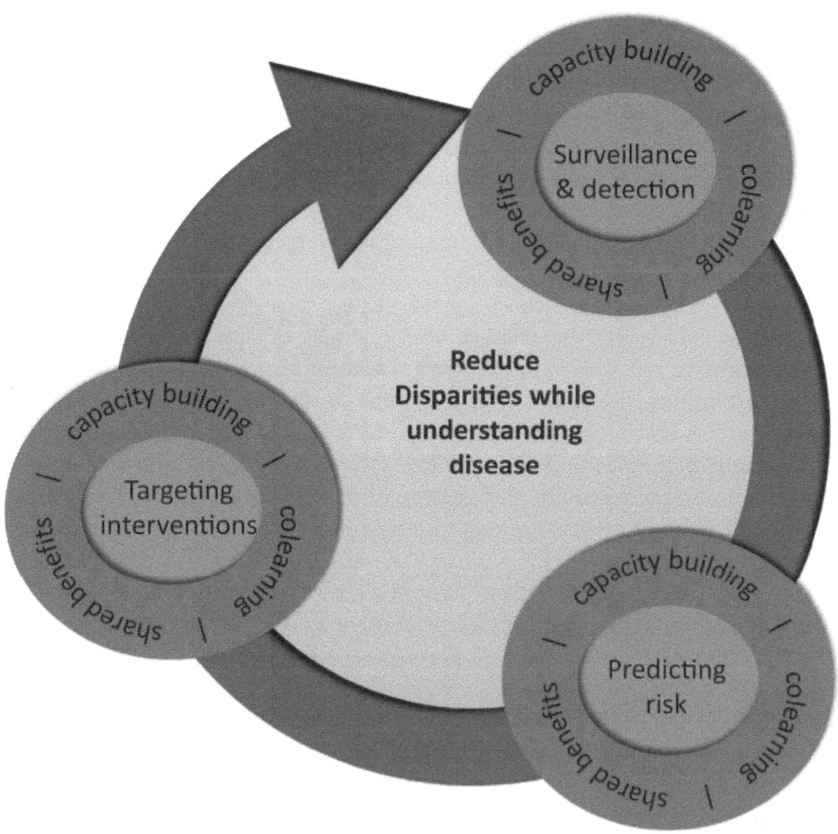

Fig. 1. PPH framework.

outcomes. Questions regarding the populations of interest, useful geography (eg, neighborhoods vs zip codes), and key assets (eg, housing, schools, pharmacies) are best answered in partnership with the community to ensure that the platform built and implemented is relevant and effective. Initial partnerships between researchers and the community could begin with an offer of *capacity building*. Capacity building could include building a biomedical understanding of asthma and enhancing knowledge about different data collection tools, like geocoding and mapping and their respective strengths and limitations. In turn, both researcher and community members work together and begin a *colearning* process to identify common priorities. Each can draw on their spheres of expertise and, together, identify how these assets do or do not work together to mitigate asthma's impact on children. Future linkage of data between disparate data sources, such as health, schools, housing, and pharmacy sectors, for full surveillance detection will ultimately require that mutual benefits to researchers and community stakeholders are compelling and clear.

PREDICTING RISK

The second stage in understanding disease involves developing a better understanding of its determinants, which includes the CBPR principles of *capacity building*, *colearning*, and *shared benefits*. For instance, through *capacity building*, communities can improve prediction of asthma risk by sharing archival data and current data collection tools. In addition, capacity building can help build community trust and enrollment in broader surveys, in-home sampling of environmental triggers, or participation in air sampling techniques. Such efforts would help PPH better detect the neighborhoods most at risk for asthma by improving survey response rates, by targeting a broader range of the population, and by increasing the validity and richness of data collected. *Colearning* can also improve risk prediction because the community can impart knowledge on why certain neighborhoods might be more at risk (eg, cockroach infestation) or point to risks that might be missed (eg, idling school buses). Both researchers and community members can experience *shared benefits* in asthma research. Results from the data can help researchers understand current data trends and gain fresh insight into why some communities are doing better than they predicted (eg, a "bright spot"). Community members can better understand which children may be at higher risk and why and be better positioned to inform city developers in the future (eg, school placement and walking routes that avoid high-traffic areas).

TARGETING INTERVENTIONS

In the final stage of understanding asthma, *capacity building*, *colearning*, and *shared benefits* are critical to successfully targeting interventions. The community can help *capacity building* by linking researchers with venues that would be most receptive for intervention. Alternatively, they may be able to share staff and funding for delivering the asthma intervention. Researchers can teach community members methods in which to manage and treat childhood asthma. In contrast, the community can share with the researchers the barriers (eg, transportation) to receiving that treatment. Targeted interventions also encompass shared benefits in their results. For instance, results may demonstrate that an intervention had different effectiveness across ethnic groups even though the individual patients were in the same neighborhood. Such results help researchers understand that interventions may need to be adapted to certain groups within a community. These heterogeneous effects from an intervention also help the community understand the anticipated effectiveness across their community to aid planning for future resource investment.

In the PPH framework (see Fig. 1), each PPH activity undergoes a distinct process by which CBPR concepts are embedded to enhance the quality of data collection and use of data through partnerships. More importantly, each PPH activity should be thought of in a cyclical process for continued refinement. Once a targeted intervention is disseminated, continued surveillance checks should be made to monitor the progress of the disease and whether disparities are being mitigated. If progress is not made, the partnership should reassess the current community needs, data validity, and the chosen logic model. When successful, lessons can be learned from the PPH approach to help predict risk and scale target interventions in other communities based on generalizable elements.

THE ROLE OF ACADEMIC INSTITUTIONS

Academic medical centers and university systems are beginning to create infrastructures and programs that align their precision health sciences, such as epidemiology and data analytics, with community-based research priorities. Distinct from the community outreach goal of recruiting diverse study populations or the patient advisory council goal of improving clinical performance, the idea of community advisory research boards is to partner with communities "upstream" in the research process and to cocreate research priorities and approaches. Academic institutions that have a mission to improve the health of their local environment should adopt the PPH framework for strategic planning and scientific development. Integrating the PPH framework will help to build trust and engage community members as partners rather than subjects. As described above, this approach is most authentic and effective in addressing health disparities when partnerships are developed before research design and the establishment of hypotheses. However, these partnerships require institutional culture change, infrastructure, and support [7,35].

For example, the University of Illinois Cancer Center has combined their population level data on cancer outcomes in the city of Chicago with the creation of a "patient brigade." By using CBPR and patient outcomes research, this patient brigade integrates itself with each research and community initiative in search of better treatments and potential disease cures. Similarly, with funding from the Patient-Centered Outcome Research Institute, the University of California San Francisco (UCSF) Child Health Equity Initiative launched the Transforming Research as Usual for Equity (TRUE) program to build institutional infrastructure for sustained community-partnered child health research. Over 2 years, TRUE developed consensus around child health research priorities for San Francisco. These priorities were then disseminated to more than 100 local, multisector stakeholders to inform their efforts to improve child health and reduce health disparities. These programs serve a critical role in providing the institutional infrastructure to support community-partnered approaches to PPH efforts.

In addition, motivated in part by the move toward value-based care and accountable care organizations, health systems and academic health institutions also are increasingly developing units to improve the health of populations. Southern Illinois University School of Medicine, a community-based medical school in Springfield, Illinois, has recently launched an entire department dedicated to bridging population health analytics and CBPR. Organized around Divisions of Epidemiology and Biostatistics, Human and Community Development, and Health System Science, this Department of Population Science and Policy is built around a social mission that recognizes that data should be collected by the people and for the people to design sustainable community-driven programs and interventions that improve the health of children and families. Similarly, UCSF has had a long-standing interest in PPH as a part of its precision medicine initiatives and has fostered discussions about how advances in the current environment can be used to improve prevention, population health, and health equity [36]. In 2016, UCSF hosted the Precision Public Health Conference sponsored by the White House Office of Science and Technology Policy and the Bill & Melinda Gates Foundation focused on the First 1000 Days of life. UCSF also has an ongoing Population Health Data Initiative that includes collaboration between the UCSF Health Office of Population and Accountable Care and various units in the UCSF School of Medicine on the role of data to improve population health.

Precision population health framework: ethical considerations and challenges

With the PPH framework (see Fig. 1), the authors aim to highlight the critical role of community partnerships in PPH efforts to reduce disparities and understand disease. Their proposed framework, however, does not avoid some of the pitfalls of PPH. The potential for data misuse forces researchers to acknowledge and consider the ethical issues of their work. Implications exist for health information privacy, data security, informed consent, and even discrimination [37].

The current technological infrastructure allows for the storage and linkage of unprecedented amounts of data from an increasingly diverse array of sources, including an individual's genetic code as well as their smart devices, text messages, credit card purchases, online activity, electronic medical records, use of public programs, and global positioning system data [38,39]. The linking of this information offers researchers and private and public interests unique opportunities to understand attitudes, behaviors, and disease states. However, when consenting to the sharing of data, researchers and participants alike are not likely to understand the extent of data being shared or the full implications of sharing the data [38–41]. Greater attention will need to be placed in understanding the agendas of both the researchers and funders. As the ability to understand the nuanced behaviors of certain communities and even certain segments of those communities becomes clearer, the potential exists to use this information to stigmatize or bias vulnerable communities in subtle ways that are not protected by the existing antidiscrimination laws and regulations. For example, interventions or services could be targeted for or against individuals living in certain zip codes, which could be proxy measures for protected classes such as race or religion. "Big data" also poses risks to individuals by uncovering potentially negative or discriminatory information that may not have even been considered in their initial intent of the research. For example, case managers review individual purchase data from electronic benefit transfer cards to identify fraud. Otherwise data are used to create algorithms to predict a child's risk for maltreatment, including prior referrals to child protective services, which introduces substantive risk in perpetuating systemic biases, racism, and inequities [37].

Finally, PPH requires that academic health institutions substantively commit to new institutional practices, such as research ethic boards and institutional review boards that are equipped to handle the complexities of "big data" and PPH endeavors. In addition, community partnerships to support PPH require a long-time horizon with sustained institutional investments. Traditional models of investigator-driven research grants are generally counterproductive, perpetuating short-term goals and challenging environments for building community trust [35]. To impact the health of populations, institutions need to invest in a sustainable infrastructure to support capacity building, colearning, and shared benefits that is on par with investments made to the traditional tripartite mission areas of patient care, research, and education.

MOVING FORWARD

The evolution of applying precision science to improve the health of populations offers the exciting possibility of addressing health inequities amid the growing evidence of widening disparities. This promise of PPH requires the collaboration of multiple sectors and, in particular, the partnership of communities most at risk for and most impacted by health inequities. The authors believe that established research practices for community collaboration, such as CBPR, should serve as core competencies of precision health efforts to reduce disparities and understand disease. PPH should also pay heed to important lessons and barriers to academic and multisector partnerships that can perpetuate inequities. Research and health institutions also must invest in infrastructure to sustain community-partnered precision health. The PPH framework illustrates the integration of CBPR into common PPH activities and highlights the iterative learning and implementation nature of this approach. It is the powerful combination of precision science with approaches like CBPR that deepen the understanding of the root causes of disparities and that can lead to identifying and addressing systemic inequities.

Acknowledgments

The authors acknowledge Deja Webster, BS, UCSF Child Health Equity Intern for technical assistance.

References

[1] Papanicolas I, Woskie LR, Jha AK. Health care spending in the United States and other high-income countries. JAMA 2018;319(10):1024–39.

[2] Metro Map: New Orleans, LA - Infographic. RWJF. 2013. Available at: https://www.rwjf.org/en/library/infographics/new-orleans-map.html. Accessed November 29, 2018.

[3] Center for Disease Control and Prevention. Infant mortality rates, by race: United States, selected years 1950–2014. 2015. Available at: https://www.cdc.gov/nchs/data/hus/2015/011.pdf. Accessed November 10, 2018.

[4] Beck AF, Cohen AJ, Colvin JD, et al. Perspectives from the Society for Pediatric Research: interventions targeting social needs in pediatric clinical care. Pediatr Res 2018;84:10–21.

[5] Cottrell EK, Gold R, Likumahuwa S, et al. Using health information technology to bring social determinants of health into primary care: a conceptual framework to guide research. J Health Care Poor Underserved 2018;29(3):949–63.
[6] Burwell SM. Setting value-based payment goals — HHS efforts to improve U.S. health care. N Engl J Med 2015;372(10):897–9.
[7] Roper WL, Newton WP. The role of academic health centers in improving health. Ann Fam Med 2006;4(Suppl 1):55–60.
[8] Collins FS, Varmus H. A new initiative on precision medicine. N Engl J Med 2015;372(9): 793–5.
[9] Chowkwanyun M, Bayer R, Galea S. "Precision" public health — between novelty and hype. N Engl J Med 2018;379(15):1398–400.
[10] Ramaswami R, Bayer R, Galea S. Precision medicine from a public health perspective. Annu Rev Public Health 2018;39(1):153–68.
[11] Lyles CR, Lunn MR, Obedin-Maliver J, et al. The new era of precision population health: insights for the All of Us Research Program and beyond. J Transl Med 2018;16(211):1–4.
[12] McGrath C, Palmarella G, Solomon S, et al. Precision prevention and public health. CPHI Data Briefs 2017;4:1–4.
[13] National Research Council. Toward precision medicine: building a knowledge network for biomedical research and a new taxonomy of 82 disease. Washington, DC: The National Academies Press; 2011.
[14] Forrest SJ, Geoerger B, Janeway KA. Precision medicine in pediatric oncology. Curr Opin Pediatr 2018;30(1):17–24.
[15] Loth E, Murphy DG, Spooren W. Defining precision medicine approaches to autism spectrum disorders: concepts and challenges. Front Psychiatry 2016;7(188):1–8.
[16] White house precision medicine initiative. 2015. Available at: https://obamawhitehouse.archives.gov/precision-medicine. Accessed December 10, 2018.
[17] National Academies of Sciences, Engineering, and Medicine; Health and Medicine Division; Board on Population Health and Public Health Practice; Committee on Community-Based Solutions to Promote Health Equity in the United States. In: Baciu A, Negussie Y, Geller A, et al, editors. Communities in Action: Pathways to Health Equity. Washington (DC): National Academies Press (US); 2017.
[18] Artiga S. Beyond health care: the role of social determinants in promoting health and health equity. The Henry J Kaiser Family Foundation. Available at: https://www.kff.org/disparities-policy/issue-brief/beyond-health-care-the-role-of-social-determinants-in-promoting-health-and-health-equity/. Accessed December 4, 2018.
[19] Magnan S. Social determinants of health 101 for health care: five plus five. NAM perspectives. Discussion Paper, National Academy of Medicine. Washington, DC, October 9, 2017.
[20] Khoury MJ, Bowen MS, Clyne M, et al. From public health genomics to precision public health: a 20-year journey. Genet Med 2018;20(6):574–82.
[21] Dowell SF, Blazes D, Desmond-Hellmann S. Four steps to precision public health. Nature 2016;540(7632):189–91.
[22] Beck AF, Huang B, Chundur R, et al. Housing code violation density associated with emergency department and hospital use by children with asthma. Health Aff (Millwood) 2014;33(11):1993–2002.
[23] Butler B. Predictive analytics in healthcare and criminal justice: three case studies. Oakland (CA): Community Oriented Correctional Health Services; 2015. p. 1–14.
[24] Dolley S. Big data's role in precision public health. Front Public Health 2018;6:68.
[25] Israel BA, Schulz AJ, Parker EA, et al. Review of community-based research: assessing partnership approaches to improve public health. Annu Rev Public Health 1998;19(1): 173–202.
[26] Wallerstein NB, Duran BD. Using community-based participatory research to address health disparities. Health Promot Pract 2006;7(3):312–23.

[27] Holkup PA, Tripp-Reimer T, Salois EM, et al. Community-based participatory research: an approach to intervention research with a Native American community. ANS Adv Nurs Sci 2004;27(3):162–75.

[28] Israel BA, Schulz AJ, Par E. Community-based participatory research: policy recommendations for promoting a partnership approach in health research. Educ Health (Abingdon) 2001;14(2):182–97.

[29] Wallerstein NB, Duran BD. The theoretical, historical, and practice roots of CBPR. In: Minkler M, Wallerstein NB, editors. Community-based participatory research for health from process to outcomes. 2nd edition. San Francisco (CA): John Wiley & Sons; 2008. p. 25–39.

[30] Ferreira MP, Gendron F. Community-based participatory research with traditional and indigenous communities of the Americas: historical context and future directions. International Journal of Critical Pedagogy 2011;3(3):153–68.

[31] Israel BA, Schulz AJ, Parker EA, et al. Critical issues in developing and following community based participatory research principles. In: Minkler M, Wallerstein N, editors. Community based participatory research for health. San Francisco (CA): Jossey-Bass; 2003. p. 53–76.

[32] Corbie-Smith G, Bryant AR, Walker DJ, et al. Building capacity in community-based participatory research partnerships through a focus on process and multiculturalism. Prog Community Health Partnersh 2015;2(9):261–73.

[33] Jolly P. Diversity of U.S. medical students by parental income. Analysis in Brief, vol. 8. Association of American Medical Colleges; 2008 (1): 1–2.

[34] Muhammed M, Garzón C, Reyes A, The West Oakland Environmental Indicators Project. Understanding contemporary racism, power, and privilege and their impacts on CBPR. In: Wallerstein N, Duran B, Oetzel J, et al, editors. Community-based participatory research for health: advancing social and health equity. San Francisco (CA): Jossey-Bass; 2018. p. 47–59.

[35] Siegel B, Erickson J, Milstein B, et al. Multisector partnerships need further development to fulfill aspirations for transforming regional health and well-being. Health Aff 2018;37(1): 30–7.

[36] Precision Medicine at UCSF. Available at: https://precisionmedicine.ucsf.edu/programs/precision-population-health. Accessed December 10, 2018.

[37] Eubanks V. Automating Inequality: how high-tech tools profile, police, and punish the poor. New York: Picador; 2018.

[38] Bechmann A. Non-informed consent cultures: privacy policies and app contracts on Facebook. Journal of Media Business Studies 2014;11:21–38.

[39] Salerno J, Knoppers BM, Lee LM, et al. Ethics, big data and computing in epidemiology and public health. Ann Epidemiol 2017;27(5):297–301.

[40] Gerber N, Reinheimer B, Volkamer M. Home sweet home? Investigating users' awareness of smart home privacy threats. Paper presented at the UNENIX Symposium on Usable Privacy and Security (SOUPS). Baltimore, MD, August 12, 2018.

[41] Liang Y, Cai Z, Yu J, et al. Deep learning based inference of private information using embedded sensors in smart devices. IEEE Netw 2018;32(4):8–14.

Advances in Pediatrics 66 (2019) 15–35

ADVANCES IN PEDIATRICS

The Need to Integrate Sex and Gender Differences into Pediatric Pedagogy

Janice L. Werbinski, MD, NCMP[a,*], Mary K. Rojek, PhD[b], Maria Demma I. Cabral, MD[c]

[a]Department of Obstetrics and Gynecology, Western Michigan University Homer Stryker MD School of Medicine, 1000 Oakland Drive, Kalamazoo, MI 49008-1284, USA; [b]Sex and Gender Health Collaborative, American Medical Women's Association, 1100 Woodfield Rd. #350, Schaumburg, IL 60173, USA; [c]Department of Pediatric and Adolescent Medicine, Western Michigan University Homer Stryker MD School of Medicine, 1000 Oakland Drive, Kalamazoo, MI 49008-1284, USA

Keywords

• Medical education • Sex and gender differences • Pediatric education
• Sex and gender based medicine

Key points

- Despite including women in research over the past 25 years, only a fraction of that research has been translated into curricula for medical students, residents, or practicing physicians.
- Tens of thousands of articles document that diseases and conditions differ between women and men, boys and girls, in terms of biology, prevention, clinical signs, therapeutic approach, prognosis, and psychological and social impact.
- A 2001 Institute of Medicine report indicated that "every cell has a sex," and knowledge of sex and gender differences would lead to improved clinical care for women and men.
- There are sex differences that begin with the fetus, and sex and gender differences throughout infancy, childhood, and adolescence that have implications for clinical care.
- Women/girls and men/boys are sometimes harmed when their unique presentation, metabolism, size, and reactions are not considered in their health care plan.

Disclosure Statement: The authors have nothing to disclose.

*Corresponding author. 10073 Woodlawn Drive, Portage, MI 49002. *E-mail address:* dr.janwerbinski@gmail.com

https://doi.org/10.1016/j.yapd.2019.03.001

INTRODUCTION

Sex and gender based medicine (SGBM) is a lens or framework with which to consider sex and gender based differences between men/women and boys/girls. It applies to all patients. It is similar to the social determinants of health in that both sex and gender have an influence on health and illness. However, it also incorporates the social and cultural context that influences access to care, resources, opportunities, among other factors that affect health. Ignoring sex and gender can lead to bias in health care (often unconscious) and may harm patients.

SGBM evolved from the Women's Health Movement of the 1990s when research demonstrated that there were substantial differences in women's health compared with men's health that were relevant to all disciplines. SGBM emerged so that the similarities and differences between men and women would be explicitly considered to improve both women's and men's health. SGBM has progressed over the last 2 decades and has the potential to transform not only medicine, but also other interprofessional disciplines [1]. This article shows that the knowledge of sex and gender differences in adults also applies to the discipline of pediatrics.

EVERY CELL HAS A SEX AND EVERY PERSON HAS A GENDER

"Every cell has a sex," and all bodies are influenced by gender. *Sex* refers to a patient's biology, whereas *gender* refers to the sociocultural factors that influence both a patient's presentation and how society responds to an individual [2,3].

As a biological variable, sex refers to the patient's chromosomes, genes, hormones, and reproductive anatomy. Given that chromosomes and genes are present in all cells, and cells are influenced by hormones, every cell has a sex. Gender is a sociocultural variable that applies to the individual and to society. Individuals adopt roles, behaviors, and identities, and they express their gender. On a societal level, there are gendered expectations and opportunities that influence how individuals will and/or can express their gender. For example, access to a specific treatment may depend on a patient's sex and gender, which can influence insurance, ability to travel, childcare, socioeconomic status, a health provider's correct diagnosis, research conducted about the condition in the relevant population, and so forth.

SEX AND GENDER TERMINOLOGY

The appropriate terminology for sex is male/female/intersex, whereas for gender it is man/woman, boy/girl, masculine/feminine, cisgender/transgender, and other gendered expressions. Cisgender refers to gender expression and birth sex being congruent (most people), and transgender refers to gender expression differing from birth sex. Although sex and gender can be examined individually in terms of health, they also interact via epigenetic processes and may influence health [3]. Box 1 summarizes sex and gender terminology.

Box 1: Sex and gender terminology

	Sex	Gender
Variable type	Biological variable	Sociocultural variable
Terms	Female, male, intersex	Woman/man Girl/boy Feminine/masculine Cisgender/transgender Other
Components	Chromosomes, genes, hormones, organs	Roles, behaviors, identities, expressions, opportunities, expectations
Levels	Organism, organ, cell	Both individual and societal

WHAT SEX AND GENDER BASED HEALTH IS NOT

Most casual observers of SGBM incorrectly confuse sexuality with gender. *Sexuality* refers to heterosexual, lesbian, gay, bisexual, asexual, and pansexual. It refers to sexual attractions, identities, and practices. *Gender identity* refers to how individuals see themselves as a man or a woman. The term *queer* refers to a chosen identity adopted by those who reject the binary distinctions regarding both sexuality and gender. Although sexuality is relevant to health, it is not the same as gender [3].

IMPLICIT BIAS IN PRACTICE

Health care providers already consider sex and gender in their practices, but they often do so unknowingly. They make assumptions about patients and interpret symptoms based on preconceived ideas about how a patient presents [4]. For example, pain is often interpreted differently in men and women. A stoic man may be assumed to be legitimately experiencing pain, whereas a stoic woman may be assumed to be experiencing little pain. Alternatively, a man complaining of severe pain will be assumed to be in great distress, whereas a woman complaining of severe pain may be interpreted as being emotional or responding to stress in her life. Such implicit bias can lead to inappropriate treatment. When that is coupled with limited research on sex and gender differences in health, it can lead to suboptimal care and outcomes [3].

SEX AND GENDER BASED HEALTH

The study and practice of sex and gender differences is referred to as sex and gender based health (SGBH). SGBH denotes that it is interprofessional and includes medicine, whereas SGBM applies solely to medicine. SGBH focuses on biological sex and sociocultural gender. It requires recognizing that every person has a sex and a gender, and both influence health. The basic differences between XX and XY must be researched and appreciated, and the health implications of the interrelationship between the two must be understood.

From the embryo to the grave, sex and gender have undeniable effects on a person's health. Diseases and conditions differ between women and men in terms of biology, prevention, clinical signs, therapeutic approach, prognosis, and psychological and social impact. Traditional medical textbooks and curricula still tend to approach health and diseases from a standard perspective largely based on research performed on male animals, cells which do not denote sex of source, and the 70-kg human man [5–7].

THE SEX AND GENDER BASED HEALTH DIFFERENCES MOVEMENT

The roots of studying sex differences between women and men are in the women's health movement [1]. In 1990, Congress passed the Women's Health Equity Act (WHEA), establishing the Office of Research on Women's Health (ORWH) at the National Institutes of Health (NIH), to ensure the inclusion of women in all NIH-funded research where appropriate. Before this time, the Food and Drug Administration (FDA) had banned the participation of women of childbearing age in clinical research. Since passage of the WHEA, and despite nearly 30 years of research that finally included women, outcomes are often not reported by sex. The lack of reporting by sex leaves outcomes in the less-studied sex (women) invisible, while muddying the data about outcomes in men. Only a small fraction of sex-specific research has been translated into curricula for medical students, residents, or practicing physicians [7,8].

The Women's Health Movement was inspired in large part by 2 momentous and pivotal research revelations:

1. The *Physicians' Health Study* of 1989 [9], showed that daily aspirin decreased the risk of a first heart attack in male physicians. More than 20,000 male physicians (but no women) were included in the study. Arguably, this became more infamous for its exclusion of women than its epidemiologic findings.
2. Results from the *Women's Health Initiative*, which had been launched in 1991, clearly showed that there were existing common medical practices that harmed some women [10,11]. For instance, hormone replacement therapy was discovered to be harmful to some women's cardiac health. Subsequent research has shown that coronary artery disease differs in women compared with men in terms of pathogenesis, symptoms, and prognosis [12].

More recent research has shown that the cardiac symptoms that are more typical in women can also occur in some men. This knowledge may help to improve clinical care not only for women at risk, but also for men [13]. This research led to the understanding that women (and men) are sometimes actually harmed when their unique presentation, metabolism, size, and reactions are not considered. There are known differences in pharmacokinetics and pharmacodynamics that matter. Whether a cell contains an XX or XY chromosome may have an impact on everything from phenotype to regulation of metabolism to the gut microbiome [10,14].

Since the 1990 WHEA legislation, a succession of events has moved us toward considering sex and gender differences in research, education, legislation, and publication. Table 1 depicts a timeline chronicling this activity.

Lay women have also become aware that women's health issues have received inadequate attention. Advocates have published books, articles, and opinion editorials about "*miss-diagnoses*" and the harm women have experienced. Maya Dusenbery's 2018 book, *Doing Harm: The Truth About How Bad Medicine and Lazy Science Leave Women Dismissed, Misdiagnosed, and Sick* [15], attempts to bring this issue to public attention. The Coalition for Women's Health Equity, a program of Hadassah, advocates for gender equity in medical prevention, research, funding, and quality of care, and raises awareness about how health inequities adversely affect women and families throughout the United States [16].

More recent legislative action has seen the introduction of the "Research 4 All Act of 2015" requiring the inclusion of both male and female cells, tissues, and animals in all human and pharmaceutical research, ordering the disaggregation of data analysis by sex, and mandating that sex differences be examined and analyzed [17]. It also directs the NIH to update its guidelines about the inclusion of women and minorities in research. Although this bill was introduced in the House of Representatives on a bipartisan basis in 2015, at the time of this writing, it has not been given a vote.

WHAT DOES THIS HAVE TO DO WITH PEDIATRICS?

It is the responsibility of the health care system to provide care to all populations equally, and it is the responsibility of doctors and doctors in training to be exposed to the health care needs of all populations. Medical training should include children as a special population. The specialty of Pediatrics was first proposed by Abraham Jacobi, who became the first president of the American Pediatric Society in 1888. Jacobi advocated for doctors to consider differences in metabolism, dosages, and therapeutics when treating children [18].

The phrase "children are not just small adults" [19] was coined, and yet it was another 45 years before the American Board of Pediatrics became a certifying body of the American Board of Medical Specialties. It is now known that there are many differences in health between men and women as well as between boys and girls. Just as it has come to be accepted that there are differences between children and adults, it must also be acknowledged that there are differences between boys and girls.

FETAL DEVELOPMENT AND HORMONES: A REVIEW OF HUMAN EMBRYOLOGY

Complex mechanisms are responsible for the development of the phenotypic differences between male and female humans from an undifferentiated zygote. It has long been recognized that testicular determination is initiated with the expression of the SRY (Sex Determining Region) gene on the Y chromosome. Once testes are developed, they begin to produce testosterone and

Table 1
Sex and gender timeline

Year	Research	Clinical	Legislation: national and international initiatives	Educational
1985	US Public Health Service task force finds exclusion of women from research negatively impacts women's health			
1990	The Society for Women's Health Research is founded		WHEA passed, establishing the ORWH at NIH	Publication of *Women's Health Issues* journal
1991	Women's Health Initiative is funded and launched in 1991		Office of Women's Health is established at US Department of Health & Human Service	
1992				Publication of the first issue of *Journal of Women's Health*
1993	NIH Revitalization Act requires that women be included in all research			The Advanced Curriculum on Women's Health is created by the AMWA
1994			Office of Women's Health is established at the FDA	
1995			National Centers of Excellence in Women's Health are funded	The Council on Graduate Medical Education calls for expanded education in women's health beyond reproductive health
1996				Publication of *Women's Health in the Curriculum: A Resource Guide for Faculty* The American College of Women's Health Physicians is founded
1998				Publication of *Textbook of Women's Health* by Dr Lila Wallis

1999		Publication of *Guide to Preventive Cardiology for Women* by Dr Lori Mosca		
2000	NIH ORWH Building Interdisciplinary Research Careers in Women's Health grants program is established for faculty in women's health and sex differences research		National Community Centers of Excellence in Women's Health is funded	Women's Health Core Competencies are developed by Association of Professors of Gynecology and Obstetrics to create women's health curriculum Publication of *Academic Medicine* special issue on sex, gender, & women's health in medical education
2001	Institute of Medicine (IOM) report published: "Exploring the Biological Contributions to Human Health: Does Sex Matter?"	US Government Accountability Office (GAO) report: 80% of market-withdrawn drugs show adverse effects in women		
2002	Women's Health Initiative study on hormone replacement therapy halted due to breast/cardiac adverse events			
2004				Publication of *Principles of Gender-Specific Medicine* by Dr Marianne Legato
2005	Scientific Group on Methodologies for the Safety Evaluation of Chemicals (SGOMSEC) concludes that sex differences are essential to the study of toxicology	Aspirin is found to decrease risk of stroke but not first myocardial infarction (MI) in women		
2006	Founding of the Foundation for Gender-Specific Medicine and the Organization for the Study of Sex Differences			

(*continued on next page*)

Table 1
(*continued*)

Year	Research	Clinical	Legislation: national and international initiatives	Educational
2007	Advancing Novel Science in Women's Health Research grant established		National Centers of Excellence in Women's Health is defunded	Laura W. Bush Institute for Women's Health is established at TTUHSC
2010	IOM report finds lack of reporting and analysis of research data by sex		Women's Health Office Act establishes Offices of Women's Health in 5 federal agencies	Publication of *Biology of Sex Differences* Journal
2011	FDA releases guidance on the role of sex difference in determining safety and effectiveness of medical devices	Publication of Update: Guidelines for the Prevention of Cardiovascular Disease in Women		Division of Sex and Gender in Emergency Medicine is established at Warren Alpert Medical School, Brown University
2012	ApoEε4 in Alzheimer disease found to cause changes in brain activity in healthy adult women but not in men			The Sex & Gender Women's Health Collaborative is established More publications: *Sex and Gender Aspects in Clinical Medicine; Handbook of Clinical Gender Medicine; Sex and Gender Differences in Pharmacology* Mayo Clinic conference: *Embedding Sex and Gender Health Differences into Medical Curricula*
2013		Zolpidem: First drug designated for different dosing in women by the FDA		

2014	FDA releases guidelines for sex-specific patient enrollment and reporting for medical device applications	Research for All Act introduced in Congress for equity in basic and clinical research	
2015	NIH dictates that all federally funded cellular and animal research must include both sexes of cells and animals		First Sex and Gender Medical Education Summit held at the Mayo Clinic
2016			Publication of textbook *Sex and Gender in Acute Care Medicine* Publication of new journal *Gender and the Genome*
2017			Publication of third edition of *Principles of Gender-Specific Medicine* by Dr Legato
2018			First Sex and Gender Health Education Summit held at the University of Utah

Adapted from: American Medical Women's Association. SGBH timeline. 2018. Available at: https://www.amwa-doc.org/sghc/sgbh-timeline. Accessed November 13, 2018; with permission.

Anti-Mullerian Hormone, which lead to the development of the typical male phenotype through the mesonephric (Wolffian) ductal system. If testes do not develop, no testosterone is produced, and female internal and external phenotype develops through the paramesonephric (Mullerian) ductal system. Although female somatic sex does not depend on endocrine activity, androgenic steroids will lead to irreversible downstream expression of the male phenotype. Thus, without testosterone, the resulting embryo develops, by default, the female phenotype [20].

Uniparental disomy is the situation in which 2 copies of a chromosome come from the same parent. When a deletion occurs on the long arm of chromosome 15, if the 2 X's come from the mother, the offspring develops Prader-Willi syndrome. When the identical deletion is contributed by the father, the child has Angelman syndrome. These genetic conditions have very recognizable, yet drastically different resulting phenotypes. Indeed, this phenomenon would suggest that even each chromosome has a sex, likely due to methylation patterns specific to the mother's or the father's chromosomes [21].

Parental manipulation of postnatal survival is a deplorable example of using sex difference knowledge in utero to orchestrate the "desired" sex of offspring by using selective abortion or infanticide. Studies show that 9% of the world's cultures still adhere to this practice. In 97% of those countries, the male offspring is considered more desirable. These are clear examples of societal misogyny [22].

SEX DIFFERENCES IN THE BRAIN

Several sex-specific genes not dependent on sex steroids are expressed differently in male and female human brains. Structural sex differences in the brain begin to become recognizable by age 2. There are also differences in adult male and female brains. The size and shape of some areas of the corpus callosum are larger in women. The fascicles connecting each hemisphere internally are larger in men [23]. Certain hypothalamic nuclei are larger in men, and the gonadotropin feedback response to estradiol differs by sex. Even at the cellular level (dendrites, axons, astrocytes, microglia, and synapses), differences between male and female brains have been identified [23].

SEX AND GENDER DIFFERENCES IN ADULTS

There are tens of thousands of articles that document sex and gender differences in adults. German researchers have developed a comprehensive library [24] of these differences. The Sex and Gender Health Collaborative website [25] is a resource to access current research information about sex and gender differences in adults across disciplines. The Laura W. Bush Institute for Women's Health [26] developed a journal article search tool, which is available at https://www.sexandgenderhealth.org/resources.html. Table 2 provides a representative list highlighting a few of the differences between the 2 sexes in adults, presented by organ system and discipline.

Table 2
Sample sex and gender differences in adults by organ system and discipline

Organ system and discipline	Adult sex and gender differences
Cardiovascular	Women are more likely to have "atypical" (ie, unlike men's) symptoms of *heart attacks* and *strokes* than men [27].
	Women who suffer *MI* are more likely to show *no* blockage in the heart arteries (coronary microvascular dysfunction) [28].
	Women <50 y old have 24% higher mortality from *MI* than men of the same age [29].
	Women are less likely than men to receive cardiopulmonary resuscitation when experiencing a *heart attack* [30].
	Women are referred 3 times less frequently for catheter ablation of *atrial fibrillation* [31].
Gastrointestinal	Women *metabolize alcohol* more slowly than men, leading to more cognitive impairment, motor vehicle accidents, and liver disease [32].
	When undergoing surgery for presumed *appendicitis*, men show more severe pathologic condition [33].
	Incidence of *Crohn disease* varies by sex and age (higher in women age 25–29 and >35, but higher in men >45) [34].
Immunology	Women are twice as likely to contract *human immunodeficiency virus* from intercourse than men [35].
	In the 2014 *Ebola* outbreak in Liberia, 75% of the people who contracted the virus were women [36].
	Myasthenia gravis is more prevalent in women <40 y old, but more prevalent in men from ages 40 to 70 [37].
	Women require only half of the men's dose of *vaccine* to be protected from the flu [38].
Musculoskeletal	Women have different outcomes resulting from military-related *extremity trauma* [39].
	A man is more likely to die the year following an *osteoporotic hip fracture* than a woman [40].
	Women runners are twice as likely to suffer from *patellofemoral pain syndrome* [41].
	Women have a higher risk of *osteoarthritis* [42].
Neurology	Women are 20% to 30% less likely to receive tissue plasminogen activator for treatment of *acute stroke* [43].
	Aspirin prevents *stroke* but not primary MI in women, whereas it prevents MI but not stroke in men [44].
	Women have higher incidence (and differing manifestations) of *concussion* given the same level of impact [45].
	Premenopausal oophorectomy is associated with a 70% increased risk of *Alzheimer disease* [46].
	Women >65 y old are more likely to develop *Alzheimer disease* due to increased likelihood of having the APOE E4 gene [47].
	Parkinson's disease is more common in men, but women have more highly disabling complications and less chance of receiving effective treatment [48].

(*continued on next page*)

Table 2
continued

Organ system and discipline	Adult sex and gender differences
Oncology	A man is more likely to die following a diagnosis of *breast cancer* [49]. Women have higher levels of DNA in their *mitochondria* [50]. More than 70% of *oropharyngeal cancer* in men is associated with the human papilloma virus (HPV), whereas 98% of cervical cancer in women is associated with HPV [51]. *Lung cancer* is the leading cancer killer of women [53]. Women with *lung cancer* are more likely to be non-smokers than men with lung cancer [54].
Psychiatry	Women are more likely to attempt *suicide*, but men are more likely to be successful at it [55]. *Depression* is twice as common in women [56]. Office *depression screening tests* often omit common questions that would identify depression in men (anger, violence, substance abuse) [56]. Men are diagnosed with *Schizophrenia* more often, and at an earlier age than women [57].
Pulmonary	40% of women have exacerbation of *asthma* symptoms premenstrually [58]. Women with chronic obstructive pulmonary disease (*COPD*) report greater breathlessness and depression than men, largely due to anatomically smaller airway lumen and thicker airway walls [59]. Women who smoke are up to 70% more likely to develop *COPD* than men who smoke [52].
Pharmacology	Women reach maximum blood levels of *Zolpidem* 8 h after dose (45% greater than in men), leading to impaired driving [60]. In 2013, the FDA *revised the dosage* recommendation of Zolpidem to one-half for women due to impaired driving [61]. *Adverse drug reactions* are 60% more frequent in women than men [62]. In a 2011 GAO audit, 80% of *drugs withdrawn* from the market in a 10-year period were due to side effects in women [63].
Radiology	In the Emergency Department, women are more likely than men to have a diagnostic procedure that includes *radiation* [64]. Women are more susceptible to the *dangers of radiation* (eg, breast cancer) than men [64]. Women are more likely than men to develop *cancer* associated with ionizing radiation [65].

WHAT IS KNOWN ABOUT SEX DIFFERENCES IN PEDIATRICS?

Using a basic search tool developed by the Laura W. Bush Institute for Women's Health [66], a PubMed search of information related to sex and gender differences in children and adolescents detected more than 9000 articles. Unfortunately, these results are not organized in a way that can be easily categorized by disease or organ. There is no organized reference available yet that addresses pediatric and adolescent sex and gender differences. However, there are several textbooks, journal special editions, and popular books published that categorize and organize research in adults into structured study references.

To emphasize the need to recognize such differences in pediatrics, a case of fever without source (FWS) is presented in Box 2. Knowing sex differences in urinary tract infections (UTI) will allow for prompt diagnosis and management, preventing severe complications such as septicemia.

More conditions showing sex and gender differences in embryology, fertilization, preterm infants, infancy, childhood, and adolescents are presented in Tables 3 and 4, as found using the sex and gender specific health PubMed search tool [66].

Box 2: Pediatric case of fever without source

	Case presentation
Pertinent medical history:	11-month-old female infant with 3-d history of fever
Medications:	None, except vitamin D and omega-3 in formula
Relevant vital signs:	Blood pressure: 100/70; heart rate: 130 bpm; O_2 saturation 98%; rectal temperature: 39.5°C
Laboratory tests:	Catheterized urine shows positive nitrites and >20 white blood cells per high-power field
Physical examination:	Crying but consolable The rest of the examination is unremarkable
Assessment/ testing:	FWS in female infant <2 y old with leukocytosis in catheterized urine sample
Discussion:	FWS is more commonly due to UTI in girls and women, as compared with boys and men (unless uncircumcised or with ureteral reflux). The most sensitive predictors of UTI in febrile girls: 1. White race 2. Age <12 mo 3. Fever >39°C 4. Fever >2 d 5. Absence of other sources of fever These risk factors have been validated as a screening tool and were adapted by the American Academy of Pediatrics [67].
Conclusion:	FWS in children <2 y of age is more commonly found in girls (8%–9%) than boys (3%–4%) [68]. Vesicoureteral reflux and *Escherichia coli* have been found to be more prevalent in girls compared with boys in children <18 y old [68].

Adapted from Canares T, Franco M, Lazarus G. Special populations. In: McGregor AJ, Choo E, Becker B, editors. Sex and gender in acute care medicine. Cambridge (Unite Kingdom): Cambridge University Press; 2016. p. 193–215; with permission.

Table 3
Sample sex and gender differences in infants and children

Stages	Pediatric sex and gender differences
Conception, embryo, and fetus	The maternal oviduct can influence which sperm, X or Y, is successful at penetrating the ovum. This is known as "*Cryptic Female Choice*" [20]. Toxins or stress in men can result in decreased *viability* of their Y, but not X, spermatozoa [20]. *Embryonic viability*, after a catastrophic event (eg, 9/11, earthquakes), more male embryos die in utero [20]. Famine and severe stress during the first trimester are more likely to cause future *addiction* problems *in male* offspring, but *schizophrenia in female* offspring [20]. Female fetal lungs produce more surfactants at an earlier time than male fetal lungs, making *respiratory distress syndrome* more prevalent in preterm male infants [20]. *Cardiovascular system birth defects in male embryos* are more likely to be coarctation, single ventricle, or hypoplastic left ventricle, but in female embryos, atrioventricular septal defects, tricuspid atresia, or truncus arteriosus are more prevalent [20].
Preterm infants	Male preterm babies are at higher risk than female preterm babies for *later adverse respiratory illness* [20]. In low-birth-weight infants, *causation of preterm birth in male infants* is more likely due to abruptio placenta, UTI, or maternal hemorrhage, but in female infants, preeclampsia or intrauterine growth restriction is more likely the cause [20]. Preterm hyperglycemic female babies have higher *insulin secretion levels* than preterm hyperglycemic male babies [69].
Infants and children	When supplemented with fish oil, male infants showed greater increase in *insulin-like growth factor* than female infants [70]. Female, but not male, offspring are protected from *maternal hypertension-induced sensitization of angiotensin II* in pregnancy [71]. *Autism diagnostic guidelines* reflect boys' lower functional levels and may lead to missed diagnoses in girls [72]. Boys under age 12 have higher *pain tolerance* than girls [73]. Boys under age 12 are more likely than girls to experience *major depression* [74]. Severity of most *infectious diseases* is higher in boys due to sex hormone effect on T cells [75]. Before puberty, *asthma* is 16% greater in boys, but in adulthood, it is 62% greater in women [76]. In children under age 2, girls are twice as likely as boys to have UTI as the cause of FWS [67]. *Developmental dysplasia of the hip* is 4 times more common in girls [77]. In families with *multiple childhood cancer* cases, girls predominate [78].

WHERE TO GO WHEN YOU WANT TO KNOW

There is a growing list of resources available to those who are interested in finding information about sex and gender differences. The NIH ORWH has a 3-part Continuing Medical Education course that delivers this content and assesses one's knowledge in the field [101]. ORWH also maintains a

Table 4
Sample sex and gender differences in adolescents by organ system and discipline

Organ system and discipline	Adolescent sex and gender differences
Cardiovascular	Pubertal boys have a stronger *cardiovascular response* to caffeine than girls [79].
Gastrointestinal	Pubertal girls, when challenged with indomethacin, are more susceptible than boys to inflammatory bowel syndrome, ulcerative colitis, and celiac disease [80].
	Boys are more likely than girls to develop *Helicobacter pylori* and its related outcomes [81].
Endocrinology	Girls exhibit a greater *insulinemic response* to meals than boys despite similar glycemic responses [82].
Immunology	*Immunization response,* girls require only half the dose of influenza vaccine for the same response [83].
	Autoimmune disease may be more prevalent in girls due to testosterone downregulation of a cytokine known as *BAFF* [84].
	Eligible boys are less likely than girls to receive the *HPV vaccine* [85].
Musculoskeletal	Female athletes sustain more *concussions* and have more severe symptoms [86].
	Anterior cruciate ligament injury is up to 8 times more prevalent in female adolescent athletes [87].
	Patellofemoral pain and instability in adolescents are more prevalent in girls [88].
	Adolescent idiopathic *scoliosis* is twice as common in girls [89].
	Ankle sprains and bunions are more prevalent in adolescent girls [90].
	The *female athlete triad* (athlete energy imbalance) is also found in boys. Both can result in hypothalamic hypogonadism, osteoporosis, and fatigue [91]
Neurology	*Catamenial epilepsy,* up to 70% of girls with epilepsy have exacerbations premenstrually [92].
	Migraine, but not other severe headaches, is more prevalent in girls after puberty [93].
Psychiatry	Adolescent girls are more likely than boys to benefit from *suicide prevention programs* [94].
	Although 60% of adolescents are exposed to traumatic events, more girls than boys develop related *posttraumatic stress disorder* [95].
	Depressive symptoms in boys are associated with long-term cortisol concentration in hair, whereas *anxiety symptoms* in girls are associated with hypothalamic-pituitary-adrenal axis hypoactivity [82].
	Watching television increases *self-esteem* in white boys, but decreases it in white girls and black girls and boys [96].
	Adolescent girls are more susceptible to *addiction* to cannabis than boys [97].
	Substance abuse in sports in adolescents is more likely to be diuretics in girls (30% vs 14%) and anabolic steroids in boys (20% vs 11%) [98].
Respiratory	Adolescent girls with *cystic fibrosis* have worse prognosis and lower median survival [99].
	Globally, predominance of *allergic rhinitis* in boys changes to predominance in women after adolescence [100].

website that contains policy statements, research guidelines, and notices of webinars and other educational programs [102]. The Laura W. Bush Institute of Women's Health at Texas Tech University Health Sciences Center (TTUHSC) has many educational resources that are now open access for educators and students. These resources include a slide library, case studies, the PubMed search tool, learning modules, and a wide collection of resources to educate about sex and gender-specific management of various conditions [26]. They have begun to use these materials to weave SGBM knowledge into all 4 years of medical education at TTUHSC. It is also being integrated into the curricula of other medical schools. It is important to note that this does not require adding a new department or division. It only requires some faculty development and adding this knowledge to already existing curricula.

The Sex and Gender Health Collaborative, an initiative of the American Medical Women's Association (AMWA), hosts a digital library that contains many resources, including teaching tools, clinical cases, and marketing materials for researchers, educators, students, and residents [25]. Dr Alyson McGregor's edited textbook for emergency physicians, *Sex and Gender in Acute Care Medicine*, has a chapter addressing pediatric patients [64]. *Sex and Why* is an Internet site hosted by Dr Jeannette Wolf, who created a Jeopardy Game with Sex and Gender Difference topics. The game was a joint project with The Society for Academic Emergency Medicine (SAEM) Sex and Gender in Emergency Medicine's Interest Group, the Academy of Inclusion and Diversity in Emergency Medicine, and The Academy of Women in Academic Emergency Medicine [103]. Dr Marianne Legato, considered the "Mother of the Sex and Gender Based Medicine Movement," has published the third edition of her textbook, *Principles of Gender-Specific Medicine: Gender in the Genomic Era* [20] and is also editor of the journal, *Gender and the Genome* [104].

WHAT CAN YOU DO RIGHT NOW?

The minimum that should be done in any educational experience, be it a lecture, team-based learning, clinical case, or journal article, is to ask 2 simple questions:

1. How would this appear in the other sex?
2. Were women/girls included in this study, and were the results reported by sex?

This alone will go a long way to advance the field of sex and gender medicine and ultimately improve the health and health care of all.

FUTURE IMPLICATIONS

We are beginning to realize that there is a growing inventory of sex and gender research available to pediatricians, but there appears to be a wide gap between research and clinical application. With the recent NIH recognition that this information is necessary for evidence-based personalized patient care, the field of pediatrics should integrate sex and gender knowledge into education and practice. The pediatric field stands to benefit immeasurably when this knowledge is applied in research, evaluation, documentation, and health care delivery. In the meantime, the least we must do as educators and clinicians is to begin to recognize that these differences exist. Just as we once recognized that children were not small adults, it is time to recognize that girls are not the same as boys. Our children's health depends on it.

References

[1] Rojek M, Jenkins M. Improving medical education using a sex- and gender-based medicine lens. J Womens Heal 2016;25(10):985–9.
[2] Wizemann TM, Pardue M-L, editors. Exploring the biological contributions to human health: does sex matter? Washington, DC: The National Academies Press; 2001.
[3] Madsen TE, Bourjeily G, Hasnain M, et al. Sex- and gender-based medicine: the need for precise terminology. Gend Genome 2017;1(3):122–8.
[4] Chapman E, Kaatz A, Carnes M. Physicians and implicit bias: how doctors may unwittingly perpetuate health care disparities. J Gen Intern Med 2013;28(11):1504–10.
[5] National Institutes of Health: Office of Research on Women's Health. NIH policy on sex as a biological variable. 2018. Available at: https://orwh.od.nih.gov/sex-gender/nih-policy-sex-biological-variable. Accessed November 20, 2018.
[6] Henrich JB, Viscoli CM. What do medical schools teach about women's health and gender differences? Acad Med 2006;81(5):476–82.
[7] Jenkins MR, Herrmann A, Tashjian A, et al. Sex and gender in medical education: a national student survey. Biol Sex Differ 2016;7(Suppl 1):45.
[8] Henrich JB. Women's health education initiatives: why have they stalled? Acad Med 2004;79(4):283–8.
[9] Steering Committee of the Physicians' Health Study Research Group. Final report on aspirin component of the ongoing physician health study. N Engl J Med 1989;321:129–35.
[10] National Institutes of Health: Office of Research on Women's Health. Sex/gender influences in health and disease. 2018. Available at: https://orwh.od.nih.gov/sex-gender/sexgender-influences-health-and-disease. Accessed November 20, 2018.
[11] McDonough PG. The randomized world is not without its imperfections: reflections on the women's health initiative study. Fertil Steril 2002;78(5):951–6.
[12] Bellasi A, Raggi P, Bairey Merz N, et al. New insights into ischemic heart disease in women. Cleve Clin J Med 2007;74(8):585–94.
[13] Rojek MK. Historical perspective. 2018. Available at: https://www.amwa-doc.org/sghc/sex-and-gender-health-historical-perspective/. Accessed November 18, 2018.
[14] Edogawa S, Peters S, Jenkins G, et al. Sex differences in NSAID-induced perturbation of human intestinal barrier function and microbiota. FASEB J 2018;fj201800056.
[15] Dusenbery M. Doing harm. New York: Harper Collins Publishers; 2017.
[16] Coalition for Women's Health Equity. 2018. Available at: http://www.hadassah.org/advocate/coalition-for-womens-health.html. Accessed November 18, 2018.
[17] Research for All Act of 2015. 2015. Available at: https://www.congress.gov/bill/114th-congress/house-bill/2101. Accessed November 18, 2018.
[18] Ligon-Borden BL. Abraham Jacobi, MD: father of American pediatrics and advocate for children's health. Semin Pediatr Infect Dis 2003;14(3):245–9.
[19] Gillis J, Loughlan P. Not just small adults: the metaphors of paediatrics. Arch Dis Child 2007;92(11):946–7.
[20] Legato MJ, editor. Principles of gender-specific medicine: gender in the Genomic Era. 3rd edition. Maryland Heights (MO): Elsevier Academic Press; 2017.
[21] Freeborn D, Haldeman-Englert C. Uniparental disomy: Prader-Willi syndrome, Angelman syndrome. 2018. Available at: https://www.urmc.rochester.edu/encyclopedia/content.aspx?ContentTypeID=90&ContentID=P02159. Accessed November 20, 2018.
[22] Pollard TM, Hyatt SB, editors. Sex, gender and health. Cambridge (United Kingdom): Cambridge University Press; 1999.

[23] Mccarthy M. Sex differences in the brain. The scientist: exploring life, inspiring innovation. 2015. Available at: https://www.the-scientist.com/features/sex-differences-in-the-brain-34758. Accessed November 22, 2018.
[24] Oertelt-Prigione S, Gohlke B, Dunkel M, et al. GenderMedDB: an interactive database of sex and gender-specific medical literature. Biol Sex Differ 2014;5:7.
[25] American Medical Women's Association. Sex and Gender Health Collaborative. 2018. Available at: https://www.amwa-doc.org/sghc/. Accessed November 18, 2018.
[26] Laura W. Bush Institute for Women's Health. Sex and gender specific health. 2018. Available at: https://www.sexandgenderhealth.org/. Accessed November 18, 2018.
[27] Bairey Merz C, Regitz-Zagrosek V. The case for sex- and gender-specific medicine. JAMA Intern Med 2014;174(8):1348–9.
[28] Safdar B, Spatz E, Dreye R, et al. Presentation, Clinical profile, and prognosis of young patients with Myocardial Infarction With Nonobstructive Coronary Arteries (MINOCA): results from the VIRGO Study. J Am Heart Assoc 2018;7(13); https://doi.org/10.1161/JAHA.118.009174. pii: e009174.
[29] Vaccarino V, Krumholz H, Berkman L, et al. Sex differences in mortality after myocardial infarction: Is there evidence for an increased risk for women? Circulation 1995;91(6):1861–71.
[30] Blewer A, McGovern S, Schmicker R, et al. Gender disparities among adult recipients of bystander cardiopulmonary resuscitation in the public. Circ Cardiovasc Qual Outcomes 2018;11(8):e004710.
[31] Dugo D, Bordignon S, Perrotta L, et al. Catheter ablation of atrial fibrillation in females. J Atr Fibrillation 2013;6(1):893.
[32] National Institutes of Health: National Institute on Alcohol Abuse and Alcoholism. Are women more vulnerable to alcohol's effects? Alcohol alert. 1999. Available at: https://pubs.niaaa.nih.gov/publications/aa46.htm. Accessed November 20, 2018.
[33] Stein GY, Rath-Wolfson L, Zeidman A, et al. Sex differences in the epidemiology, seasonal variation, and trends in the management of patients with acute appendicitis. Langenbecks Arch Surg 2012;397(7):1087–92.
[34] Shah S, Khalili H, Gower-Rousseau C, et al. Sex-based differences in incidence of inflammatory bowel diseases-pooled analysis of population-based studies from western countries. Gastroenterology 2018;155(4):1079–89.
[35] Griesbeck M, Scully E, Altfeld M. Sex and gender differences in HIV-1 infection. Clin Sci 2016;130(16):1435–51.
[36] Ebola outbreak takes its toll on women. UN Women. 2014. Available at: http://www.unwomen.org/en/news/stories/2014/9/ebola-outbreak-takes-its-toll-on-women. Accessed November 22, 2018.
[37] Asmail A, Kesler A, Kolb H, et al. A tri-modal distribution of age-of-onset in female patients with myasthenia gravis is associated with the gender-related clinical differences. Int J Neurosci 2019;129(4):313–9.
[38] Furman D, Hejblum B, Simon N, et al. Systems analysis of sex differences reveals an immunosuppressive role for testosterone in the response to influenza vaccination. Proc Natl Acad Sci U S A 2014;111(2):869–74.
[39] Roy T, Piva S, Christiansen B, et al. Description of musculoskeletal injuries occurring in female soldiers deployed to Afghanistan. Mil Med 2015;180(3):269–75.
[40] Center J, Nguyen T, Schneider D, et al. Mortality after all major types of osteoporotic fracture in men and women: an observational study. Lancet 1999;353(9156):878–82.
[41] Boling M, Padua D, Marshall S, et al. Gender differences in the incidence and prevalence of patellofemoral pain syndrome. Scand J Med Sci Sports 2010;20(5):725–30.
[42] O'Connor M. Osteoarthritis of the hip and knee: sex and gender differences. Orthop Clin North Am 2006;37(4):559–68.
[43] Reeves M, Bhatt A, Jajou P, et al. Sex differences in the use of intravenous rt-PA thrombolysis treatment for acute ischemic stroke: a meta-analysis. Stroke 2009;40(5):1743–9.

[44] Ridker P, Cook N, Lee I, et al. A randomized trial of low-dose aspirin in the primary prevention of cardiovascular disease in women. N Engl J Med 2005;352(13):1293–304.
[45] Mollayeva T, El-Khechen-Richandi G, Colantonio A. Sex & gender considerations in concussion research. Concussion 2018;3(1):CNC51.
[46] Zeydan B, Tosakulwong N, Schawarz C, et al. Association of bilateral salpingo-oophorectomy before menopause onset with medial temporal lobe neurodegeneration. JAMA Neurol 2019;76(1):95–100.
[47] Ungar L, Altmann A, Greicius M. Apolipoprotein E, gender, and Alzheimer's disease: an overlooked, but potent and promising interaction. Brain Imaging Behav 2015;8(2): 262–73.
[48] Picillo M, Nicoletti A, Fetoni V, et al. The relevance of gender in Parkinson's disease: a review. J Neurol 2017;264(8):1583–607.
[49] Nemchek L. Male breast cancer: examining gender disparity in diagnosis and treatment. Clin J Oncol Nurs 2018;22(5):E127–33.
[50] Knez J, Winckelmans E, Plusquin M, et al. Correlates of peripheral blood mitochondrial DNA content in a general population. Am J Epidemiol 2016;183(2):138–46.
[51] Pytynia K, Dahlstrom K, Sturgis E. Epidemiology of HPV-associated oropharyngeal cancer. Oral Oncol 2014;50(5):380–6.
[52] Gan W, Man S, Postma D, et al. Female smokers beyond the perimenopausal period are at increased risk of chronic obstructive pulmonary disease: a systematic review and meta-analysis. Respir Res 2006;7:52.
[53] Torre L, Siegel R, Jemal A. Lung cancer statistics. Adv Exp Med Biol 2016;893:1–19.
[54] Eldridge L. Lung cancer in women. Verywell health. 2017. Available at: https://www.verywellhealth.com/lung-cancer-in-women-2249402. Accessed November 22, 2018.
[55] Jack S, Petrosky E, Lyons B, et al. Surveillance for violent deaths - National Violent Death Reporting System, 27 States, 2015. MMWR Surveill Summ 2018;67(11):1–32.
[56] Martin L, Neighbors H, Griffith D. The experience of symptoms of depression in men vs women. JAMA Psychiatry 2013;70(10):1100–6.
[57] Riecher-Rössler A. Oestrogens, prolactin, hypothalamic-pituitary-gonadal axis, and schizophrenic psychoses. Lancet Psychiatry 2017;4(1):63–72.
[58] Gibbs C, Coutts I, Lock R, et al. Premenstrual exacerbation of asthma. Thorax 1984;39(11):833–6.
[59] Martinez F, Curtis J, Sciurba F, et al. Sex differences in severe pulmonary emphysema. Am J Respir Crit Care Med 2007;176:243–52.
[60] Kesselheim A, Donneyong M, Dal Pan G, et al. Changes in prescribing and healthcare resource utilization after FDA Drug Safety Communications involving zolpidem-containing medications. Pharmacoepidemiol Drug Saf 2017;26(6):712–21.
[61] United States Department of Health and Human Services. FDA drug safety communication: FDA approves new label changes and dosing for zolpidem products and a recommendation to avoid driving the day after using Ambien CR. 2017. Available at: https://www.fda.gov/Drugs/DrugSafety/ucm352085.htm. Accessed November 30, 2018.
[62] Martin R, Biswas P, Freemantle S, et al. Age and sex distribution of suspected adverse drug reactions to newly marketed drugs in general practice in England: analysis of 48 cohort studies. Br J Clin Pharmacol 1998;46(5):505–11.
[63] United States General Accounting Office. Drug safety: most drugs withdrawn in recent years had greater health risks for women. GAO-01-286R. 2001. Jan 19. https://www.gao.gov/products/GAO-01-286R. Accessed April 8, 2019.
[64] McGregor A, editor. Sex and gender in acute care medicine. Cambridge (United Kingdom): Cambridge University Press; 2016.
[65] Narendran N, Luzhna L, Kovalchuk O. Sex difference of radiation response in occupational and accidental exposure. Front Genetics 2019;10:260. https://www.frontiersin.org/articles/10.3389/fgene.2019.00260/abstract. Accessed April 8, 2019.

[66] Song MM, Simonsen CK, Wilson JD, et al. Development of a PubMed based search tool for identifying sex and gender specific health literature. J Womens Heal 2016;25(2):181–7.
[67] Subcommittee on Urinary Tract Infection, Steering Committee on Quality Improvement and Management, Roberts KB. Urinary tract infection: clinical practice guideline for the diagnosis and management of the initial UTI in febrile infants and children 2 to 24 months. Pediatrics 2011;128(3):595–610.
[68] Canares T, Franco M, Lazarus G. Special populations. In: McGregor AJ, Choo E, Becker B, editors. Sex and gender in acute care medicine. Cambridge (United Kingdom): Cambridge University Press; 2016. p. 193–215.
[69] Dickson J, Chase J, Pretty C, et al. Hyperglycaemic preterm babies have sex differences in insulin secretion. Neonatology 2015;108(2):93–8.
[70] Damsgaard C, Harsløf L, Andersen A, et al. Fish oil supplementation from 9 to 18 months of age affects the insulin-like growth factor axis in a sex-specific manner in Danish infants. Br J Nutr 2016;115(5):782–90.
[71] Xue B, Beltz T, Guo F, et al. Sex differences in maternal gestational hypertension-induced sensitization of angiotensin II hypertension in rat offspring: the protective effect of estrogen. Am J Physiol Regul Integr Comp Physiol 2018;314(2):R274–81.
[72] Kirkovski M, Enticott P, Fitzgerald P. A review of the role of female gender in autism spectrum disorders. J Autism Dev Disord 2013;43(11):2584–603.
[73] Boerner K, Birnie K, Caes L, et al. Sex differences in experimental pain among healthy children: a systematic review and meta-analysis. Pain 2014;155(5):983–93.
[74] Douglas J, Scott J. A systematic review of gender-specific rates of unipolar and bipolar disorders in community studies of pre-pubertal children. Bipolar Disord 2014;16(1):5–15.
[75] Muenchhoff M, Goulder P. Sex differences in pediatric infectious diseases. J Infect Dis 2014;209(Suppl):S120–6.
[76] Kynyk J, Mastronarde J, McCallister J. Asthma the sex difference. Curr Opin Pulm Med 2011;17(1):6–11.
[77] Kotlarsky P, Haber R, Bialik V, et al. Developmental dysplasia of the hip: what has changed in the last 20 years? World J Orthop 2015;6(11):886–901.
[78] Stjernfelt K, Von Stedingk K, Wiebe T, et al. Predominance of girls with cancer in families with multiple childhood cancer cases. BMC Cancer 2017;17(1):868.
[79] Temple J, Ziegler A, Graczyk A, et al. Cardiovascular responses to caffeine by gender and pubertal stage. Pediatrics 2014;134(1):e112–9.
[80] Federation of American Societies for Experimental Biology. The FASEB Journal: gender-specific differences in intestinal lining. EurekAlert 2018. Available at: https://www.eurekalert.org/pub_releases/2018-06/foas-tfj061918.php. Accessed November 22, 2018.
[81] Ibrahim A, Morais S, Ferro A, et al. Sex-differences in the prevalence of Helicobacter pylori infection in pediatric and adult populations: systematic review and meta-analysis of 244 studies. Dig Liver Dis 2017;49(7):742–9.
[82] Lu Q, Pan F, Ren L, et al. Sex differences in the association between internalizing symptoms and hair cortisol level among 10-12 year-old adolescents in China. PLoS One 2018;13(3): e0192901.
[83] Engler R, Nelson M, Klote M, et al. Half- vs full-dose trivalent inactivated influenza vaccine (2004-2005): age, dose, and sex effects on immune responses. Arch Intern Med 2008;168(22):2405–14.
[84] Wilhelmson A, Rodriguez M, Stubelius A, et al. Testosterone is an endogenous regulator of BAFF and splenic B cell number. Nat Commun 2018;9(1):2067.
[85] Beavis A, Krakow M, Levinson K, et al. Reasons for lack of HPV vaccine initiation in NIS-Teen over time: shifting the focus from gender and sexuality to necessity and safety. J Adolesc Health 2018;63(5):652–6.
[86] Dougan B, Horswill M, Geffen G. Athletes' age, sex, and years of education moderate the acute neuropsychological impact of sports-related concussion: a meta-analysis. J Int Neuropsychol Soc 2014;20(1):64–80.

[87] Templeton KJ, Hame SL, Hannafin JA, et al. Sports injuries in women: sex-and gender-based differences in etiology and prevention. Instr Course Lectures 2008;57:539–52.
[88] Stracciolini A, Casciano R, Levey Friedman H, et al. Pediatric sports injuries: a comparison of males versus females. Am J Sports Med 2014;42(4):965–72.
[89] Luan FJ, Zhang J, Hai-Qiang W. Epidemiological study of adolescent idiopathic scoliosis using low/non-radiation screening methodology. J Rehabil Med 2018;50:765–6.
[90] Omey M, MIcheli L. Foot and ankle problems in the young athlete. Med Sci Sports Exerc 1999;31(7 Suppl):S470–86.
[91] Hooper D, Tenforde A, Hackney A. Treating exercise-associated low testosterone and its related symptoms. Phys Sportsmed 2018;46(4):427–34.
[92] Case A, Reid R. Effects of the menstrual cycle on medical disorders. JAMA Intern Med 1998;158(13):1405–12.
[93] Buse D, Loder E, Gorman J, et al. Sex differences in the prevalence, symptoms, and associated features of migraine, probable migraine and other severe headache: results of the American Migraine Prevalence and Prevention (AMPP) Study. Headache 2013;53(8): 1278–99.
[94] Hamilton E, Klimes-Dougan B. Gender differences in suicide prevention responses: implications for adolescents based on an illustrative review of the literature. Int J Environ Res Public Health 2015;12(3):2359–72.
[95] Garza K, Jovanovic T. Impact of gender on child and adolescent PTSD. Curr Psychiatry Rep 2017;19(11):87.
[96] Martins N, Harrison K. Racial and gender differences in the relationship between children's television use and self-esteem: a longitudinal panel study. Communication Research 2012;39(3):338–57.
[97] Struik D, Sanna F, Fattore L. The modulating role of sex and anabolic-androgenic steroid hormones in cannabinoid sensitivity. Front Behav Neurosci 2018;12:249.
[98] Kuhn C. Emergence of sex differences in the development of substance use and abuse during adolescence. Pharmacol Ther 2015;153:55–78.
[99] McIntyre K. Gender and survival in cystic fibrosis. Curr Opin Pulm Med 2013;19(6): 692–7.
[100] Pinart M, Keller T, Reich A, et al. Sex-related allergic rhinitis prevalence switch from childhood to adulthood: a systematic review and meta-analysis. Int Arch Allergy Immunol 2017;172(4):224–35.
[101] National Institutes of Health: Office of Research on Women's Health. Online courses on sex/gender differences. 2018. Available at: https://orwh.od.nih.gov/sex-gender/online-courses-sex-gender-differences. Accessed November 18, 2018.
[102] National Institutes of Health: Office of Research on Women's Health. Sex & gender. 2018. Available at: https://orwh.od.nih.gov/sex-gender. Accessed November 18, 2018.
[103] Wolfe J. Sex & why. 2018. Available at: https://www.sexandwhy.com/basics/. Accessed November 18, 2018.
[104] Legato M. Gender and the genome: a new journal for the 21st century. Gend Genome 2016;1(1):1–3.

Advances in Pediatrics 66 (2019) 37–54
ADVANCES IN PEDIATRICS

Gene Therapy

Current Applications and Future Possibilities

David H.M. Steffin, MD[a,b], Emily M. Hsieh, MD[a,b], Rayne H. Rouce, MD[a,b,*]

[a]Center for Cell and Gene Therapy, Baylor College of Medicine, Houston Methodist Hospital and Texas Children's Hospital, Houston, TX, USA; [b]Texas Children's Cancer and Hematology Centers/Baylor College of Medicine, One Baylor Plaza, Houston, TX 77030, USA

Keywords

• Gene therapy • Immunotherapy • CAR T cell • Human genome editing • CRISPR-Cas9

Key points

- Early clinical trials of gene therapy, despite mixed outcomes, solidified the use of viral vectors to transmit genetic material and paved the way for current clinical applications.
- Gene therapy has demonstrated success in inherited and acquired pediatric diseases including immunodeficiencies, inherited retinal disorders, neurologic disorders, blood disorders, and cancer.
- Chimeric antigen receptor (CAR) T cells targeting CD19 expressed on B-ALL, the most common childhood cancer, have induced complete remissions in refractory patients, leading to recent FDA approval.
- Novel gene-editing techniques such as CRISPR-Cas9 offer precise mechanisms of human genome modification, a technique that will be tested in upcoming clinical trials.

INTRODUCTION

Gene therapy encompasses multiple approaches to manipulate genetic material in an effort to treat specific diseases, including replacing a mutated or defective gene with a healthy one, introducing a new gene to help fight disease, or editing an existing gene to change its function [1]. From a clinical perspective, gene therapy has the potential to reverse the clinical sequelae of a condition, a

*Corresponding author. Center for Cell and Gene Therapy, Feigin Center, 1102 Bates Street, 17th Floor, Houston, TX 77030, USA. *E-mail address:* rhrouce@gmail.com

https://doi.org/10.1016/j.yapd.2019.04.001
0065-3101/19/

concept that was long met with understandable skepticism. In pediatrics, these strategies hold special promise, because many childhood diseases were considered incurable before recent innovations in gene therapy.

Although gene therapy has been studied for decades, the last few years have yielded some of the most exciting clinical advances in the treatment of inherited and acquired diseases. The road to translating these therapies to the clinic has been a perilous one, although positive results in some rare diseases have contributed to optimism in the field. Nevertheless, concerns over safety and appropriate clinical applications have arisen, highlighting the importance of careful regulation and monitoring of in-human use.

Here, we will briefly review types of gene therapy and their potential uses, before highlighting recent advances in gene therapy for pediatric disorders. We will focus on therapies that have been translated to the clinic. We will also discuss current safety and ethical guidelines that must be considered when using gene therapy, as well as what the future holds for this promising therapy.

SUCCESSFUL EXAMPLES OF GENE THERAPY USED TO TREAT DISEASES

Gene therapy is typically divided into 2 main types: germ line and somatic. In somatic gene therapy, genes are introduced into somatic cells or patients, and thus therapy is limited to the individual patient and cannot be inherited or passed on. Germ line gene therapy involves introducing a new gene into sperm or egg cells, which allows the introduced changes to be heritable and therefore passed on [1]. Germ line therapy is less common, and more technically and ethically challenging because of the ability of therapeutic effects to be passed on. Thus, somatic gene therapy has had the most clinical success to date and is the main focus of this review.

Despite years of preclinical work, it was not until the early 1990s that the first gene therapies were studied in humans, albeit with mixed results. The first clinical trial to gain approval for transfer of a foreign gene into humans was conducted at the National Cancer Institute in Bethesda, Maryland, in 1990. This trial used a retroviral vector to insert the gene encoding the cytokine, inteleukin-2 (IL-2) into patient-derived tumor-infiltrating lymphocytes (TILs). The genetically modified TILs were then infused back into patients with advanced melanoma. Although the efficacy results were disappointing–all 5 patients treated ultimately died of progressive disease–TILs from 4 of 5 patients displayed in vivo expansion without significant toxicity [2].

That same year, the first gene therapy trial targeting an inherited immunodeficiency, severe combined immunodeficiency (SCID), was performed. Again, a retroviral vector was used to insert the gene encoding adenosine deaminase (ADA), the enzyme deficient in patients with SCID, into patient T cells. These genetically modified T cells were then given back to 2 patients with SCID, one of whom demonstrated an increase in ADA activity that may have been attributable to the therapy, although the patient was concurrently receiving an enzyme replacement therapy, thus confounding results [3].

The early clinical applications of cell therapy, while demonstrating safety and feasibility, unfortunately resulted in limited efficacy. More than 100 clinical trials of various gene therapies were developed in the 1990s. Despite their mixed outcomes, one concept solidified by these early gene therapy trials was the use of viral vectors to transfer genetic material. Therefore the promise of adoptively transferring cells genetically modified in the laboratory using viral vectors, once considered myth, became reality [4].

Despite a plateau in clinical progress in the 1990s, over the last 20 years there has been a resurgence of research committed to improving cell therapies, with significant progress (Fig. 1). Since the 2000s, there have been successes in the manipulation and use of a variety of vectors, namely retro and lentiviral ones, which has directly correlated with enhanced clinical translation.

GENE THERAPY FOR HEREDITARY DISEASES

Gene therapy has been particularly useful in the treatment of inherited diseases whereby there is often a nonfunctional or dysfunctional gene product. These approaches also provide an alternative, less-toxic, but potentially curative therapy to hematopoietic stem cell transplant (HSCT), which has historically been the only therapeutic option to reverse some inherited diseases.

Inherited immunodeficiencies

As mentioned in the preceding section, one of the first diseases successfully treated with gene therapy was SCID, an inherited combined immunodeficiency resulting from several gene deletions. Patients with these gene deletions lack functional B, T, and natural killer (NK) cells, and thus are very susceptible to life-threatening bacterial, viral, and fungal infections [5]. HSCT is the only known cure, but is associated with its own short- and long-term toxicities. Following the initial gene therapy trials for SCID in the 1990s, a significant breakthrough in gene therapy for SCID due to ADA deficiency was reported

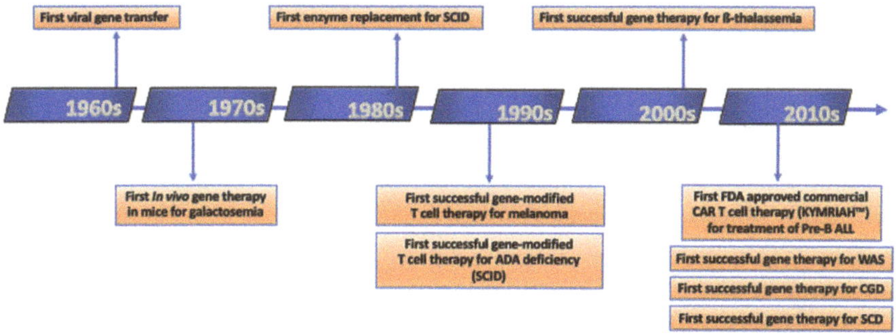

Fig. 1. Timeline depicting key milestones in preclinical research and clinical trials in gene therapy from the 1960s to the present day. CGD, Chronic granulomatous disease; SCD, sickle cell disease; WAS, Wiskott-Aldrich syndrome.

in 2002. The first clinical study using gene transfer into HSCs was completed at Hadassah Hospital in Israel (NCT00598481) [6]. This study inserted a functional ADA gene into a retroviral vector, then transferred this vector into HSCs of patients with SCID. The study evaluated 18 patients from 2000 to 2014 with a primary endpoint of safety and secondary endpoint of efficacy. All 18 patients underwent initial conditioning treatment with busulfan, followed by infusion of the genetically modified therapy. Overall, the intervention was safe, with all patients surviving to the last follow-up in 2014. The treatment was well tolerated with most adverse events being cytopenias, increased transaminases, and hypertension, symptoms that resolved in all patients and were thought to be related to busulfan conditioning rather than the gene therapy itself. Most importantly, 15 of the 18 patients developed increased ADA levels, increased lymphocyte counts, sustained immune reconstitution, and sustained humoral and cellular immune responses [6,7], indicating the efficacy of this therapeutic approach. None of these patients developed evidence of myelodysplasia or leukemia at any point during follow-up, which is notable given that this long-term toxicity has occurred as a result of other gene therapies, as discussed in the safety section below.

The success in SCID paved the way for attempts to correct genetic impairments in other inherited immunodeficiencies. Chronic granulomatous disease (CGD) is a debilitating immunodeficiency that occurs as a result of mutations in the CYBB gene. CGD is characterized by a decrease in oxidase-positive neutrophils, resulting in an inability to respond to bacterial and fungal infections [8]. The identified isolated CYBB mutation in CGD makes it an ideal target for gene therapy.

There has been extensive preclinical research demonstrating success for gene therapy in CGD [9,10]. Based on these promising data, a phase 1 clinical trial (NCT02234934) was opened in January 2015 in 3 locations: Boston Children's Hospital, University of California, LA, and the NIH [11]. The study used a lentiviral vector to insert a functional CYBB gene into patient HSCs. Recently reported interim data on 7 pediatric patients with a 12-month follow-up showed patients have tolerated the therapy well so far. Aside from one infusion-related inflammatory syndrome that resolved with steroid supplementation, there have been no reported significant adverse events. Six of 7 patients had an increased percentage of oxidase-positive neutrophils (range 16%–46%) from baseline (notably, at least 10% oxidase-positive neutrophils are necessary for normal neutrophil function). All 6 responding patients demonstrated persistent peripheral blood copies of the lentiviral vector expressing the CYBB gene, even at 12 months postinfusion [12]. Further, all patients were able to discontinue prophylactic antimicrobials.

Gene therapy for Wiskott-Aldrich syndrome (WAS) has also demonstrated promising results. WAS is an X-linked disorder characterized by a mutation in the WAS protein (WASP) gene leading to thrombocytopenia and immunodeficiency. As a result, patients suffer from eczema, inability to fight infections, and have a significant risk of bleeding [13]. Recently, a phase 1/2 clinical trial

(NCT01347242) started in March 2019, at the Great Ormond Street Hospital for Children in London, demonstrated promising interim results of 7 pediatric patients treated with ex vivo gene-modified CD34+ stem cells encoding a lentiviral vector with a functional WASP gene. One patient died from a preexisting drug-resistant herpes infection. Of the remaining 6 patients, all had immune constitution with corrected lymphoid cells, and all 6 patients had resolution of bleeding episodes and eczema [14].

Leber congenital amaurosis

One of the earliest successes in gene therapy came in the treatment of Leber congenital amaurosis, which is an early and irreversible cause of blindness. There are no supportive treatments for the disease, which typically occurs in the first 2 decades of life. Once researchers, in 1988, discovered hereditary mitochondrial DNA mutations as the primary defect leading to congenital amaurosis, the possibility arose of reversing this devastating cause of blindness with targeted gene therapy [15]. In 2007, 3 groups treated patients in early clinical trials in the United States and United Kingdom. In 1 phase 1 clinical trial, 3 patients (21–24 years) underwent unilateral intraretinal injections of an adenoviral-associated vector (AAV) carrying a functional copy of RPE65, known to be deficient in Leber congenital amaurosis. Treatment was well tolerated with no significant adverse events reported. All 3 patients noted significant improvement in visual acuity in the treated eye, prompting a cascade of gene therapy clinical trials in the field [16]. The exciting results ultimately led to US Food and Drug Administration (FDA) approval of the gene therapy, Luxturna, in 2017 [17].

Neurologic disorders

Identification of the precise causative mutations for most neurologic disorders has aided in the ability of researchers to develop targeted gene therapies to combat them. AAV gene therapy enables both gene replacement to address loss-of-function mutations and gene silencing to address gain-of-function mutations. Both strategies have been used in preclinical and clinical studies for neurologic diseases. For example, survival motor neuron (SMN) protein has been replaced to treat spinal muscular atrophy (SMA) [1,2,3], while superoxide dismutase 1 has been silenced to treat amyotrophic lateral sclerosis [4,5,6], as has Huntington for Huntington disease [7,8,9] [18]. The FDA recently approved the drug Spinraza, which increases production of SMN protein, after it showed promising results in patients with SMA. In an expanded access program in Europe, 61 children with SMA were treated with Spinraza and experienced substantial improvement in motor function after only 6 months [19]. Another gene therapy drug for SMA type 1 called Zolgensma, which provides a normal copy of the SMA1 gene, also showed great promise in early clinical trials and is currently pending FDA approval [20].

X-linked myotubular myopathy is another rare neuromuscular disorder caused by a mutation in the myotubularin gene and characterized by progressive muscle weakness and respiratory failure [21]. A recent clinical trial testing a gene therapy called AT132, composed of an AAV encoding the functional copy of the myotubularin gene has reported early success (NCT03199469). Interim results from 7 patients enrolled in an AT123 trial showed that 3 patients attained ventilator independence at 48 weeks follow-up, demonstrating their rapid improvement in muscle function [22].

Lysosomal storage diseases

Targeting causative gene mutations in lysosomal storage diseases may also provide promising therapeutic options. Fabry disease is caused by a mutation in the α-galactosidase A gene, which produces galactosidase A. A recent phase 1 clinical trial (NCT02800070) performed ex vivo transduction of CD34+ stem cells with a lentiviral vector containing a normal copy of the human α-Gal A gene with the intention to determine the safety and toxicity, as well as any potential benefit in adult patients. The trial began in 2017, operating at 3 centers in Canada. Six patients have been enrolled thus far. Interim data report no adverse effects, and 1 patient demonstrated engraftment and generation of galactosidase A activity at 2 years follow-up [23]. Promising data also have been reported for ex vivo clinical gene therapies as treatment of mucopolysaccharoidosis (MPS), Gaucher disease, and Hurler syndrome. In 2018, a phase 1 clinical trial (NCT02702115) was opened also using ex vivo transduction of CD34+ stem cells with an AAV to insert a corrected gene copy expressing iduronidase, a liver enzyme deficient in MPS1. The first patient was recently enrolled with, results pending [24,25].

Inherited hematologic diseases

Gene therapy has become a viable therapeutic option for several inherited hematologic diseases. β-Thalassemia major, characterized by loss of 3 copies of the β-globin gene, leads to severe anemia, growth and developmental delay, and complications of transfusion dependence often leading to liver and heart failure. The incidence of β-thalassemia is 1/100,000 worldwide and HSCT is the only curative therapy [26]. Recently, 2 phase 1/2 gene therapy trials have entered the spotlight after demonstrating success [25,27]. In both trials, CD34-mobilized stem cells were transduced in vitro with a lentiviral vector encoding HbA, the normal hemoglobin that is missing in patients with β-thalassemia major. Twenty-two patients (aged 12–35 years of age) received busulfan as preconditioning chemotherapy, followed by infusion of the gene-modified stem cell product. Thirteen of the patients had a mild phenotype characterized by residual function of the β-globin gene, while 9 had a severe phenotype. Twelve of the 13 patients with the mild phenotype stopped requiring red blood cell (RBC) transfusions at a median of 26 months after treatment. Moreover, of the 9 patients with the completely nonfunctional phenotype, the mean transfusion volume per year was reduced by 73%, allowing discontinuation in 3 of the patients. Neither study resulted in significant toxicities, although 9 of 22 patients suffered minor adverse events consistent with side effects related to busulfan [28].

The exciting results in β-thalassemia paved the way for the use of gene therapy in other hemoglobinopathies. Worldwide, approximately 250,000 babies are born every year with sickle cell disease (SCD) and 95,000 people are living with SCD in the United States [29]. SCD is the result of a single-nucleotide mutation in the SCD β-globin chain that leads to a substitution of glutamic acid to valine. This mutation results in an unstable hemoglobin, producing the classic "sickled" RBCs, which, despite modern treatment modalities can become trapped, leading to several complications including significant anemia, veno-oclussive crisis, infection, stroke, organ failure, and decreased lifespan [30]. Conventional treatment has consisted of supportive care including prophylactic antibiotics to protect from encapsulated bacteria. More recently, therapeutic options such as hydroxyurea have emerged. Hydroxyurea stimulates the production of fetal hemoglobin (HbF), thus minimizing the production of sickled RBCs.

Despite recent advances, SCD remains one of the most challenging inherited disorders to treat, with HSCT being the only curative option. However, the less than ideal outcomes following HSCT for SCD largely related to lack of ideal donor sources, have resulted in significant focus being placed on gene therapy [31]. Clinical trials conducted at 3 different centers have reported exciting results to date. Bluebird Bio (Cambridge, MA) is treating patients with SCD on an ongoing phase 1/2 trial (NCT02140554) that is enrolling patients at multiple sites in the United States. In this trial, patient CD34+ stem cells are collected and undergo lentiglobin gene therapy to insert a normal β-globin gene. Before infusion of these gene-modified HSCs, patients are treated with busulfan conditioning therapy [32]. Early results from 7 patients treated with this therapy revealed improvements in hemoglobin in 4 of them after 6 months of follow-up. No veno-occlusive crises were reported, and laboratory values commonly used to follow SCD were improved compared with baseline levels in all patients. These clinical improvements correlated with a quantitative reduction in mutated globin chain β^S in all treated patients [32].

Other groups have explored mechanisms to increase HbF production, as opposed to repairing the β-globin gene. In a phase 1/2 clinical trial at Cincinnati Children's (NCT02186418), CD34+ stem cells were collected by way of marrow harvest or pheresis, followed by in vitro transduction of HSCs with a lentiviral vector encoding a modified γ-globin chain encoding for HbF. Patients subsequently underwent conditioning with melphalan before product infusion. Preliminary results demonstrate an acceptable safety profile and prompt count recovery. Two patients have been treated thus far, both experiencing significant improvement in chronic pain and reduction in sickling events [33].

With regard to the inherited bleeding disorders hemophilias A and B (Factor VIII and IX deficiency, respectively), there are several phase 1 and 2 clinical trials that are ongoing or were recently completed. Despite recombinant factor replacement and vigilant treatment, patients with hemophilia often experience significant and repeated bleeding into joints, muscles, or intracranially, leading to considerable morbidity and mortality [34]. Several groups have explored the use of AAV as a means of correcting the deficiencies in hemophilia A and B. Because the mutations associated with the hemophilias are complex–due to either inversions, missense, or small/large deletions [35]–researchers have focused on providing a functional copy of the gene encoding the absent factor.

Despite promising preclinical results, the clinical translation of gene therapy for the hemophilias remains challenging. For one, there are constraints limiting the use of viral vectors as modes of gene transfer: gene insertions must be relatively small to ensure that the gene is inserted properly, efficiently transferred to the patient, and that its expression is maintained on infusion. As the size of the insert increases, successful gene therapy becomes more challenging. This concept is especially relevant for factor VIII, which is quite large [36]. Factor IX (FIX) gene therapy has yielded more success. Recently, a phase 1 clinical trial (NCT03307980) conducted by Pfizer at multiple centers in the United States and Australia treated 10 patients with severe FIX deficiency with an AAV-transduced FIX gene product. The product was well tolerated, yielding a mean increase in FIX activity of 33.8% $\pm$ 18.1% (mean $\pm$ SD) [37]. Table 1 summarizes gene therapies for heritable conditions to date [38].

NONVIRAL GENE THERAPIES: CYSTIC FIBROSIS AS A MODEL

Early attempts at gene therapy in cystic fibrosis (CF) were hindered by the limited ability of viral vectors to effectively deliver gene-modified therapies from the luminal surface to the respiratory epithelium. More recently, nonviral gene transfer (using plasmids, for example) has arisen as a potential therapeutic option for patients with CF.

CF is a heritable disease due to a mutation in the CFTR gene that leads to worsening respiratory function, infections, and high rates of mortality at an early age. Most current treatments are primarily supportive, focused on respiratory support and antimicrobial therapy [39]. One challenge distinct to gene therapy products for CF is the requirement to localize to the respiratory epithelium to ensure maximal therapeutic effect while minimizing inflammation, which is an already prominent feature of the disease [40]. Recently, a phase 1/2 trial (NCT01621867) across 18 CF centers evaluated directed lung delivery (via nebulization) of a plasmid DNA encoding the functional CFTR gene. One hundred and forty patients $\geq$12 years old were randomized to receive either placebo or the nebulized product monthly over a 1-year period (n = 78 in treatment group). Using a primary endpoint of percentage predicted forced expiratory volume, the treatment group was noted to have significantly improved lung function compared with the placebo group [41]. This important study provided the first proof-of-concept of nonviral gene therapy specifically designed to improve lung disease.

GENE THERAPY FOR ACQUIRED DISEASES

A genetic engineering strategy that has gained substantial attention over the past 10 years because of its widespread success, predominantly in treating

Table 1
Summary of recently completed and/or recruiting clinical trials (as indicated by NCT no.) for patients with heritable diseases

Gene therapies for heritable disease				
Disease Treated	Intervention	Location/Year Initiated	Clinicaltrials.gov ID	Outcomes Reported
X-linked SCID	Retroviral gene transfer to insert a functional copy of ADA	NIH, Bethesda, USA/2001	NCT00028236	n/a
MPS type III A; Sanfilippo disease type A	AAV transfer of human SGSH and SUMF1 cDNAs	Hôpital Bicêtre – Assistance Publique, Paris, France/2011	NCT01474343	n/a
WAS	Lentiviral-mediated HSC gene transfer of a functional WAS gene	Children's Hospital Boston, Boston, USA/2011	NCT01410825	n/a
CGD, X-linked	Lentiviral-mediated viral transfer of the human CGD gene (G1XCGD)	UCLA, LA; NIH, Bethesda, Boston Children's, Boston, USA/2018	NCT02234934	n/a
MPS II (Hunter syndrome)	AAV transfer of iduronate-2-sulfatase (IDS) gene	UPMC, Pittsburgh, USA/2018	NCT03566043	n/a
CF	Liposomal transfer of pGT-1 gene lipid complex	University of Alabama, Birmingham, AL, USA/1999	NCT00004471	n/a
CALD	Lentiviral transfer of gene encoding the human ALD protein	Boston Children's Hospital, Boston, USA/2013	NCT01896102	n/a
LCA, hereditary retinal diseases	AAV gene transfer of RPE65	Moorfields Eye Hospital, London, UK/2016	NCT02946879	n/a
SCD	Lentiviral-transduced CD34+ HSC targeting BCL11a	Boston Children's Hospital, Boston, USA/2017	NCT03282656	n/a
SMA1-1	AAV transfer to insert functional copy of SMN (AVXS-101)	Nationwide Children's, Columbus, USA/2014	NCT02122952	15/15 patients alive and event free at 20 mo out, compared with 8% in control

Abbreviations: AAV, adenovirus-associated vector; CALD, cerebral adrenoleukodystrophy; CGD, chronic granulomatous disease; NCT, Clinicaltrials.gov identifier; CF, cystic fibrosis; LCA, Leber congenital amaurosis; MPS, mucopolysaccharidosis; n/a, not applicable; RPE65, retinal pigment epithelium 65; SCID, severe combined immunodeficiency; SCD, sickle cell disease; SMA, spinal muscular atrophy; WAS, Wiskott-Aldrich syndrome.

cancer, is the combination of cellular and gene therapy. This combination, often known simply as "cellular immunotherapy," typically involves immune effector cells collected from a patient and genetically manipulated in the laboratory. These cells are then expanded to a specified dose and returned to the patient. Similar to other forms of gene therapy, the most commonly used gene transfer vectors include adenoviral vectors, retroviral and lentiviral vectors, and naked plasmids. Although most trials to date have used T cells, genetically modified NK and NK-T cells have also been used in clinical trials.

Success in treating cancer

Cellular immunotherapies have been most successful against cancer. In fact, cancer is the most common disease treated by gene therapy, comprising 66% of all ongoing clinical gene therapy trials worldwide [42]. The most successful cellular immunotherapy to date are T cells genetically modified to express chimeric antigen receptors that target cancer antigens (CAR T cells). CAR T cells are manufactured in the laboratory to combine the antigen-recognition capabilities of a monoclonal antibody with the signaling and killing capacity of the T cell. CAR T cells typically contain 4 major components: the antigen-recognition component that is derived from a single-chain variable fragment of a monoclonal antibody; a linker or transmembrane domain; an endodomain that is, responsible for providing the T-cell activation signal; an additional costimulatory domain responsible for enhanced in vivo persistence. These artificial CAR receptors can therefore be designed to recognize almost any antigen on the surface of a cancer cell, then introduced into the patient's own T cells, typically using a retroviral or lentiviral vector. One of the primary advantages of CAR T cells is that they bypass the requirement of antigen presentation by major histocompatibility complex molecules and thus have human leukocyte antigen-independent killing [43].

Whereas CAR T-cell therapy has been clinically studied in a variety of malignancies, it has been most effective in hematologic malignancies, presumably because of the accessibility of leukemic blasts in bone marrow/blood of affected patients and widespread antigen availability. The most successful CAR T cell by far has been the CD19-CAR T cell, targeting the CD19 antigen expressed on the vast majority of B-cell malignancies. Lymphodepleting chemotherapy followed by a single infusion of autologous CD19-CAR T cells to patients with refractory acute lymphoblastic leukemia ([ALL], the most common childhood cancer) has had resounding success (>70% responses) in heavily pretreated patients with limited treatment options [44]. This groundbreaking therapy led to recent FDA approval of the first cellular gene therapy, a CD19-CAR T cell, by the company Novartis (Kymriah [tisagenlecleucel]), approved for the treatment of pediatric B-ALL that is refractory or in second or greater relapse [43]. There are numerous ongoing early-phase clinical trials of CAR T cells targeting other childhood and adult hematologic malignancies, some of which are highlighted in Table 2.

Table 2
Summary of recently completed and/or recruiting clinical trials (as indicated by NCT no.) for children with hematologic malignancies, solid tumors, and brain tumors

Cancer type	Target Antigen	Clinicaltrials.gov ID
T-cell malignancies	CD5	NCT03081910
AML, blastic plasmacytoid dendritic cell neoplasm		NCT02159495
Lymphoma	CD30	NCT02663297
Liver neoplasms	Glypican 3	NCT02932956
Neuroblastoma	GD2	NCT03294954
GD2+ sarcoma and neuroblastoma	GD2	NCT01953900
Sarcoma and central nervous system tumors	Human epidermal growth factor receptor 2 + tumor cells	NCT00902044 NCT02442297
Malignant glioma	Tumor-associated antigen interleukin-13 receptor α2	NCT02208362

Extending the success of CAR T cells to the treatment of solid and brain tumors has proven more difficult because of difficulties in navigating the hostile tumor microenvironment. Several studies have shown that CAR T cells targeting solid tumors, once infused into patients, face inhibitory signals, immunosuppressive cell populations, and a hypoxic, nutrition-depleted environment that can impair T-cell function [45]. These factors limit T-cell activation, expansion, and persistence, which translates to limited antitumor activity [46,47]. Box 1 shows actively enrolling clinical trials of CAR T cells for solid and brain tumors registered on clinicialtrials.gov as of February 2019.

GENE EDITING AND GENE THERAPY OF THE FUTURE

As gene therapy efforts have become more sophisticated over the past few years, much of the field has focused on refining tools to offer more elegant and precise methods of treating genetic diseases. Gene editing has generated enthusiasm for its promise in achieving these goals. In genome editing, a double-strand break is created using engineered nucleases that modify the genome in a site-specific manner. Whereas several artificial nuclease systems have been developed for genome editing, including protein-guided DNA cleavage systems of zinc-finger nucleases (ZFNs) and transcription activatorlike effector nucleases, the CRISPR/CRISPR-Cas9 system has shown most promise and earned most media attention of late. CRISPR relies on small RNA for sequence-specific cleavage, enabling researchers to precisely manipulate specific genomic elements to achieve a therapeutic effect [48] A schematic of CRISPR-Cas9 gene editing is shown in Fig. 2.

The first clinical trial showing feasibility of gene editing was published in 2014. In an effort to render CD4 T cells from patients with human immunodeficiency virus (HIV) resistant to infection with the virus, researchers used ZFNs to disrupt or "knock out" the gene that encodes a cellular co-receptor

Box 1: List of indications and potential ethical considerations for heritable genome editing.

Regulatory Framework for Clinical Trials That Use Heritable Genome Editing

1. Absence of reasonable alternatives
2. Restriction to preventing a serious disease or condition
3. Restriction to editing genes that have been convincingly demonstrated to cause or strongly predispose to the disease or condition
4. Restriction to converting such genes to version that are prevalent in the population and are known to be associated with ordinary health with little or no evidence of adverse effects
5. Availability of credible preclinical and/or clinical data on risks and potential health benefits of the procedures
6. Ongoing, rigorous oversight during clinical trials of the effects of the procedure on the health and safety of the research participants
7. Comprehensive plans for long-term, multigenerational follow-up that still respect personal autonomy
8. Maximum transparency consistent with patient privacy
9. Continued reassessment of health and societal benefits and risks
10. Reliable oversight mechanisms to prevent extension to uses other than preventing a serious disease or condition

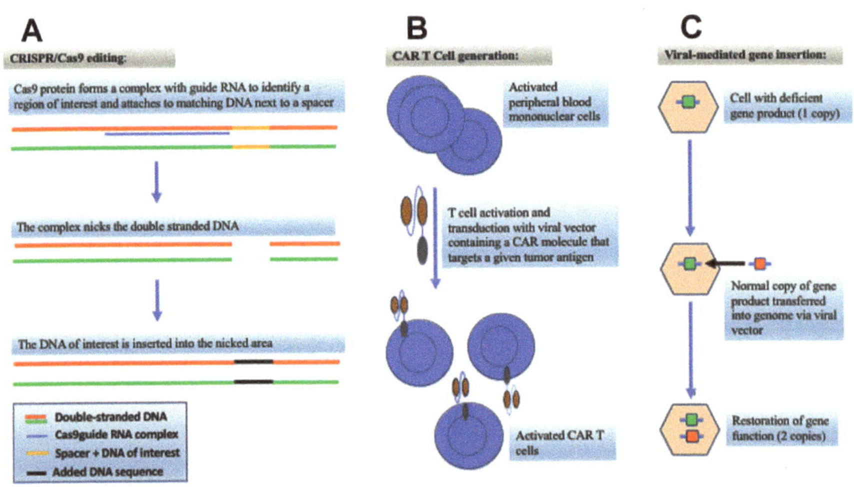

Fig. 2. Schematic of gene therapy techniques. (*A*) CRISPR-Cas9 gene editing. (*B*) Transduction of T cells with chimeric antigen receptor (CAR) to create CAR T cells. (*C*) Example of ex vivo viral insertion of a functional gene copy before insertion in a patient.

for HIV, CCR5 [49]. These patient-specific T cells were manipulated in the laboratory before re-infusion. The study revealed the safety, tolerability, and persistence of CCR5-modified CD4-T cells on treatment. During periods of viremia, the decline in circulating CCR5-modified cells was significantly less than the decline in unmodified cells, indicating that the modified cells were protected from infection. Despite the limited therapeutic effect of this treatment, the trial paved the way for the clinical application of ex vivo gene-editing strategies [50,51].

As mentioned above, much of the gene-editing field recently has shifted to exploring the use of CRISPR-Cas9 because of its ability to precisely manipulate genes. There are currently 11 actively recruiting clinical trials that use CRISPR-Cas9 to address several hereditary and acquired diseases, including β-thalassemia, SCD, solid tumors, and multiple myeloma [51–54]. Our group is exploring methods to use CRISPR-Cas9 to edit T cells engineered with CAR molecules targeting a pan-T cell antigen. This approach (NCT03690011) should protect the CAR T cells from targeting themselves, allowing them to expand before infusion into patients with refractory T-cell malignancies [55].

In addition, upcoming clinical trials using CRISPR-Cas9 to treat β-thalassemia have gained recent approval in the United States (NCT03655678, NCT03728322). Based on demonstration of therapeutic benefit in mouse models for Duchenne muscular dystrophy [56] and hereditary tyrosinemia [57], clinical trials using genetic-editing techniques have been submitted for regulatory approval for these and many other diseases.

SAFETY

As with most innovative strategies, gene therapy is not without safety concerns. As the feasibility and applicability of gene therapy has grown over the past few years, more data on real and theoretic safety concerns have come to light. As illustrated in the previous sections, most clinical gene therapy strategies use viral, specifically retroviral, vectors.

Genotoxicity due to retroviral vectors

Several reports of T-cell leukemia occurring in patients with immunodeficiencies receiving genetically modified stem cell products in the initial trials rocked the field in the late 1990s and shed important light on the necessity of long-term follow-up. In these early trials, retroviral vectors were transferred to HSCs to correct inherited immunodeficiencies. However, despite the clinical activity discussed in preceding sections, several years after treatment, a subset of patients receiving gene therapy for SCID, CGD, and WAS developed acute leukemias owing to activation of proto-oncogenes adjacent to proviral insertions [58,59]. These toxicities led to the adoption of enhancer-deleted lentiviral or retroviral vectors for HSC clinical gene therapies. Up to now, these newer vectors have ameliorated disease without causing genotoxicity [60].

Retroviral transduction results in new, random integrations in host cell DNA, which infrequently may cause abnormal or uncontrolled proliferation. Moreover, this effect is much more common with replication-competent retrovirus (RCR), whereby each cell receives multiple additions. Clinical trials regulated by the FDA are required to test transduced cells and postinfusion samples for RCR, and to exclude any RCR-containing products from clinical use. More recently, several publications have reviewed the extensive and long-term data on RCR monitoring in gene-modified T cells immediately after gamma retroviral transduction and in follow-up patient samples. Importantly, in over 1000 patients treated with gene-modified T cells, no evidence for RCR has been identified, demonstrating the safety of genetic modification of T cells [61–63].

A separate concern that is discussed in the Ethics section below is the modification of germline genetic material, which is potentially heritable [9,10].

Inflammatory responses to chimeric antigen receptor T cells

The promising clinical responses observed with CAR T cells in pediatric leukemia have not come without concern. In fact, in all CD19 CAR T-cell trials demonstrating clinical responses, serious toxicities have also been reported. The most frequent toxicity occurring after infusion of CD19 CAR T cells is cytokine release syndrome (CRS). Cytokine release syndrome is a commonly occurring systemic inflammatory response that can range from a mild syndrome requiring supportive care alone (antipyretics, IV fluids, close monitoring) to symptoms resembling sepsis, systemic inflammatory response syndrome, and hemophagocytic lymphohistiocytosis and requiring intensive care intervention [64]. The symptoms of CRS correspond with peripheral expansion of the infused CAR T cells, and are typically more severe in patients with larger disease burden. Identification of IL-6 as the most prominent cytokine responsible for the symptomatology led to adoption of the anti-IL-6R antibody tocilizumab as the treatment of choice in patients with more severe symptoms. Standardized grading algorithms based on clinical and laboratory features have streamlined CRS identification and management, ensuring that patients treated with this promising therapy are managed safely [64,65].

Neurologic toxicity has also occurred following infusion of CD19 CAR T cells, and can range from somnolence to seizure activity and cerebral edema. Whereas the cause of CAR-related neurotoxicity, sometimes known as cytokine release encephalopathy syndrome, is less clear than that of CRS, endothelial activation and disruption of the blood-brain barrier seems to play a role, and symptoms typically are self-limited requiring supportive care, including empiric antiepileptics, although therapy with steroids is sometimes required [64,65].

ETHICS

As developments in gene therapy and human genome editing continue to evolve, so have ethical concerns surrounding these advancements. Many of these concerns are focused specifically on newer genome-editing tools, which have yet to be used in humans, thus safety and efficacy data do not exist.

In response to these growing ethical concerns, The US National Academy of Sciences and the National Academy of Medicine convened a multidisciplinary, international committee to review the current status of human genome editing and make recommendations. The final report was published in February of 2017 [66], with specific recommendations regarding regulation of clinical trials using heritable genome editing as detailed in Box 1.

Ethical concerns regarding genome editing largely surround its use in correcting germ line mutations. Germ line editing is highly contentious because the resulting genetic changes could be inherited by offspring, thus broadening the scope of concern beyond the individual being treated. The result is a complex situation whereby the appropriateness of genome-editing interventions and their potential effects on individuals and society must be considered.

Aside from obvious concerns that a heritable gene edit could do harm (to the individual and their progeny), some have cited potential for misuse of this technology for state-imposed eugenic applications [67]. As gene therapy continues to push the boundaries of science and technology, bioethics experts continue to struggle to ensure that the ethical use of these procedures occurs and that ethical concerns are taken into account.

FUTURE DIRECTIONS

In summary, this is an exciting time for the ever-growing field of gene therapy. Successful translation of preclinical discoveries to clinical trials has yielded promising results in several historically devastating diseases. Although some techniques are in their third decade of use and require only optimization, others such as genome editing are in their infancy. Like many novel therapies, the future of gene therapy requires a revisit of the past–attention to safety, efficacy, cost, and ethical concerns must be addressed in order for the promise of this therapy to become reality.

References

[1] Verma IM, Naldini L, Kafti T, et al. Gene therapy: promises, problems and prospects. In: Boulyjenkov V, Berg K, Christen Y, editors. Genes and Resistance to Disease. Berlin, Heidelberg: Springer; 2000. p. 147–57.

[2] Rosenberg SA, Aebersold P, Cornetta K, et al. Gene transfer into humans—immunotherapy of patients with advanced melanoma, using tumor-infiltrating lymphocytes modified by retroviral gene transduction. N Engl J Med 1990;323:570–8.

[3] Blaese RM, Culver KW, Miller AD, et al. T lymphocyte-directed gene therapy for ADA–SCID: initial trial results after 4 years. Science 1995;270:475–80.

[4] Lenzi RN, Altevogt BM, Gostin LO. Oversight and review of clinical gene transfer protocols: assessing the role of the recombinant DNA advisory committee. Washington, DC: National Academies Press; 2014.

[5] Cavazzana-Calvo M, Hacein-Bey S, de Saint Basile G, et al. Gene therapy of human severe combined immunodeficiency (SCID)-X1 disease. Science 2000;288:669–72.

[6] Aiuti A, Slavin S, Aker M, et al. Correction of ADA-SCID by stem cell gene therapy combined with nonmyeloablative conditioning. Science 2002;296:2410–3.

[7] Cicalese MP, Ferrua F, Castagnaro L, et al. Update on the safety and efficacy of retroviral gene therapy for immunodeficiency due to adenosine deaminase deficiency. Blood 2016;128:45–54.
[8] Keller MD, Notarangelo LD, Malech HL. Future of care for patients with chronic granulomatous disease: gene therapy and targeted molecular medicine. J Pediatric Infect Dis Soc 2018;7:S40–4.
[9] Kawai T, Okamura K, Yagita M, et al. A gene therapy clinical study of a patient with X-linked chronic granulomatous disease. Mol Ther 2016;24:S87–8.
[10] Kang HJ, Bartholomae CC, Paruzynski A, et al. Retroviral gene therapy for X-linked chronic granulomatous disease: results from phase I/II trial. Mol Ther 2011;19:2092–101.
[11] Brendel C, Rothe M, Santilli G, et al. Non-clinical efficacy and safety studies on G1XCGD, a lentiviral vector for ex vivo gene therapy of X-linked chronic granulomatous disease. Hum Gene Ther Clin Dev 2018;29:69–79.
[12] Orchard therapeutics presents clinical proof-of-concept data for OTL-102 for the treatment of X-CGD. Available at: https://globenewswire.com/news-release/2019/02/25/1741442/0/en/Orchard-Therapeutics-Presents-Clinical-Proof-of-Concept-Data-for-OTL-102-for-the-Treatment-of-X-CGD.html. Accessed February 2, 2019.
[13] Ochs HD, Thrasher AJ. The Wiskott-Aldrich syndrome. J Allergy Clin Immunol 2006;117: 725–38.
[14] Abina SH-B, Gaspar HB, Blondeau J, et al. Outcomes following gene therapy in patients with severe Wiskott-Aldrich syndrome. JAMA 2015;313:1550–63.
[15] Feuer WJ, Schiffman JC, Davis JL, et al. Gene therapy for Leber hereditary optic neuropathy: initial results. Ophthalmology 2016;123:558–70.
[16] Zhang Y, Tian Z, Yuan J, et al. The progress of gene therapy for Leber's optic hereditary neuropathy. Curr Gene Ther 2017;17:320–6.
[17] Smalley E. First AAV gene therapy poised for landmark approval. Nat Biotechnol 2017;35: 998–9.
[18] Deverman BE, Ravina BM, Bankiewicz KS, et al. Gene therapy for neurological disorders: progress and prospects. Nat Rev Drug Discov 2018;17:641.
[19] Scoto M, Main M, Munot P, et al. G299 Nusinersen (spinraza) is the first drug approved for spinal muscular atrophy (sma): initial experience in patients with sma type 1 treated in the expanded access program (eap). Archives of Disease in Childhood 2018;103:cA122.
[20] Althoff E, Speer F. Novartis announces FDA filing acceptance and priority review of AVXS-101, a one-time treatment designed to address the genetic root cause of SMA type 1. Available at: http://www.novartis.com/news/media-releases/novartis-announces-fda-filing-acceptance-and-priority-review-avxs-101-one-time-treatment-designed-address-genetic-root-cause-sma-type-1. Accessed February 2, 2019.
[21] Amburgey K, Tsuchiya E, de Chastonay S, et al. A natural history study of X-linked myotubular myopathy. Neurology 2017;89:1355–64.
[22] Kuntz N, Shieh P, Smith B, et al. New therapeutic approaches and their readout: O. 17ASPIRO phase 1/2 gene therapy trial in X-linked myotubular myopathy: preliminary safety and efficacy findings. Neuromuscul Disord 2018;28:S91.
[23] Medin JA, Khan A, Huang J, et al. FACTs Fabry gene therapy clinical trial: two-year data. Mol Genet Metab 2019;126:S99.
[24] Gonzalez EA, Baldo G. Gene therapy for lysosomal storage disorders: recent advances and limitations. J Inborn Errors Metab Screen 2017;5:2326409816689786.
[25] Poswar F, Baldo G, Giugliani R. Phase I and II clinical trials for the mucopolysaccharidoses. Expert Opin Investig Drugs 2017;26:1331–40.
[26] Galanello R, Origa R. beta-Thalassemia. Orphanet J Rare Dis 2010;5:11.
[27] Hacein-Bey-Abina S, Pai SY, Gaspar HB, et al. A modified γ-retrovirus vector for X-linked severe combined immunodeficiency. New England Journal of Medicine 2014;371(15): 1407–17.

[28] Thompson AA, Walters MC, Kwiatkowski J, et al. Gene therapy in patients with transfusion-dependent β-thalassemia. N Engl J Med 2018;378:1479–93.
[29] Ribeil JA, Hacein-Bey-Abina S, Payen E, et al. Gene therapy in a patient with sickle cell disease. N Engl J Med 2017;376:848–55.
[30] Ware RE, de Montalembert M, Tshilolo L, et al. Sickle cell disease. Lancet 2017;390:311–23.
[31] Matte A, Zorzi F, Mazzi F, et al. New therapeutic options for the treatment of sickle cell disease. Mediterr J Hematol Infect Dis 2019;11.
[32] Kanter J, Walters MC, Hsieh M, et al. Initial results from study Hgb-206: a phase 1 study evaluating gene therapy by transplantation of autologous CD34+ stem cells transduced ex vivo with the lentiglobin BB305 lentiviral vector in subjects with severe sickle cell disease. Blood 2015;126:3233.
[33] Malik P, Grimley M, Quinn CT, et al. Gene therapy for sickle cell anemia using a modified gamma globin lentivirus vector and reduced intensity conditioning transplant shows promising correction of the disease phenotype. Blood 2018;132:1021.
[34] Nienhuis AW, Nathwani AC, Davidoff AM. Gene therapy for hemophilia. Mol Ther 2017;25:1163–7.
[35] Melchiorre D, Linari S, Castaman G. The higher prevalence of missense mutations in hemophilia B compared to hemophilia A could be important in determining a milder clinical phenotype in patients with severe hemophilia B. Haematologica 2016;101:e429.
[36] Doshi BS, Arruda VR. Gene therapy for hemophilia: what does the future hold? Ther Adv Hematol 2018;9:273–93.
[37] High KA, George LA, Eyster ME, et al. A Phase 1/2 Trial of Investigational Spk-8011 in Hemophilia a Demonstrates Durable Expression and Prevention of Bleeds. Blood 2018;132:487.
[38] Flinn AM, Gennery AR. Adenosine deaminase deficiency: a review. Orphanet J Rare Dis 2018;13:65.
[39] Rey MM, Bonk MP, Hadjiliadis D. Cystic fibrosis: emerging understanding and therapies. Annu Rev Med 2019;70:197–210.
[40] Castellani S, Conese M. Lentiviral vectors and cystic fibrosis gene therapy. Viruses 2010;2:395–412.
[41] Alton EW, Armstrong DK, Ashby D, et al. Repeated nebulisation of non-viral CFTR gene therapy in patients with cystic fibrosis: a randomised, double-blind, placebo-controlled, phase 2b trial. Lancet Respir Med 2015;3:684–91.
[42] Ginn SL, Alexander IE, Edelstein ML, et al. Gene therapy clinical trials worldwide to 2012–an update. J Gene Med 2013;15:65–77.
[43] Rouce RH, Sharma S, Huynh M, et al. Recent advances in T-cell immunotherapy for haematological malignancies. Br J Haematol 2017;176:688–704.
[44] Maude SL, Teachey DT, Porter DL, et al. CD19-targeted chimeric antigen receptor T-cell therapy for acute lymphoblastic leukemia. Blood 2015;125:4017–23.
[45] Kakarla S, Gottschalk S. CAR T cells for solid tumors: armed and ready to go? Cancer J 2014;20:151.
[46] Newick K, Moon E, Albelda SM. Chimeric antigen receptor T-cell therapy for solid tumors. Mol Ther Oncolytics 2016;3:16006.
[47] Gilham DE, Debets R, Pule M, et al. CAR-T cells and solid tumors: tuning T cells to challenge an inveterate foe. Trends Mol Med 2012;18:377–84.
[48] Wang H, La Russa M, Qi LS. CRISPR/Cas9 in genome editing and beyond. Annu Rev Biochem 2016;85:227–64.
[49] Tebas P, Stein D, Tang WW, et al. Gene editing of CCR5 in autologous CD4 T cells of persons infected with HIV. N Engl J Med 2014;370:901–10.
[50] Yi G, Choi JG, Bharaj P, et al. CCR5 gene editing of resting CD4+ T cells by transient ZFN expression from HIV envelope pseudotyped nonintegrating lentivirus confers HIV-1 resistance in humanized mice. Mol Ther Nucleic Acids 2014;3:e198.

[51] Baylis F, McLeod M. First-in-human phase 1 CRISPR gene editing cancer trials: are we ready? Curr Gene Ther 2017;17:309–19.
[52] Dever DP, Bak RO, Reinisch A, et al. CRISPR/Cas9 β-globin gene targeting in human haematopoietic stem cells. Nature 2016;539:384.
[53] Xie F, Ye L, Chang JC, et al. Seamless gene correction of β-thalassemia mutations in patient-specific iPSCs using CRISPR/Cas9 and piggyBac. Genome Res 2014;24:1526–33.
[54] Rupp LJ, Schumann K, Roybal KT, et al. CRISPR/Cas9-mediated PD-1 disruption enhances anti-tumor efficacy of human chimeric antigen receptor T cells. Sci Rep 2017;7:737.
[55] Silva D, Tashiro H, Srinivasan M, et al. Am Soc Hematology 2016.
[56] Nelson CE, Schumann K, Roybal KT, et al. In vivo genome editing improves muscle function in a mouse model of Duchenne muscular dystrophy. Science 2016;351:403–7.
[57] Yin H, Song CQ, Dorkin JR, et al. Therapeutic genome editing by combined viral and non-viral delivery of CRISPR system components in vivo. Nat Biotechnol 2016;34:328.
[58] Hacein-Bey-Abina S, Garrigue A, Wang GP, et al. Insertional oncogenesis in 4 patients after retrovirus-mediated gene therapy of SCID-X1. J Clin Invest 2008;118:3132–42.
[59] Stein S, Ott MG, Schultze-Strasser S, et al. Genomic instability and myelodysplasia with monosomy 7 consequent to EVI1 activation after gene therapy for chronic granulomatous disease. Nat Med 2010;16:198.
[60] Dunbar CE, High KA, Joung JK, et al. Gene therapy comes of age. Science 2018;359 [pii:eaan4672].
[61] Heslop HE, Brenner MK. Seek and you will not find: ending the hunt for replication-competent retroviruses during human gene therapy. Mol Ther 2018;26:1–2.
[62] Marcucci KT, Jadlowsky JK, Hwang WT, et al. Retroviral and lentiviral safety analysis of gene-modified T cell products and infused HIV and oncology patients. Mol Ther 2018;26: 269–79.
[63] Lyon D, Lapteva N, Gee AP. Absence of replication-competent retrovirus in vectors, T cell products, and patient follow-up samples. Mol Ther 2018;26:6–7.
[64] Lee DW, Gardner R, Porter DL, et al. Current concepts in the diagnosis and management of cytokine release syndrome. Blood 2014;124:188–95.
[65] Rouce RH, Heslop HE. Forecasting cytokine storms with new predictive biomarkers. Cancer Discov 2016;6:579–80.
[66] Scheufele DA, Xenos MA, Howell EL, et al. US attitudes on human genome editing. Science 2017;357:553–4.
[67] Coller BS. Ethics of human genome editing. Annu Rev Med 2019;70:289–305.

Advances in Pediatrics 66 (2019) 55–85

ADVANCES IN PEDIATRICS

Pediatric Telehealth

Approaches by Specialty and Implications for General Pediatric Care

Alan Tomines, MD[a,b,c,d,*]

[a]Department of Pediatrics, UCLA Geffen School of Medicine, Los Angeles, CA, USA; [b]Enterprise Information Services, Cedars-Sinai Medical Center, Los Angeles, CA, USA; [c]Harbor-UCLA Medical Center, Torrance, CA, USA; [d]Department of Health Policy and Management, UCLA Fielding School of Public Health, Los Angeles, CA, USA

Keywords

• Telehealth • Telemedicine • Pediatrics • Informatics • mHealth • Teleconsultation • Telepractice • Telecare

Key points

- Telehealth is the use of electronic information and telecommunication technologies to support clinical care and public health, and to promote patient education and professional development.
- Advances in technology, access to care, service reimbursement, and consumer demand are primary drivers for pediatric telehealth.
- The effectiveness and applicability of a telehealth approach may vary by pediatric specialty, care delivery setting, and patient preference.
- The expanding demand for real-time telemedicine services may have disruptive effects on the practice of pediatrics.

INTRODUCTION

Telehealth is the use of electronic information and telecommunication technologies to support clinical care and public health, and to promote patient education and professional development [1]. Telehealth technologies run the gamut from telephones and e-mail, to transmitted images, to real-time videoconferencing and robotic surgery. Telehealth has been an area of formal informatics research for more than 2 decades [2], and has recently generated broader

*6500 Wilshire Boulevard #200, Los Angeles, CA 90048. *E-mail address:* atomines@ucla.edu

https://doi.org/10.1016/j.yapd.2019.04.005

interest as an alternative mode of health care delivery that can cost-effectively expand access to care. In pediatrics, telehealth has found success in specialty niches, but remains mostly unproven as a model for general pediatric care. Understanding the effectiveness of telehealth approaches by specialty and context may provide guidance on how best to apply telehealth to present and future challenges in the pediatric health care landscape.

Terminology

The term telemedicine is often used interchangeably with telehealth, as it was once the all-encompassing term for the use of remote communication technologies in health care. Under Medicaid, telemedicine is not recognized as a distinct service from telehealth; rather, it has been redefined as a narrowly-focused subset of telehealth: Telemedicine is the use of 2-way, real-time interactive audio and video communication between a patient at an originating (or "spoke") site and a physician or a practitioner at a distant (or "hub") site [3]. This administrative definition provides a reference point for an expansive nomenclature (Table 1) that better differentiates by characteristics (Table 2) the breadth of applications of telehealth in pediatrics.

Telemedicine uses 2-way, real-time (or synchronous) videoconferencing to transmit clinical information for interactive assessment. By contrast, telehealth embraces both synchronous and asynchronous (not real-time) modes. Sometimes referred to as "store and forward," asynchronous technologies involve the acquisition, storage, and transmission of clinical information (whether data, images, or other multimedia) from originating to distant site for remote interpretation at a later time.

Table 1
Telehealth and subordinate categories

Telehealth	The use of electronic information and telecommunication technologies to support and promote long-distance clinical health care, patient and professional health-related education, public health and health administration, using technologies including video conferencing, the Internet, store-and-forward imaging, streaming media, and terrestrial and wireless communications
Telemedicine	The use of 2-way, real-time interactive audio and video communication between a patient and a physician or a practitioner at a distant site
Teleconsultation	The synchronous or asynchronous use of information communication technologies between practitioners to guide the diagnosis or care of a patient
Telepractice	The synchronous or asynchronous use of information communication technologies between a patient and a practitioner
Telecare	The use of information, communication, and monitoring technologies to remotely evaluate health status, give educational intervention, or deliver health and social care to patients in their homes
Tele-education	The provision of remote training to health practitioners to improve knowledge and skills, and for continuing education or maintenance of certification

Table 2
Telehealth terminology

Asynchronous ("store and forward")	The acquisition, storage, and transmission of clinical information (including data and multimedia) from one site to another for remote assessment
Synchronous	The transmission of clinical information in real time for remote assessment
Originating ("spoke") site	The location of the patient at the time of the telemedicine service
Distant ("hub") site	The location of the practitioner at the time of the telemedicine service
Telemedicine platform	Software that a practitioner uses to interact with patients
mHealth	An abbreviation for "mobile health"—the use of mobile device technology in health care
Remote patient monitoring (RPM)	The use of technology to capture physiologic or behavioral data outside of the traditional clinical care setting
Direct-to-consumer (DTC) telehealth	A form of telehealth, often delivered using an mHealth device, that is marketed directly to patients with service initiated by patients

In addition, telemedicine focuses specifically on communication between a patient and a practitioner but does not explicitly acknowledge the use of technologies between practitioners to provide consultation. To that end, the terms telepractice and teleconsultation are well suited to characterize other pediatric telehealth activities [4]. Telepractice here refers to the synchronous or asynchronous use of information communication technologies between a patient and a practitioner, building on the formal definition of telemedicine and allowing for the use of asynchronous applications, such as e-mail or store-and-forward imaging. Teleconsultation here refers to the synchronous or asynchronous use of information communication technologies between practitioners to guide the diagnosis or care of a patient.

Although telepractice or teleconsultation may extend traditional paradigms of physician-patient or physician-physician interaction, they do not generally gather information or provide intervention outside of the formal health care setting. Telecare is the use of technologies to remotely evaluate a patient's health status or to provide educational, health, or social interventions to patients in their life environment [5], conceptually extending the medical home to a "health home" to periodically or continuously monitor for disease risk factors or aggravators and provide intervention as needed [6]. Telecare may use remote patient monitoring (RPM) to capture physiologic, behavioral, social, or environmental data about a patient outside of the health care setting. The use of smartphones, or other portable communication or monitoring devices, to enable RPM and provide education or other interventions, is sometimes referred to as mobile health (mHealth).

Although tele-education is sometimes used in the context of telecare, to refer to remote health education provided to patients, the term tele-education generally refers to the provision of remote training to health practitioners to improve knowledge and skills, or to participate in continuing education or maintenance of certification.

Drivers

Advances in information and communication technology, barriers in access to care, evolving policies in service reimbursement, and expanding consumer demand are the principal drivers that have fostered interest and innovation in pediatric telehealth.

Technology

Fast and reliable broadband Internet is a foundation of effective telehealth. At the advent of the telemedicine era, prevailing Internet bandwidth allowed for asynchronous transmission and display of static images but limited the quality of real-time video interactions; present-day Internet speed and capacity, coupled with high-definition videoconferencing equipment, have made real-time interactive audio and video synonymous with telemedicine. Although scarce and sluggish Internet access has limited telehealth opportunities in rural and underserved areas, the debut and expansion of 5G wireless networks may reduce infrastructure barriers.

The cost-prohibitive acquisition and maintenance of high-definition equipment once limited videoconferencing technology to large health care networks and academic centers that were able to host patient-convenient originating sites. Now, vendors of telemedicine platforms are marketing software to small and solo practices that allows practitioners to interact with patients using consumer-oriented devices, such as smartphones and tablets. These mHealth technologies may readily support both telemedicine and telecare scenarios: The integration of patient surveys and environmental or physiologic sensors into mobile devices may allow the medical home to continuously monitor risk factors, including social determinants of health, and provide for real-time interventions, such as medication reminders or videoconference consultations, which can be delivered when and where needed to prevent problems or mitigate further harm.

Electronic health records (EHRs) may not immediately come to mind as a telehealth technology, but it may be convenient to think of an EHR as a "store-and-forward" repository for clinical information that may be reviewed and interpreted remotely by a practitioner participating in a patient's care. As of 2017, more than 90% of hospitals [7] and nearly 90% of physician offices [8] had access to EHRs. In a teleconsultation scenario, a physician could use the EHR to transmit relevant documentation or studies to a specialist for assessment; if the specialist has shared access to the patient's EHR the process of transmitting information can be bypassed, further expediting the process. An EHR patient portal may allow practitioners and patients to exchange messages securely and asynchronously; additional patient portal resources may provide patient education and self-triage, and other tools to support scheduling of in-person or telemedicine visits. A patient being seen by a practitioner outside of their medical home, perhaps even via a telemedicine visit, may be able to provide their acute care practitioner with "break-the-glass" access to their electronic records, allowing for a more complete review of history than the patient may be able to recall or express.

Provider access

Inability to access pediatric specialty care may be a conflation of several issues, including absolute shortages of specialists and their geographic concentration: Since the American Academy of Pediatrics (AAP) Future of Pediatric Education (FOPE II) workforce survey in 1998, pediatric subspecialists are working fewer hours and spending less time in direct patient care, and practicing in academic medical centers in greater proportion [9]. Differential access to pediatric specialists in rural or underserved areas may create disparities that contribute to poorer health outcomes [10].

Telehealth strategies may improve pediatric subspecialty access [11]. These strategies may leverage readily available technologies, such as e-mail and telephone consultations, or specialist access to remote EHRs; other strategies may require significant technology investment, including videoconferencing equipment, or mHealth devices for patients, or even establishing broadband Internet access in a community. Although investment in new technologies may be initially cost prohibitive, with sufficient volume to justify infrastructure commitments, telehealth services can be a cost-effective alternative to in-person care, particularly when time and effort for patient travel is considered [12]. In addition, when remote subspecialty care is made available in originating settings that are convenient for patients, such as primary care offices or community hospitals, pediatric patients in rural and underserved areas are more likely to receive and adhere to evidence-based care [13]. Telehealth may even support the role of nonphysician intermediaries in nonclinical settings, such as school nurses, to increase access to primary pediatric care [14].

Families are interested in telehealth opportunities, independent of specific clinical problems, disease severity or chronicity, or distance from hospital [15], although for ongoing specialty care beyond an initial assessment, the use of telehealth should complement existing relationships [16].

Reimbursement

Evidence for telehealth has often come from pilot projects, many of which have been grant funded. For example, the Health Resources and Services Administration Office for the Advancement of Telehealth has specifically supported funding opportunities to promote telehealth services in rural areas and pediatric populations [17]. However, these types of funding sources are not generally designed to sustain or expand telehealth programs over the long term. As a result, it is not surprising that, despite technology advances and inaccessibility to pediatric specialty care, the use of telehealth has remained the exception rather than the rule with larger practices (more than 50 physicians) being more likely to sustain a telemedicine program [18].

Recently, Medicaid has come to view telemedicine as a cost-effective alternative to traditional in-person care, and has provided states with the flexibility to determine which services and providers to reimburse for telemedicine care [19].

Although policies for reimbursement vary from state to state, Current Procedural Terminology codes and modifiers have been identified to support the standardized documentation of pediatric telemedicine services for Medicaid reimbursement; although the billing of private insurance for telemedicine services has not become universal, these codes provide a mechanism for private payers to cover these services [20]. At present, 37 states and the District of Columbia have parity laws that mandate private payer reimbursement for telemedicine services at the same rate as in-person care, with 2 other states having parity laws proposed or pending [21].

As telehealth services have become increasingly reimbursable, accountable care organizations and health maintenance organizations have looked to telemedicine visits as an alternative for cost-effective access to care. Likewise, employers may look to telemedicine providers as less expensive and timelier alternatives to traditional in-person office or emergency room visits.

Finally, with the Affordable Care Act having an optional Medicaid benefit for states to establish health homes, toward better coordinated care for patients with chronic conditions, telecare may become a reimbursable telehealth opportunity.

Consumer demand

Consumers highly value convenience in accessing health care, as has been seen with the increase in urgent care centers. Urgent care visits are particularly popular in the pediatric population [22], and free-standing urgent care centers have become a common source of pediatric health care outside of the traditional medical home [23]. As savvy consumers have become accustomed to having other services available on demand, such as ride sharing or food delivery, it should come as no surprise that there would be similar demand to access health care at any time and from any location [24].

This consumer interest has been reinforced by health care networks offering access to telemedicine services, and payers and employers increasing their coverage of these services. Although many physicians remain skeptical of offering telemedicine services, providing consumers with the opportunity to connect remotely to their care can promote patient satisfaction and engagement [25], potentially enhancing the physician-patient relationship.

Health care entrepreneurs are eager to fulfill unmet consumer demand for telemedicine, as several national companies have leveraged technologies of the sharing economy to connect practitioners and patients for virtual visits using direct-to-consumer (DTC) offerings. As these companies continue to expand telemedicine access outside of traditional health care networks, there will be a need for licensed physicians to staff their virtual telemedicine offices.

SELECTED EXAMPLES BY TELEHEALTH CATEGORY AND PEDIATRIC SPECIALTY

With the stage set for broader use of telehealth, it may be helpful to consider examples of telehealth in different pediatric specialties and care delivery contexts, to understand in which milieus telehealth may be effectively applied or where more study or innovation may be required.

Teleconsultations: addressing specialty access

The use of teleconsultation between practitioners may bridge gaps to timely access to pediatric specialists, and has been shown to be effective asynchronously and synchronously, where supported by appropriate infrastructure.

Cardiology

The use of telehealth in pediatric cardiology consultations and specialty care has been well studied for nearly 30 years [26], with significant applications in evaluating congenital heart disease, murmurs, and arrhythmias.

Echocardiography is a safe and cost-effective modality that makes use of noninvasive ultrasound images to assess the anatomy and function of the heart, and its use in teleconsultations is now considered routine. An asynchronous approach has traditionally been used to obtain, transmit, and interpret echocardiogram images. From a remote workstation, a pediatric cardiologist can accurately confirm or exclude congenital heart disease with comparable accuracy and improved timeliness over bedside interpretation [27]. Improvements in Internet bandwidth and videoconference quality have allowed for the evaluation of echocardiograms remotely in real time. In a Brazilian study, neonatologists performed echocardiograms with remote video supervision by a cardiologist, resulting in improved detection of congenital heart disease than without consultation [28]. In another study, real-time video was successfully used remotely by pediatric cardiologists to evaluate echocardiograms, consult with referring physicians, and provide direct education to the family on the need for surgery [29].

Although echocardiography for congenital heart disease has been the most common use of pediatric cardiology telemedicine consultation, the evaluation of a heart murmur remains the most common reason for referral to a pediatric cardiologist. Echocardiography has been evaluated for acute evaluation of murmur [30], although this modality may not be available in many ambulatory settings. Tele-auscultation (the electronic capture of heart sounds, asynchronously or in real time, for remote interpretation) has generated some interest as an alternative teleconsultation approach, and has been shown to allow reliable differentiation between innocent and pathologic murmurs [31], although the technology is best reserved for purposes of screening and referral [32]. However, as digital signal analysis of transmitted heart sounds is improved, there may be a future role for artificial intelligence in distinguishing between murmurs to improve the diagnostic utility of tele-auscultation [33].

Although the evidence of its effectiveness in this area is not yet well established, RPM may be well suited to some pediatric cardiology applications. Remote monitoring of implantable pediatric cardiovascular devices, such as pacemakers, improves the detection of adverse events [34], with a cardiologist or care nurse able to analyze transmitted data and contact patients or families if action is required. Remote electrocardiographic monitoring via wearable devices (such as smartwatches and biomedical shirts) has the potential to provide continuous recording and visualization of data, which may be monitored in real time or evaluated asynchronously [35]; though not adding significant information to what may be offered via traditional Holter monitoring options, these wearable devices may offer additional convenience and acceptability for patients, with implications for both telemedicine diagnosis and home monitoring telecare.

Ophthalmology

The use of telehealth in pediatric ophthalmology has been best studied in the context of retinopathy of prematurity (ROP). Ophthalmologic teleconsultations may support both diagnosis and monitoring of ROP in neonatal intensive care units (NICUs), reducing the need for in-person examination and minimizing exposure of the neonate.

Although direct fundoscopic examination is considered the gold standard, asynchronous screening of high-definition retinal images can provide accurate and timely feedback to determine whether an in-person neonate examination is necessary [36], and has been shown to be a viable option when access to an ophthalmologist is limited [37]. However, this image-centered approach is constrained by the cost of technology investment as well as the risk of capturing less detailed information to stage the extent of ROP [38]. For example, the sensitivity of ROP detection is reduced when a full set of 5 retinal images cannot be obtained [39]; furthermore, the quality of ROP grading using images is subject to reviewer variability, indicating the importance of standardized approaches and protocols [40].

Looking to the future, specific characteristics detected in retinal images may be suggestive as predictors for ROP [41]; although this finding requires additional validation, it may have implications for using imaging informatics tools and artificial intelligence to enhance the predictive ability of using retinal images for diagnosis and referral [42].

Nephrology

Like cardiology and ophthalmology, pediatric nephrology is an example of successfully implemented specialty teleconsultation: relevant medical information and digital images can generally be exchanged asynchronously, mitigating the need for investment in real-time audiovisual equipment. This application of teleconsultation has proven to be cost-effective, timely, and convenient for diagnosing congenital anomalies of the kidney and urinary tract, nephrotic syndrome, urinary tract infections, and the need for kidney transplant, without requiring in-person evaluation [43]. Patient and provider reception to this use of telehealth for pediatric nephrology consultation has generally been favorable [44].

Although more relevant to telepractice and telecare than teleconsultation, nephrology care and follow-up may also be provided remotely to support patient convenience. The use of RPM to monitor blood pressure in the home setting can provide more representative status than periodic clinic measurement, and technology to transmit data via remote cuffs connected to smartphones is evolving; that said, blood pressure cuffs are not always well tolerated in children and adolescents, which may affect the suitability of this telecare adjunct [45]. Recent changes to Medicare benefits have expanded the use of telehealth services, including real-time video visits, to dialysis in the patient's home or in free-standing dialysis clinics [46]; if a similar benefit is afforded to the pediatric population, video visits could augment nurse visits to improve the effectiveness and convenience of home dialysis [47].

Dermatology

The reliance on visual observation, sometimes to the exclusion of what the patient has to say, has made teleconsultation a natural match for dermatology [48]. Although most evidence for the use of dermatology teleconsultation has been in adults, there is evidence of its effectiveness in the pediatric population [49].

For example, parental use of smartphones can capture images with quality so high that, even when parents are provided little or no instruction, there is high concordance between diagnosis using smartphone images and in-person assessment [50]. The use of live video transmitted via a mobile phone, when compared with transmitted images, has been shown to be a reliable method for evaluating pediatric nevi [51]; however, although high-resolution video can approach traditional store-and-forward image interpretation or in-person evaluation for diagnostic accuracy, video resolution may be compromised by bandwidth constraints, making in-person evaluation the preferred approach [52].

Emergency medicine

In addition to the previous examples of consultations with pediatric subspecialists, teleconsultation can bring general pediatric and subspecialty expertise to adult settings. Although an in-person assessment is always preferred, and consultation via telephone may be useful in some instances, the use of real-time videoconferencing to consult on ill children has been shown to be effective in adult or after-hours emergency department (ED) settings.

When evaluating respiratory distress, there is excellent agreement between bedside and remote video observers on measures such as respiratory rate, retractions, and dyspnea [53]; this concurrence has likewise been demonstrated on febrile children in respiratory distress [54]. If a pediatric intensive care unit (PICU) admission becomes necessary, the use of pediatric teleconsultation in the ED setting has been associated with illness of lower severity at the time of PICU admission and lower mortality rates [55]. The use of pediatric video consultations in rural EDs has also resulted in fewer medication errors than telephone consultation [56].

Despite these effective uses, few EDs nationally use teleconsultation to assist in pediatric evaluation, and those that do are primarily consulting for patient placement or transfer coordination [57]. Among the identified challenges to implementing teleconsultation in the ED setting is the difficulty in incorporating virtual consultations into the ED physician's workflow in comparison with an in-person consultation.

In some instances general pediatric expertise may be available in the ED setting, but additional subspecialty consultation is required, particularly with pediatric imaging in the management of trauma. Remote radiography consultation via tablet devices has been effective in reducing in-person orthopedic consultation for children with suspected bone fractures [58], facilitating determination of whether urgent surgical management is necessary. As specialists are increasingly able to access digitized images remotely in EHRs, the tie to a specific tablet-device scenario may be unnecessary. Even photographs of radiographic images taken via cellphone and transmitted via e-mail have a high concurrence with expert image evaluation [59], although this approach should be limited to ad hoc assessment when the formal digital image is not accessible remotely. In an example from another imaging modality, ED pediatricians guided in ultrasonography by an expert radiologist using videoconferencing were able to produce reliable and timely diagnoses in the evaluation of abdominal trauma and nonspecific abdominal pain, when compared with an in-person assessment conducted by a radiologist [60].

Surgery

Remote surgery is a form of telepractice that uses medical robotics and real-time video communication. The particulars of telesurgery are beyond the scope of this review; however, some aspects of presurgical evaluation and postsurgical follow-up are amenable to teleconsultation.

In surgical telementoring, one surgeon provides teleconsultation to another surgeon remotely; this is generally reserved for a procedure that would require patients to travel for consultation. The evaluation of images and video of a lesion, paired with telephone consultation, can provide definitive diagnosis in some instances and may avoid unnecessary referrals [61]. In some instances, telementoring (using real-time videoconferencing) may extend to guidance during the surgical procedure. In a survey regarding surgical telementoring for the pediatric population, this form of teleconsultation was acceptable to nearly half of parental respondents; however, a desire for an in-person consultation, and concern regarding physician competence, were cited as reasons against surgical telementoring [62].

Telecare: managing chronic conditions

The use of telehealth technologies to connect with the pediatric patient in the home environment has had mixed results, but the advent of mHealth has the potential to passively monitor status and actively modify behaviors to improve health outcomes, particularly for chronic conditions.

Asthma

Asthma is the most common pediatric illness in the United States, disproportionately burdening families of lower socioeconomic status [63]. Using telecare to deliver asthma education and case management to improve behavioral outcomes is an area of great interest, although the evidence for effectiveness of telecare in improving asthma outcomes is limited.

Among the shortcomings of asthma telecare has been the need for the pediatric patient, or patient and family, to be actively engaged with Web-based interventions. For example, online asthma communities may provide helpful supportive benefits but do not necessarily improve asthma medication adherence [64] or reinforce ongoing engagement with the online communities. Providing a layer of patient-specific self-management may personalize and enhance Web-based telecare: The use of nurse-mediated telephone case management, when combined with Web-based self-management tools, improved overall pediatric asthma control, although medication adherence did not improve [65]. In another study, online asthma self-management was associated with a higher quality of life, but not necessarily improvement of asthma control [66].

The use of mobile technology has been posited as an approach to make asthma telecare more convenient for the patient than Web-based interventions, although it may be insufficient alone as a motivator. In one large trial, the use of mobile devices for active self-management was comparable to paper-based protocols in asthma control and self-management, although the associated technology investments were found not to be cost-effective [67].

The use of mobile devices to make participation in telecare interventions more passive shows promise for the future of asthma self-management, when incorporating RPM and alerts. In one study, plan-based medication and trigger reminders were more likely to result in reporting improved asthma management, although it did not significantly decrease asthma-related ED visits or hospitalizations [68]. The use of mobile or wearable devices with environmental sensors may be the next major step in asthma telecare: Analysis of sensor data may allow temporal correlation of environmental triggers (such as weather or air quality) with asthma symptoms to provide more specific and timely assessment of asthma risk [69] and better predict when a need-based (rather than schedule-based) medication reminder is needed [70]. Further personalization of reminders, integrating patient-centered messages of encouragement, may also improve their effectiveness [71].

Risk factors for overweight

Adolescent behaviors related to unhealthful diet and physical inactivity can contribute to overweight and obesity that may lead to chronic disease in the future. The evidence that telecare interventions may mitigate behavioral risk factors for overweight is mixed.

There is evidence that behavioral group intervention can be an effective use of telecare. In one study treating pediatric obesity for families living in rural areas, both video and telephone-only interventions were shown to be effective and acceptable methods for group intervention delivery, and there were no differences in the video and telephone groups on primary outcomes [72].

Telecare studies that have focused on individual management of risk factors for overweight have often used Web sites to directly engage with patients. Web-site interventions that made significant change in risk behaviors were generally associated with multidimensional approaches, including education, goal-setting, self-monitoring, and parental involvement as intervention strategies [73]. However, maintaining active patient engagement with a telecare intervention remains a significant barrier to effecting weight-change outcomes [74].

Mobile applications directed at intervening in behavioral risk factors for chronic disease in youth have shown some promise in maintaining engagement, using text messages, games, e-mails, and social media to promote active and ongoing participation. Within mHealth, the need for parental involvement is less clear: In one study, parent-focused mHealth interventions for adolescent obesity and overweight did not demonstrate a reliable impact on patients' dietary or physical outcomes [75], although another study implementing a caregiver strengthened the effect over communications to child patients alone [76].

Diabetes mellitus

Because some of the risk factors for managing overweight overlap with the risk factors for managing insulin-dependent diabetes mellitus (IDDM), those lessons may be transferable in effective diabetes telecare. In addition, there is diabetes-specific evidence that a telemedicine visit does not show significant difference from an in-person visit in managing behavioral aspects of IDDM [77].

Where behavior management for IDDM may differ from overweight is the opportunity for remote physiologic monitoring. In one study, patients and their families manually documented and e-mailed readings from a glucose monitor 5 times daily, receiving text messages or e-mails if values were critically out of range: This intervention resulted in decreased hemoglobin A1c levels and improved diabetes control, although the manual data entry was difficult for patients and families to adhere to [78]. In another study the use of continuous glucose monitoring, mediated by an insulin pump that concurrently alerted the patient and notified the treatment team of out-of-range values while simultaneously managing the correction, led to overall improvement in diabetes control that was safe and well accepted by patients [79].

Oncology

The role of telecare in improving outcomes for pediatric oncology patients has likewise been explored. These patients often experience mental and physical fatigue during and after chemotherapy treatments, and telecare technologies may have a role in supporting and empowering patients to better manage their care.

A survey of oncologists generally favored the idea of telecare, and the specific use of mobile oncology applications by patients, as a mechanism for monitoring side effects of chemotherapy and providing quicker response from the oncology team, while limiting patient inconvenience [80]. The use of an electronic checklist to support symptom identification and management was found to be associated with increased patient-clinic communication and satisfaction, and was strongly correlated with improved outcomes, without increasing costs

[81]. One study found that more than half of patients reported taking their scheduled medication immediately on receipt of a reminder from a smartphone-based application [82]. However, the evidence that real-time monitoring of symptoms decreases morbidity and unplanned admissions is limited and anecdotal [83].

Real-time video telephony has been suggested as a cost-effective and convenient means for providing clinical and psychosocial support for pediatric oncology patients [84]. In a Brazilian study on telecare for patients with acute lymphoblastic leukemia, implementation of an online meeting program resulted in decreases in overall mortality, early death, and relapses [85].

In areas of future interest, the use of video, electronic games, and mobile health applications are speculated to have a neurobiological role in encouraging resilience and empowerment in pediatric patients with cancer [86], and the use of mHealth technology for e-learning, promoting exercise, tracking behaviors, and supportive gaming are areas of promise [87].

Telehealth in public health: protecting populations

An important focus of public health is the protection of populations from disease and disability. Specific to child health, public health may include educating patients and families, screening for preventable or correctable conditions, and protection from infectious diseases.

Audiometric screening

Telehealth for audiometric screening is not well explored in the United States, where most newborns receive a hospital-based screening at birth, and screening for acquired hearing loss is available as a Medicaid-covered benefit through the Early and Periodic Screening, Diagnosis, and Treatment (EPSDT) Program, as well as through school-based programs. However, teleaudiometry–generally the use of a computer-based or tablet-based application to administer a hearing screening–is of significant interest internationally, where access to formal audiometric screening is limited, and often relies on questionnaire-based parental assessments [88].

Teleaudiometry is comparable in effectiveness with sweep audiometry in detecting hearing deficit, and may be feasible and cost effective as an initial screen in remote settings [89]. The audiologist may participate directly in the screening administering the examination remotely in real time using videoconferencing [90], or via a store-and-forward model where a trained assistant mediates an otoscopic examination and audiometric testing, with results later evaluated by the audiologist [91]. Although less common, teleaudiometry has sometimes included screening for other auditory conditions, such as tinnitus [92].

When an audiologist is not available to interpret a screening, a tablet-based hearing screening test can be used effectively for initial screening [93]. Smartphone-based hearing screening has been used by community health care workers to detect unidentified hearing loss at early childhood development centers [94]. In India, remote screening via auditory brainstem response has been facilitated by trained village health workers, with detection rates comparable with in-person screening, and with improved follow-up that has been attributed to geographic convenience [95].

After a hearing deficit is identified, teleaudiometry may also be used to validate the intervention. For example, in pediatric patients with cochlear implants, several visits to the cochlear implant center are required in the first year of use, and once or twice yearly thereafter, to assure ongoing effectiveness. Real-time, videoconference-mediated testing of cochlear implants did not reveal significant differences between remote and in-person testing, although the quality of the testing equipment and environment sometimes affected speech perception remotely [96].

Dental health

Like hearing screening, dental examinations are an EPSDT benefit, although individual states vary in their coverage, and many dentists opt not to participate in EPSDT programs. Beyond the EPSDT benefit, California requires an oral health assessment to be performed by a licensed dentist or registered dental hygienist (RDH) before, or soon after, school entry. Given significant unmet demand for pediatric dentists, the use of teledentistry (a form of teleconsultation using video and information communication technologies in real time or asynchronously) may provide an opportunity for an RDH to conduct initial dental screening and consult with a dentist on the need for additional referral. Although an area of practical interest with anecdotal successes, teledentistry-assisted use of RDHs has a limited evidence base and faces opposition from other dental care providers as hurdles to wider implementation [97].

Home-visitation programs

Public health nurse home-visitation programs can protect the health and well-being of at-risk children [98], some of whom may be medically complex. These programs are often grant funded, and many are subject to resource constraints or workforce limitations to providing direct care. Although there is sparse evidence of the use of telehealth technology in home-visitation programs, there is some evidence of success with medically complex children: Nursing televisits have been shown to result in fewer unplanned clinical visits [99] and lower rates of hospitalization and greater caregiver satisfaction [100]. This effective use of telecare may be appropriate to extend the reach of public health nurse home-visitation programs that educate caregivers and monitor at-risk children. The use of real-time audio/video has been discussed as an adjunct to social worker visits, to facilitate more frequent public health nursing assessments of children in foster care [101].

Tuberculosis control

Directly observed therapy (DOT) is a public health strategy to ensure patient adherence to treatment of tuberculosis. In DOT, patients meet with health workers, daily or several times per week, at a special public health clinic or via a community worker home visit; in either setting, health workers observe patients taking tuberculosis medication and enquire about side effects. This is a resource-intensive approach for health departments and can also be inconvenient for patients.

Video DOT (VDOT) is a form of telehealth that uses video in place of in-person visits and may be conducted asynchronously or in real time. In a study in New York City, the use of real-time, scheduled VDOT permitted workers to see the same number of patients as they would have in the clinic, and twice as many as they would have seen on home visits, with similar treatment completion outcomes in both scenarios [102]. In a similar California-based study, some patients recommended (and often preferred) real-time VDOT over DOT, with VDOT having higher adherence at lower cost than DOT [103]. Asynchronous VDOT, with videos reviewed daily, has also been shown to be feasible, and have high rates of patient approval and adherence [104].

Most studies on VDOT have involved management of adult patients. However, the lessons of VDOT may also be applicable to children, with strategies focused on scheduling VDOT asynchronously or synchronously before or during school hours to better monitor compliance.

Sexual health

There is some evidence of the effectiveness of telehealth applications to improve adolescent sexual health. For example, a rural, school-based telehealth education program was found to be effective in teaching reproductive health to female students, including those engaged in high-risk sexual activity, as evidenced by the increased use of condoms and hormonal contraceptives, and increased rates of human papillomavirus vaccination [105]. In another study of patients 16 years of age or older, a telehealth program was used to confirm *Chlamydia* diagnosis and initiate treatment, including partner notification and capture of surveillance data, with treatment outcomes similar to those for in-person care [106].

Although there are some states that specifically prohibit its use for abortion, telemedicine has been used in adult populations to access medications to terminate pregnancy, with outcomes comparable with in-person care [107]. It has been proposed that this type of telemedicine could be expanded to improve access to medical termination for women living in remote areas [108], and that such access would reduce terminations in the second trimester [109]. A telemedicine visit resulting in medical abortion has been shown to have similar efficacy, with no increased risk of adverse events, when compared with in-person abortion [110]. In jurisdictions where adolescents may consent to care regarding their sexual health, these applications of telehealth may reduce barriers to intervention.

Telepractice: transforming the physician-patient relationship

The previous telehealth examples have focused on pediatric specialties, and noteworthy examples of their use of technology to support teleconsultation or telecare. Telehealth is increasingly being used to support the traditional physician-patient interaction in several pediatric specialty areas.

Neonatology

The use of telehealth in the neonatal period has been previously highlighted under cardiology and ophthalmology consultations, but the applications in neonatology span many telehealth categories and neonatal phases of care.

Neonatology has made use of asynchronous teleconsultation from the early 1990s to meet the increased demand for specialty evaluation created by conditions of prematurity [111], but synchronous teleconsultation has also been shown to be effective, with the neonatologist as either the requestor or the consultee. For example, real-time video teleconsultations, with the specialist observing remotely and the neonatologist on-site in the NICU to adjust the position of the camera or the patient, have been used to conduct genetic and neurologic evaluations, allowing identification of more than 90% of abnormalities–with implications for use as a screening, if not diagnostic, tool [112]. In the counter example, when a community hospital seeks a teleconsultation with a remote neonatologist, it is more likely to adhere to standard measures of neonatal care and have higher-quality resuscitations of preterm neonates [113]; these positive impacts have been found to be greater when the teleconsultation is used earlier in the evaluation.

Telehealth technologies are increasingly used for RPM in the practice of neonatology. The extensive use of telemetry in the NICU provides opportunities to monitor patient status remotely, and the introduction of audiovisual equipment provides opportunities for real-time observation of the neonate. In one study, robots were used to convey a live audiovisual feed to a neonatologist rounding remotely: no significant differences were noted in care or outcomes when compared with an on-site neonatologist, except for interruptions caused by the mobility of the robot or issues with the Internet connection. This use of robots was positively received by parents and NICU staff, with potential implications for the timing and frequency of daily patient rounds [114]. In another NICU study, telemedicine respiratory assessments were well correlated with in-person evaluation, and respiratory therapists found the careful use of the telemedicine technology to be acceptable, suggesting the incorporation of tele-auscultation to further augment assessments [115].

Telehealth may serve additional uses outside of the NICU. For example, after the neonate is discharged from the NICU, the use of an informational Web site and videoconferences with families was shown to decrease emergency hospital visits in this population; families expressed satisfaction with this use of telecare, and perceived that they had more scheduled appointments than necessary when compared with other families without access to telecare [116]. In another example, telehealth may have a role in the immediate prenatal period, as prenatal telemonitoring [117] and telemedicine obstetric consults [118] have both been used to decrease the incidence of very-low-birth-weight deliveries.

Neurology

Telehealth has demonstrated effectiveness across the spectrum of pediatric neurology, from diagnosis to ongoing management.

For institutions without a pediatric neurologist, teleconsultation is an important path to access this expertise. Consultation by telephone alone has proved effective to pediatricians in managing neurologic cases and reducing unnecessary admissions or transfers to tertiary care hospitals [119]. Other types of neurology consultations may be conducted effectively asynchronously or synchronously. In one study, electroencephalograms (EEGs) were made available securely over a virtual private network, expanding access to EEG review services and reducing waiting time for consultation by half, at a comparable unit cost per EEG [120]. In another study, videoconferencing was evaluated as a mechanism for physical examination to diagnose a rare neurologic condition (Batten disease): Using a standardized scale, a nonphysician in-person examination was observed by an in-person rater, and a remote rater participating via teleconference, with high inter-rater reliability [121].

For patients already under the care of a pediatric neurologist, telehealth may have a role in the management of various neurologic conditions. For example, in the management of stable epilepsy, no significant difference was noted in the number of breakthrough seizures for patients who were followed telephonically or in person, allowing telephonic review to be considered with selected patients for whom access may be an issue [122]. In a telecare example, the use of text message reminders improved the education of patients with epilepsy, and compliance with both drug-taking and clinic appointments, with high patient acceptability [123]. In the management of migraines, RPM focused on adherence to preventive treatment and lifestyle may improve outcomes: In one study, the electronic monitoring of bottle-cap opening was associated with significantly higher adolescent adherence to medication regimen than self-reported rates without monitoring (75% vs 64%) [124].

Mental health

In a study of Medicaid telemedicine claims between 2008 and 2009, nearly 95% were associated with a psychiatric or behavioral health diagnosis, mostly bipolar disorder or attention-deficit disorder [125]. As the number of child and adolescent psychiatrists, particularly in rural or underserved communities, does not meet projected needs, tele-mental health (TMH) services can be an effective approach to provide direct patient care via telephone or videoconferencing, or teleconsultation to pediatricians, with additional services as needed in other settings such as schools or home [126]. The use of TMH can improve access simply by eliminating clinician travel time, increasing the opportunities for unscheduled visits during times of urgency or crisis [127].

Therapist-guided cognitive behavioral therapy (CBT) delivered via the Internet as texts or streaming media may provide an alternative to in-person care in addressing somatic complaints such as chronic pain, and psychiatric conditions including anxiety [128] and depression [129]. More research is needed with regard to the safety, efficacy, and effectiveness of mHealth CBT applications before supporting their stand-alone use for children and adolescents, but they may have a role as extenders of relationships with mental health professionals [130].

Telehealth may have a role in supporting timely assessment of developmental disorders, whereby early intervention may be critical. For example, the mean time between evaluation, diagnosis, and intervention for autism spectrum disorder may exceed a year [131]. In one evaluation model, the use of in-home, parent-recorded video was demonstrated to be an effective complement to traditional in-office assessment of autism [132], and was speculated to improve the efficiency of diagnosis [133].

Rheumatology

There is approximately one board-certified pediatric rheumatologist for every 1000 children with a rheumatologic condition in the United States, with more than half of the states having between zero and 2 of these specialists, as many are geographically concentrated in urban centers or at academic institutions [134].

This challenge in access has generated interest in offering telemedicine as a practice option, although a survey of pediatric rheumatology practices found that only 3 of 77 had ever used telemedicine [135].

In a study comparing families seen at an in-person pediatric rheumatology clinic in Missouri with families seen at a telemedicine outreach clinic more than 150 miles away, telemedicine visits were shown to mitigate the burden of time and cost, with no change in clinical outcomes [136]. Patient preference may play an important role in the acceptability of this mode of care, as another study showed that an overwhelming majority (95%) of patients' families preferred in-person pediatric rheumatology visits to telemedicine, even when travel was noted to be inconvenient (more than 3 hours) [137]. However, in a study from Chile, where some patients with juvenile idiopathic arthritis (JIA) live in remote areas with limited access to health care of any kind, telemedicine was used as a tool to support diagnosis and ongoing follow-up, with the number of patients requiring specific referral for in-person care decreasing from 10 to 1. In contrast to the aforementioned United States findings, the advantages of this telemedicine outreach model were seen by both patients and their parents to outweigh the disadvantages [138].

The use of a single, integrated pediatric rheumatology questionnaire to track parent- and child-reported outcomes for JIA, juvenile dermatomyositis, and juvenile autoinflammatory diseases has been shown to be effective in guiding patient self-management, documentation of change in health, assessment of therapeutic interventions, and verification of satisfaction with outcomes [139]. Where telemedicine via videoconferencing is not available, this telecare approach may be a useful option to support the management of patients already under care.

Telepractice: changing the game for general pediatric care

General pediatricians have long participated in the art of telepractice: from asynchronous review and triage of telephone messages, to real-time calls back to families and phoned-in prescriptions, the concept of telehealth is not a new one. Some pediatricians may even entrust patients and families with their mobile phone numbers for on-demand, synchronous care. With the convergence of enabling technologies, increasing reimbursement opportunities, and consumer demand, the stage is set for a formal telemedicine role in general pediatrics, especially for acute care.

With the rapid proliferation of DTC telemedicine in the United States, it is natural to think about the role that telemedicine may play in pediatric urgent care visits. When compared with traditional office or ED visits, telemedicine visits have been increasingly identified and promoted as a cost-effective alternative to in-person care [140], making virtual urgent care an increasingly attractive proposition for health plans and employers. In adult studies, patients have reported high satisfaction with these visits, rating convenience and perceived quality of care as important factors [141]. Such quality of care, however, may simply be perceived.

Respiratory tract infections (RTIs) are the predominant reason for a DTC telemedicine visit: One study of RTI visit-length data found that DTC visits were shorter when antibiotics were prescribed and longer when nonantibiotics were prescribed, compared with visits with no prescriptions, suggesting that DTC prescriber incentive to increase patient volume could come at the expense of antibiotic stewardship [142]. In a follow-up study of patients surveyed for these RTI visits, patients rated DTC prescribers (whether for antibiotics or nonantibiotics) higher than DTC nonprescribers [143]. Specific to pediatrics, children seen at DTC visits for acute respiratory infections were more likely to receive antibiotics, and in a manner more likely to deviate from guidelines, than children at their primary care provider (PCP) or traditional urgent care visit [144]. More generally, when a national DTC vendor was compared with traditional physician offices, the DTC approach trailed in measures of access and quality [145].

DISCUSSION

Telehealth approaches by specialty

The effectiveness and applicability of a telehealth approach varies widely by pediatric specialty, care delivery setting, and patient preference.

Asynchronous specialty teleconsultation has long been a stalwart of pediatric telehealth, as demonstrated in cardiology, ophthalmology, nephrology, and dermatology. Real-time teleconsultation has been effective in improving outcomes in the evaluation of the acutely ill child in the ED setting as well as in the NICU.

Early efforts in managing chronic conditions via telecare have relied on active patient participation with Web sites, whereby adherence to the intervention is not readily sustained over time. The use of RPM and mHealth applications have shown some promise for telecare, as they may require less active patient engagement while providing real-time intervention in the form of education, reminders, or real-time consultations as needed.

The use of telehealth in public health has been shown to be effective in audiology screening and tuberculosis control, overcoming geographic and resource limitations to detect and treat conditions. Evidence of the effective use of telehealth in other areas of public health is limited but may be helpful in expanding the reach of dental screening and home-visitation programs, as well as providing population-based health education. The most significant constraint to the public health application of telehealth is the reliance on core public funding or external grant funding to evolve and sustain innovative programs.

Perhaps the greatest interest in telehealth is in telepractice/telemedicine, where each specialty is unique in the opportunities that it may successfully exploit. Neonatology has historically been a technologically advanced specialty, which has translated well across the spectrum of telehealth applications. The nature of observation and communication in mental health and development are amenable to the use of evidence-based screening tools and videoconferencing or even telephony. Telemedicine is effective in rheumatology practice, although this is one identified specialty with a specific patient preference for in-person visits.

Telehealth in general pediatrics

The use of DTC is more likely in nonmetropolitan communities and in children without preventive care visits, and when compared with children receiving acute care with their PCP, children with DTC visits were also more likely to have had urgent care and ED visits [146]. In an analysis of commercial claims data, it was estimated that 12% of DTC visits replaced visits to other providers, and 88% represented new utilization, without the touted decrease in overall cost [147]. The records from these visits may not be readily captured into the EHR system of the patient's medical home, if the practice is even aware that the DTC visit occurred. Given the popularity of urgent care visits in the pediatric population, as some DTC service vendors begin to establish (or partner with) brick-and-mortar urgent care centers, there is a risk that children and families may never have–or even depart from–a pediatric medical home.

The AAP supports the pediatric medical home as the optimal location for children to receive acute, nonemergent care, acknowledging that families may take advantage of other services for convenience of access or cost [148]. Digital communication has been shown to provide the most benefit when there is an existing relationship between the patient and the clinical team [149]. To maximize opportunities for families to keep care within the pediatric medical home, pediatric practices may need to establish urgent care telemedicine as a core offering. One study estimated that approximately 85% of sick visits in a pediatric practice could be completed using a telemedicine model that offers only simple office testing and albuterol administration [150], suggesting that urgent care telemedicine in the context of a pediatric medical home could be a viable alternative to in-person acute care. It has also been suggested that a robust pediatric urgent care telemedicine practice could provide teleconsultations to augment acute care needs where access to health professionals might be limited, such as athletic tournaments or at schools [151]. At present, Medicaid reimbursement for real-time telemedicine exceeds reimbursement for store-and-forward and RPM; as states expand their policies and reimbursements to specifically support telecare or asynchronous telepractice, there may be opportunities for innovation in pediatric practice to extend core telehealth offerings [152]. The AAP provides resources for practices interested in providing telehealth services [153], including practice transformation [154].

Telemedicine practice considerations

Although telemedicine platforms have become cost accessible for even smaller pediatric practices, there are numerous additional considerations before implementing telemedicine in a practice, including licensure, liability, privacy and security, technology, and workflow.

As originating and remote sites may be in different states, multistate licensure may be a consideration for practices with a catchment area that straddles state lines, or where patients travel out of state. The Interstate Medical Licensure Compact is an agreement between 29 states and 1 territory and their respective Medical and Osteopathic Boards that qualifies licensed physicians to practice medicine in participating states in the Compact, if eligibility requirements are met [155].

Although medical malpractice insurance is essential to any practice, telemedicine adds complexity to the liability coverage required. Telemedicine services may be excluded by some carriers; moreover, coverage may be defined by the state where the physician is licensed rather than the originating site, with premiums based on time worked in each state, and additional coverage for privacy and security exposure over the Internet.

Practices should resist the temptation to use social media applications as their entrée into telemedicine. Although social media may offer video-chat technologies, these applications are not usually encrypted, and are not compliant with the Health Insurance Portability and Accountability Act of 1996 (HIPAA); in addition, cloud service providers are generally not covered under HIPAA [156]. Although there are mechanisms to send encrypted e-mail to personal e-mail accounts, asynchronous communications with patients should be limited to secure messaging, preferably associated with the telemedicine platform or an EHR patient portal.

When evaluating a telemedicine platform, it would ideally integrate with the practice's EHR: lack of integration may lead to redundant documentation in separate systems, or having separate information silos for documentation, ordering, and billing for telemedicine and in-office visits.

The telemedicine platform should be suitable for a wide range of user skills, for both the physician and the patient population, to ensure that telehealth interactions are reliable, error-free, efficient, and without undue delay or interruption. In a heuristic evaluation of 4 telemedicine software platforms, 46 unique issues were uncovered for potential usability problems with existing user interfaces [157]. In offices with multiple concurrent telemedicine visits, or simply limited broadband Internet capacity, performance issues may be encountered as network-reliant applications compete for bandwidth.

Each practice should carefully consider the implications of its telemedicine scheduling structure and staffing model, as there is no one-size-fits-all model for success. With regard to scheduling, use of telemedicine may be ad hoc (akin to the model of responding to telephone messages) or have dedicated spots in the schedule. Telemedicine encounters in a general pediatrics practice should be reserved for acute care and follow-up of established patients only, with new patients having in-person visits. When visits are scheduled, some physicians may prefer dedicated blocks of telemedicine visits, whereas others may prefer virtual visits to be interspersed with in-office visits. Telemedicine visits may be an option to establish, or augment existing, urgent care hours on evenings and weekends. Depending on the videoconferencing and other technologies used, a dedicated space may be required for telemedicine visits, or may even be desired when the physician's office is in a shared, highly interruptive, or otherwise unsuitable space; if the dedicated space is an examination room, this should also be factored into scheduling.

With regard to staffing, when there are dedicated telemedicine blocks scheduled, physicians may choose to share in telemedicine responsibilities covering "shifts"; larger practices may have the flexibility to assign or dedicate certain physicians to telemedicine, especially when other physicians in the practice are not comfortable with virtual visits.

Telemedicine may provide work flexibility that supports physicians who are temporarily or permanently unable to practice medicine in a traditional setting full time, as well as moonlighting opportunities. For physicians who have become disenchanted with the practice of medicine, telemedicine may allow for reduction in workload without abandoning practice altogether. On the other hand, there may also be physicians who have no desire to practice telemedicine, but are compelled to do so by their employers or the demands of the health care environment. With cross-cutting subspecialties such as sports medicine, adolescent medicine, and even clinical informatics, some have proposed that telehealth should become its own medical specialty or subspecialty, certifying "medical virtualists" who will spend most or all of their time delivering competent and compassionate care at the "webside" [158]. More research is required to determine whether telemedicine subspecialists in the primary care disciplines can mitigate inequities in telemedicine clinical practice and outcomes.

Physicians should remain cognizant of the impact of these technologies on the physician-patient relationship, and maintaining continuity of care and minimizing the risk for patient abandonment [159]. Indiscriminate use of telehealth technologies for delicate patient revelations may result in perceptions of care as insensitive or unethical [160].

SUMMARY

Advances in technology, access to care, service reimbursement, and consumer demand have been primary drivers for pediatric telehealth. In some specialties, telehealth is used across all phases of care from diagnosis to follow-up. Teleconsultation has been successful in closing gaps in access to pediatric specialists, and telecare may create opportunities to more closely monitor and intervene in the health of the pediatric patient, extending the concept of the medical home to a patient "health home."

While there is limited, context-specific evidence that telehealth improves health outcomes when compared with direct, in-person care, the expanding consumer demand for telemedicine may have disruptive effects on the practice of pediatrics and the urgency with which practices choose to adopt telehealth technologies. The effectiveness and applicability of a telehealth approach varies by pediatric specialty, care delivery setting, and patient preference; in addition, there are licensure, liability, privacy and security, technology, and workflow considerations that may affect implementation. Whether implementing telehealth in a general or specialty pediatrics practice, the diversity of previous experiences may inform appropriate uses that are suitable for the needs of an individual practice.

References

[1] Telehealth programs. Available at: https://www.hrsa.gov/rural-health/telehealth/index.html. Accessed April 8, 2019.
[2] Masys DR. Telehealth: the need for evaluation. J Am Med Inform Assoc 1997;4(1):69–70.
[3] Telemedicine. Available at: https://www.medicaid.gov/medicaid/benefits/telemed/index.html. Accessed April 8, 2019.
[4] Burke BL, Hall RW. Telemedicine: pediatric applications. Pediatrics 2015;136(1):e293–308.
[5] Dyk LV. A review of telehealth service implementation frameworks. Int J Environ Res Public Health 2014;11(2):1279–98.
[6] Health Homes. Available at: https://www.medicaid.gov/medicaid/ltss/health-homes/index.html. Accessed April 8, 2019.
[7] Office of the National Coordinator for Health Information Technology. Percent of hospitals, by type, that possess certified health IT, Health IT Quick-Stat #52. 2018. Available at: dashboard.healthit.gov/quickstats/pages/certified-electronic-health-record-technology-in-hospitals.php. Accessed April 8, 2019.
[8] Office of the National Coordinator for Health Information Technology. Office-based physician electronic health record adoption. Health IT Quick-Stat #50. 2019. Available at: dashboard.healthit.gov/quickstats/pages/physician-ehr-adoption-trends.php. Accessed April 8, 2019.
[9] Rimsza ME, Ruch-Ross HS, Clemens CJ, et al. Workforce trends and analysis of selected pediatric subspecialties in the United States. Acad Pediatr 2018;18(7):805–12.
[10] Peltz A, Wu CL, White ML, et al. Characteristics of rural children admitted to pediatric hospitals. Pediatrics 2016;137(5):e20153156.
[11] Ray KN, Demirci JR, Bogen DL, et al. Optimizing telehealth strategies for subspecialty care: recommendations from rural pediatricians. Telemed J E Health 2015;21(8):622–9.
[12] Smith AC, Scuffham P, Wootton R. The costs and potential savings of a novel telepaediatric service in Queensland. BMC Health Serv Res 2007;7(1):35.
[13] Marcin JP, Shaikh U, Steinhorn RH. Addressing health disparities in rural communities using telehealth. Pediatr Res 2015;79(1–2):169–76.

[14] Lessard JA, Knox R. Telehealth in a rural school-based health center. J Sch Nurs 2000;16(2):38–41.
[15] Russo L, Campagna I, Ferretti B, et al. What drives attitude towards telemedicine among families of pediatric patients? A survey. BMC Pediatr 2017;17(1):21.
[16] Ray KN, Ashcraft LE, Mehrotra A, et al. Family perspectives on telemedicine for pediatric subspecialty care. Telemed J E Health 2017;23(10):852–62.
[17] HRSA Telehealth programs. Available at: https://www.hrsa.gov/rural-health/telehealth/index.html. Accessed March 7, 2019.
[18] Kane CK, Gillis K. The use of telemedicine by physicians: still the exception rather than the rule. Health Aff 2018;37(12):1923–30.
[19] Telemedicine reimbursement. Available at: https://www.medicaid.gov/medicaid/benefits/telemed/index.html. Accessed March 7, 2019.
[20] Telemedicine services. Available at: https://www.aap.org/en-us/Documents/coding_factsheet_telemedicine.pdf. Accessed March 7, 2019.
[21] State policy resource center. Available at: http://legacy.americantelemed.org/policy-page/state-policy-resource-center. Accessed April 8, 2019.
[22] Montalbano A, Rodean J, Canares T, et al. Urgent care utilization in the pediatric Medicaid population. J Pediatr 2017;191:238–43.
[23] Urgent care centers. Available at: https://www.aap.org/en-us/professional-resources/practice-transformation/economics/Pages/Urgent-Care-Centers.aspx. Accessed April 8, 2019.
[24] Grube ME, Kaufman K, Clarin D, et al. Health care on demand: four telehealth priorities for 2016. Healthc Financ Manage 2016;70(1):42–51.
[25] Kruse CS, Krowski N, Rodriguez B, et al. Telehealth and patient satisfaction: a systematic review and narrative analysis. BMJ Open 2017;7:e016242.
[26] Trippi JA, Lee KS, Kopp G, et al. Emergency echocardiography telemedicine: an efficient method to provide 24-Hour consultative echocardiography. J Am Coll Cardiol 1996;27(7):1748–52.
[27] Satou GM, Rheuban K, Alverson D, et al. Telemedicine in pediatric cardiology: a scientific statement from the American Heart Association. Circulation 2017;135(11):e648–78.
[28] Mattos SD, Hazin SM, Regis CT, et al. A telemedicine network for remote paediatric cardiology services in north-east Brazil. Bull World Health Organ 2015;93(12):881–7.
[29] Geoffroy O, Acar P, Caillet D, et al. Videoconference pediatric and congenital cardiology consultations: a new application in telemedicine. Arch Cardiovasc Dis 2008;101(2):89–93.
[30] Rose-Felker K, Kelleman MS, Campbell RM, et al. Appropriate use and clinical impact of echocardiographic "evaluation of murmur" in pediatric patients. Congenit Heart Dis 2016;11(6):721–6.
[31] Finley JP, Warren AE, Sharratt GP, et al. Assessing childrens heart sounds at a distance with digital recordings. Pediatrics 2006;118(6):2322–5.
[32] Behere S, Baffa JM, Penfil S, et al. Real-world evaluation of the Eko Electronic Teleauscultation System. Pediatr Cardiol 2018;40(1):154–60.
[33] Thompson WR, Reinisch AJ, Unterberger MJ, et al. Artificial intelligence-assisted auscultation of heart murmurs: validation by virtual clinical trial. Pediatr Cardiol 2018;40(3):623–9.
[34] Malloy LE, Gingerich J, Olson MD, et al. Remote monitoring of cardiovascular implantable devices in the pediatric population improves detection of adverse events. Pediatr Cardiol 2014;35(2):301–6.
[35] Balsam P, Lodziński P, Tymińska A, et al. Study design and rationale for biomedical shirt-based electrocardiography monitoring in relevant clinical situations: ECG-shirt study. Cardiol J 2018;25(1):52–9.
[36] Quinn GE, Ying G, Repka MX, et al. Timely implementation of a retinopathy of prematurity telemedicine system. J AAPOS 2016;20(5):425–30.

[37] Shah PK, Ramya A, Narendran V. Telemedicine for ROP. Asia Pac J Ophthalmol (Phila) 2018;7(1):52–5.
[38] Fierson WM, Capone A, American Academy of Pediatrics Section on Ophthalmology, American Academy of OphthalmologyAmerican Association of Certified Orthoptists. Telemedicine for evaluation of retinopathy of prematurity. Pediatrics 2015;35(1):e238–54.
[39] Bothun ED, Morrison D, Ying G-S, et al. Impact of number and quality of retinal images in a telemedicine screening program for ROP: results from the e-ROP study. J AAPOS 2016;20(4):481–5.
[40] Quinn GE, Ying GS, Pan W, et al. Detection of potentially severe retinopathy of prematurity by remote image grading. JAMA Ophthalmol 2017;135(9):982–6.
[41] Ying GS, Vanderveen D, Daniel E, et al. Risk score for predicting treatment-requiring retinopathy of prematurity (ROP) in the telemedicine approaches to evaluating acute-phase ROP study. Ophthalmology 2016;123(10):2176–82.
[42] Fauw JD, Ledsam JR, Romera-Paredes B, et al. Clinically applicable deep learning for diagnosis and referral in retinal disease. Nat Med 2018;24(9):1342–50.
[43] Trnka P, White MM, Renton WD, et al. A retrospective review of telehealth services for children referred to a paediatric nephrologist. BMC Nephrol 2015;16(1):125.
[44] Bello AK, Molzahn AE, Girard LP, et al. Patient and provider perspectives on the design and implementation of an electronic consultation system for kidney care delivery in Canada: a focus group study. BMJ Open 2017;7(3):e014784.
[45] Hamdani G, Flynn JT, Daniels S, et al. Ambulatory blood pressure monitoring tolerability and blood pressure status in adolescents. Blood Press Monit 2019;24(1):12–7.
[46] Lew SQ, Sikka N. Operationalizing telehealth for home dialysis patients in the United States. Am J Kid Dis 2019.
[47] Ellis EN, Blaszak C, Wright S, et al. Effectiveness of home visits to pediatric peritoneal dialysis patients. Perit Dial Int 2011;32(4):419–23.
[48] Hart J. The visual nature of dermatology is a good match for telemedicine. Telemed J E Health 2011;17(6):405–8.
[49] Naka F, Makkar H, Lu J. Teledermatology: kids are not just little people. Clin Dermatol 2017;35(6):594–600.
[50] O'Connor DM, Jew OS, Perman MJ, et al. Diagnostic accuracy of pediatric teledermatology using parent-submitted photographs. JAMA Dermatol 2017;153(12):1243–8.
[51] Karlsson M, Lindelöf B, Wahlgren C, et al. Mobile teledermatology is a valid method to estimate prevalence of melanocytic naevi in children. Acta Dermato Venereol 2015;95(3):303–6.
[52] Marchell R, Locatis C, Burges G, et al. Comparing high definition live interactive and store-and-forward consultations to in-person examinations. Telemed J E Health 2017;23(3):213–8.
[53] Gattu R, Scollan J, Desouza A, et al. Telemedicine: a reliable tool to assess the severity of respiratory distress in children. Hosp Pediatr 2016;6(8):476–82.
[54] Siew L, Hsiao A, Mccarthy P, et al. Reliability of telemedicine in the assessment of seriously ill children. Pediatrics 2016;137(3):e20150712.
[55] Dayal P, Hojman NM, Kissee JL, et al. Impact of telemedicine on severity of illness and outcomes among children transferred from referring emergency departments to a children's hospital PICU. Pediatr Crit Care Med 2016;17(6):516–21.
[56] Dharmar M, Kuppermann N, Romano PS, et al. Telemedicine consultations and medication errors in rural emergency departments. Pediatrics 2013;132(6):1090–7.
[57] Brova M, Boggs KM, Zachrison KS, et al. Pediatric telemedicine use in United States emergency departments. Acad Emerg Med 2018;25(12):1427–32.
[58] Zennaro F, Grosso D, Fascetta R, et al. Teleradiology for remote consultation using iPad improves the use of health system human resources for paediatric fractures: prospective controlled study in a tertiary care hospital in Italy. BMC Health Serv Res 2014;14(1):327.

[59] Goost H, Witten J, Heck A, et al. Image and diagnosis quality of x-ray image transmission via cell phone camera: a project study evaluating quality and reliability. PLoS One 2012;7(10):e43402.
[60] Zennaro F, Neri E, Nappi F, et al. Real-time tele-mentored low cost "point-of-care US" in the hands of paediatricians in the emergency department: diagnostic accuracy compared to expert radiologists. PLoS One 2016;11(10):e0164539.
[61] Akkoyun I. The advantages of using photographs and video images in telephone consultations with a specialist in paediatric surgery. Afr J Paediatr Surg 2012;9(2):128–31.
[62] Abdulhai S, Glenn IC, Mcninch NL, et al. Public perception of telemedicine and surgical telementoring in the pediatric population: results of a parental survey. J Laparoendosc Adv Surg Tech A 2018;28(2):215–7.
[63] Ferrante G, Grutta SL. The burden of pediatric asthma. Front Pediatr 2018;6:186.
[64] Koufopoulos JT, Conner MT, Gardner PH, et al. A web-based and mobile health social support intervention to promote adherence to inhaled asthma medications: randomized controlled trial. J Med Internet Res 2016;18(6):e122.
[65] Gustafson D, Wise M, Bhattacharya A, et al. The effects of combining web-based eHealth with telephone nurse case management for pediatric asthma control: a randomized controlled trial. J Med Internet Res 2012;14(4):e101.
[66] Ahmed S, Ernst P, Bartlett SJ, et al. The effectiveness of web-based asthma self-management system, My Asthma Portal (MAP): a pilot randomized controlled trial. J Med Internet Res 2016;18(12):e313.
[67] Ryan D, Price D, Musgrave SD, et al. Clinical and cost effectiveness of mobile phone supported self monitoring of asthma: multicentre randomised controlled trial. BMJ 2012;344:e1756.
[68] Stukus DR, Farooqui N, Strothman K, et al. Real-world evaluation of a mobile health application in children with asthma. Ann Allergy Asthma Immunol 2018;120(4):395–400.
[69] Hosseini A, Buonocore C, Hashemzadeh S, et al. Feasibility of a secure wireless sensing smartwatch application for the self-management of pediatric asthma. Sensors (Basel) 2017;17(8):1780.
[70] Chan YY, Wang P, Rogers L, et al. The Asthma Mobile Health Study, a large-scale clinical observational study using ResearchKit. Nat Biotechnol 2017;35(4):354–62.
[71] Yoo W, Kim SY, Hong Y, et al. Patient-clinician mobile communication: analyzing text Messaging between adolescents with asthma and nurse case managers. Telemed J E Health 2015;21(1):62–9.
[72] Davis AM, Sampilo M, Gallagher KS, et al. Treating rural paediatric obesity through telemedicine vs. telephone: outcomes from a cluster randomized controlled trial. J Telemed Telecare 2015;22(2):86–95.
[73] Rose T, Barker M, Jacob CM, et al. A systematic review of digital interventions for improving the diet and physical activity behaviors of adolescents. J Adolesc Health 2017;61(6):669–77.
[74] Tu AW, Watts AW, Chanoine J-P, et al. Does parental and adolescent participation in an e-health lifestyle modification intervention improve weight outcomes? BMC Public Health 2017;17(1):352.
[75] Hammersley ML, Jones RA, Okely AD. Parent-focused childhood and adolescent overweight and obesity eHealth interventions: a systematic review and meta-analysis. J Med Internet Res 2016;18(7):e203.
[76] Fedele DA, Cushing CC, Fritz A, et al. Mobile health interventions for improving health outcomes in youth. JAMA Pediatr 2017;171(5):461–9.
[77] Freeman KA, Duke DC, Harris MA. Behavioral health care for adolescents with poorly controlled diabetes via Skype: does working alliance remain intact? J Diabetes Sci Technol 2013;7(3):727–35.

[78] Peña NV, Torres M, Cardona JA, et al. Impact of telemedicine assessment on glycemic variability in children with type 1 diabetes mellitus. Diabetes Technol Ther 2013;15(2): 136–42.
[79] DeSalvo DJ, Keith-Hynes P, Peyser T, et al. Remote glucose monitoring in cAMP setting reduces the risk of prolonged nocturnal hypoglycemia. Diabetes Technol Ther 2014;16(1): 1–7.
[80] Kessel KA, Vogel MM, Schmidt-Graf F, et al. Mobile Apps in Oncology: a survey on health care professionals' attitude toward telemedicine, mHealth, and oncological apps. J Med Internet Res 2016;18(11):e312.
[81] Williams AR, Williams DD, Williams PD, et al. The development and application of an oncology Therapy-Related Symptom Checklist for Adults (TRSC) and Children (TRSC-C) and e-health applications. Biomed Eng Online 2015;14(Suppl 2):S1.
[82] Wu Y, Linder L, Kanokvimankul P, et al. Use of a smartphone application for prompting oral medication adherence among adolescents and young adults with cancer. Oncol Nurs Forum 2018;45(1):69–76.
[83] Maguire R, Fox PA, Mccann L, et al. The eSMART study protocol: a randomised controlled trial to evaluate electronic symptom management using the advanced symptom management system (ASyMS) remote technology for patients with cancer. BMJ Open 2017;7(5):e015016.
[84] Bensink M, Wootton R, Irving H, et al. Investigating the cost-effectiveness of videotelephone based support for newly diagnosed paediatric oncology patients and their families: design of a randomised controlled trial. BMC Health Serv Res 2007;7(1):38.
[85] Pedrosa F, Shaikh F, Rivera G, et al. The impact of prospective telemedicine implementation in the management of childhood acute lymphoblastic leukemia in Recife, Brazil. Telemed J E Health 2017;23(10):863–7.
[86] Govender M, Bowen RC, German ML, et al. Clinical and neurobiological perspectives of empowering pediatric cancer patients using videogames. Games Health J 2015;4(5): 362–74.
[87] Elliot DL, Lindemulder SJ, Goldberg L, et al. Health promotion for adolescent childhood leukemia survivors: building on prevention science and eHealth. Pediatr Blood Cancer 2012;60(6):905–10.
[88] Maulik PK, Darmstadt GL. Childhood disability in low- and middle-income countries: overview of screening, prevention, services, legislation, and epidemiology. Pediatrics 2007;120(Supplement):S1–55.
[89] Botasso M, Sanches S, Bento R, et al. Teleaudiometry as a screening method in school children. Clinics (Sao Paulo) 2015;70(4):283–8.
[90] Monica SD, Ramkumar V, Krumm M, et al. School entry level tele-hearing screening in a town in South India—lessons learnt. Int J Pediatr Otorhinolaryngol 2017;92:130–5.
[91] Govender SM, Mars M. Assessing the efficacy of asynchronous telehealth-based hearing screening and diagnostic services using automated audiometry in a rural South African school. S Afr J Commun Disord 2018;65(1):e1–9.
[92] Skarzyński PH, Świerniak W, Piłka A, et al. A hearing screening program for children in primary schools in tajikistan: a telemedicine model. Med Sci Monit 2016;22:2424–30.
[93] Samelli AG, Rabelo CM, Sanches SG, et al. Tablet-based hearing screening test. Telemed J E Health 2017;23(9):747–52.
[94] Hussein SY, Swanepoel DW, Mahomed F, et al. Community-based hearing screening for young children using an mHealth service-delivery model. Glob Health Action 2018;11(1):1467077.
[95] Ramkumar V, Nagarajan R, Shankarnarayan VC, et al. Implementation and evaluation of a rural community-based pediatric hearing screening program integrating in-person and tele-diagnostic auditory brainstem response (ABR). BMC Health Serv Res 2019;19(1):1.

[96] Hughes ML, Goehring JL, Baudhuin JL, et al. Use of telehealth for research and clinical measures in cochlear implant recipients: a validation study. J Speech Lang Hear Res 2012;55(4):1112–27.
[97] Summerfelt FF. Teledentistry-assisted affiliated practice dental hygiene. In: Kumar S, editor. Teledentistry. Health informatics. Cham (Switzerland): Springer; 2015. p. 43–52.
[98] Council on Child and Adolescent Health. The role of home-visitation programs in improving health outcomes for children and families. Pediatrics 1998;101(3):486–9.
[99] McKissick HD, Cady RG, Looman WS, et al. The impact of telehealth and care coordination on the number and type of clinical visits for children with medical complexity. J Pediatr Health Care 2017;31(4):452–8.
[100] Notario PM, Gentile E, Amidon M, et al. Home-based telemedicine for children with medical complexity. Telemed J E Health 2019.
[101] Health Care Program for Children in Foster Care, internal planning discussions, 2013-2017. Los Angeles (CA).
[102] Chuck C, Robinson E, Macaraig M, et al. Enhancing management of tuberculosis treatment with video directly observed therapy in New York City. Int J Tuberc Lung Dis 2016;20(5):588–93.
[103] Garfein RS, Liu L, Cuevas-Mota J, et al. Tuberculosis treatment monitoring by video directly observed therapy in 5 health districts, California, USA. Emerg Infect Dis 2018;24(10): 1806–15.
[104] Nguyen TA, Pham MT, Nguyen TL, et al. Video directly observed therapy to support adherence with treatment for tuberculosis in Vietnam: a prospective cohort study. Int J Infect Dis 2017;65:85–9.
[105] Yoost JL, Starcher RW, King-Mallory RA, et al. The use of telehealth to teach reproductive health to female rural high school students. J Pediatr Adolesc Gynecol 2017;30(2): 193–8.
[106] Aicken CR, Sutcliffe LJ, Gibbs J, et al. Using the eSexual Health Clinic to access chlamydia treatment and care via the Internet: a qualitative interview study. Sex Transm Infect 2017;94(4):241–7.
[107] Gomperts RJ, Jelinska K, Davies S, et al. Using telemedicine for termination of pregnancy with mifepristone and misoprostol in settings where there is no access to safe services. BJOG 2008;115(12):1587–8.
[108] Johns NE, Foster DG, Upadhyay UD. Distance traveled for Medicaid-covered abortion care in California. BMC Health Serv Res 2017;17(1):287.
[109] Grossman D, Grindlay K, Buchacker T, et al. Changes in service delivery patterns after launching telemedicine provision of medication abortion in Iowa. Contraception 2010;82(2):205–6.
[110] Fok WK, Mark A. Abortion through telemedicine. Curr Opin Obstet Gynecol 2018;30(6): 394–9.
[111] Gray J, Jones PC, Phillips M, et al. Telematics in the neonatal ICU and beyond: improving care for high-risk newborns and their families. Proceedings: A Conference of the American Medical Informatics Association. AMIA Fall Symposium, Nashville, TN. October 25–29, 1997. p. 413–7.
[112] Wenger TL, Gerdes J, Taub K, et al. Telemedicine for genetic and neurologic evaluation in the neonatal intensive care unit. J Perinatol 2014;34(3):234–40.
[113] Fang JL, Campbell MS, Weaver AL, et al. The impact of telemedicine on the quality of newborn resuscitation: a retrospective study. Resuscitation 2018;125:48–55.
[114] Garingo A, Friedlich P, Chavez T, et al. "Tele-rounding" with a remotely controlled mobile robot in the neonatal intensive care unit. J Telemed Telecare 2015;22(2):132–8.
[115] Bell RC, Yager PH, Clark ME, et al. Telemedicine versus face-to-face evaluations by respiratory therapists of mechanically ventilated neonates and children: a pilot study. Respir Care 2015;61(2):149–54.

[116] Robinson C, Gund A, Sjöqvist B-A, et al. Using telemedicine in the care of newborn infants after discharge from a neonatal intensive care unit reduced the need of hospital visits. Acta Paediatr 2016;105(8):902–9.
[117] Lanssens D, Vandenberk T, Thijs IM, et al. Effectiveness of telemonitoring in obstetrics: scoping review. J Med Internet Res 2017;19(9):e327.
[118] Kim EW, Teague-Ross TJ, Greenfield WW, et al. Telemedicine collaboration improves perinatal regionalization and lowers statewide infant mortality. J Perinatol 2013;33(9): 725–30.
[119] Hadjikoumi I, Ghazavi M, Fallon P, et al. Survey of telephone calls to tertiary paediatric neurology specialist registrars. Arch Dis Child 2007;92(6):561–2.
[120] Breen P, Murphy K, Browne G, et al. Formative evaluation of a telemedicine model for delivering clinical neurophysiology services part I: utility, technical performance and service provider perspective. BMC Med Inform Decis Mak 2010;10(1):48.
[121] Cialone J, Augustine EF, Newhouse N, et al. Quantitative telemedicine ratings in Batten disease: implications for rare disease research. Neurology 2011;77(20):1808–11.
[122] Bahrani K, Singh MB, Bhatia R, et al. Telephonic review for outpatients with epilepsy—a prospective randomized, parallel group study. Seizure 2017;53:55–61.
[123] Lua PL, Neni WS. Feasibility and acceptability of Mobile Epilepsy Educational System (MEES) for people with epilepsy in Malaysia. Telemed J E Health 2012;18(10):777–84.
[124] Diest A, Ramsey R, Aylward B, et al. Adherence to biobehavioral recommendations in pediatric migraine as measured by electronic monitoring: the Adherence in Migraine (AIM) study. Headache 2016;56(7):1137–46.
[125] Douglas MD, Xu J, Heggs A, et al. Assessing telemedicine utilization by using Medicaid claims data. Psychiatr Serv 2017;68(2):173–8.
[126] Gloff NE, Lenoue SR, Novins DK, et al. Telemental health for children and adolescents. Int Rev Psychiatry 2015;27(6):513–24.
[127] Neufeld J, Case R. Walk-in telemental health clinics improve access and efficiency: a 2-year follow-up analysis. Telemed J E Health 2013;19(12):938–41.
[128] Vigerland S, Lenhard F, Bonnert M, et al. Internet-delivered cognitive behavior therapy for children and adolescents: a systematic review and meta-analysis. Clin Psychol Rev 2016;50:1–10.
[129] Wozney L, Huguet A, Bennett K, et al. How do eHealth programs for adolescents with depression work? A realist review of persuasive system design components in internet-based psychological therapies. J Med Internet Res 2017;19(8):e266.
[130] Grist R, Porter J, Stallard P. Mental health mobile apps for preadolescents and adolescents: a systematic review. J Med Internet Res 2017;19(5):e176.
[131] Wiggins LD, Baio J, Rice C. Examination of the time between first evaluation and first autism spectrum diagnosis in a population-based sample. J Dev Behav Pediatr 2006;27(Supplement 2):S79–87.
[132] Nazneen N, Rozga A, Smith CJ, et al. A novel system for supporting autism diagnosis using home videos: iterative development and evaluation of system design. JMIR Mhealth and Uhealth 2015;3(2):e68.
[133] Smith CJ, Rozga A, Matthews N, et al. Investigating the accuracy of a novel telehealth diagnostic approach for autism spectrum disorder. Psychol Assess 2017;29(3):245–52.
[134] Correll CK, Spector LG, Zhang L, et al. Barriers and alternatives to pediatric rheumatology referrals: survey of general pediatricians in the United States. Pediatr Rheumatol Online J 2015;13(1):32.
[135] Riebschleger MP, Tootoo J, Mroczek A, et al. Alternative mechanisms of care delivery in pediatric rheumatology: to what extent do they expand the reach of pediatric rheumatologists? Arthritis Rheumatol 2014;66:S211.
[136] Kessler EA, Sherman AK, Becker ML. Decreasing patient cost and travel time through pediatric rheumatology telemedicine visits. Pediatr Rheumatol Online J 2016;14(1):54.

[137] Bullock DR, Vehe RK, Zhang L, et al. Telemedicine and other care models in pediatric rheumatology: an exploratory study of parents' perceptions of barriers to care and care preferences. Pediatr Rheumatol Online J 2017;15(1):55.
[138] Strickler AS, Palma J, Charris R, et al. Contribution of the use of basic telemedicine tools to the care of children and adolescents with juvenile idiopathic arthritis at the Puerto Montt Hospital, Chile. Rev Chil Pediatr 2018;89(1):59–66.
[139] Consolaro A, Morgan EM, Giancane G, et al. Information technology in paediatric rheumatology. Clin Exp Rheumatol 2016;34(5):S11–6.
[140] Gordon AS, Adamson WC, Devries AR. Virtual visits for acute, nonurgent care: a claims analysis of episode-level utilization. J Med Internet Res 2017;19(2):e35.
[141] Polinski JM, Barker T, Gagliano N, et al. Patients' satisfaction with and preference for telehealth visits. J Gen Intern Med 2015;31(3):269–75.
[142] Martinez KA, Rood M, Jhangiani N, et al. Antibiotic prescribing for respiratory tract infections and encounter length: an observational study of telemedicine. Ann Intern Med 2019;170:275–7.
[143] Martinez KA, Rood M, Jhangiani N, et al. Association between antibiotic prescribing for respiratory tract infections and patient satisfaction in direct-to-consumer telemedicine. JAMA Intern Med 2018;178(11):1558–60.
[144] Ray KN, Shi Z, Gidengil CA, et al. Antibiotic prescribing during pediatric direct-to-consumer telemedicine visits. Pediatrics 2019;143(5).
[145] Uscher-Pines L, Mulcahy A, Cowling D, et al. Access and quality of care in direct-to-consumer telemedicine. Telemed J E Health 2016;22(4):282–7.
[146] Ray KN, Shi Z, Poon SJ, et al. Use of commercial direct-to-consumer telemedicine by children. Acad Pediatr 2019.
[147] Ashwood JS, Mehrotra A, Cowling D, et al. Direct-to-consumer telehealth may increase access to care but does not decrease spending. Health Aff 2017;36(3):485–91.
[148] Conners GP, Kressly SJ, Perrin JM, et al. Nonemergency acute care: when it's not the medical home. Pediatrics 2017;139(5).
[149] Griffiths F, Bryce C, Cave J, et al. Timely digital patient-clinician communication in specialist clinical services for young people: a mixed-methods study (The LYNC Study). J Med Internet Res 2017;19(4):e102.
[150] McConnochie KM, Conners GP, Brayer AF, et al. Effectiveness of telemedicine in replacing in-person evaluation for acute childhood illness in office settings. Telemed J E Health 2006;12(3):308–16.
[151] Raskas MD, Gali K, Schinasi DA, et al. Telemedicine and pediatric urgent care: a vision into the future. Clin Pediatr Emerg Med 2017;18(1):24–31.
[152] Utidjian L, Abramson E. Pediatric telehealth: opportunities and challenges. Pediatr Clin North Am 2016;63(2):367–78.
[153] AAP Section on telehealth care. Available at: https://www.aap.org/en-us/about-the-aap/Sections/Section-on-Telehealth-Care/Pages/SOTC.aspx. Accessed April 8, 2019.
[154] Telehealth care and after hours care. Available at: https://www.aap.org/en-us/professional-resources/practice-transformation/managing-patients/telehealth-care/Pages/telehealth-advocacy-and-policy.aspx. Accessed April 8, 2019.
[155] The IMLC. Available at: https://imlcc.org/. Accessed April 8, 2019.
[156] Guidance on HIPAA & cloud computing. Available at: https://www.hhs.gov/hipaa/for-professionals/special-topics/cloud-computing/index.html. Accessed April 8, 2019.
[157] Agnisarman S, Narasimha S, Chalil Madathil K, et al. Toward a more useable home-based video telemedicine system: a heuristic evaluation of the clinician user interfaces of home-based video telemedicine systems. JMIR Hum Factors 2017;4(2):e11.
[158] Nochomovitz M, Sharma R. Is it time for a new medical specialty? The medical virtualist. JAMA 2018;319(5):437–8.

[159] Chaet D, Clearfield R, Sabin JE, et al. Ethical practice in telehealth and telemedicine. J Gen Intern Med 2017;32(10):1136–40.
[160] Advisory daily briefing: this man was told he didn't have long to live—via video screen, family says. Available at: https://www.advisory.com/daily-briefing/2019/03/12/kaiser-telemedicine. Accessed April 8, 2019.

Advances in Pediatrics 66 (2019) 87–110

ADVANCES IN PEDIATRICS

Health Considerations for Immigrant and Refugee Children

Abigail L.H. Kroening, MD[a,*],
Elizabeth Dawson-Hahn, MD, MPH[b]

[a]Division of Developmental and Behavioral Pediatrics, Golisano Children's Hospital, University of Rochester, 601 Elmwood Avenue Box #671, Rochester, NY 14623, USA; [b]Division of General Pediatrics, University of Washington, 6200 Northeast 74th Street Suite 110, Seattle, WA 98115-81860, USA

Keywords

• Immigrant • Refugee • Children • Health • Development • Behavior • Education • Trauma

Key points

- Immigrant and refugee children are at increased risk for physical, developmental, and behavioral health challenges.
- Health considerations for immigrant and refugee children should be framed within an ecological context that includes considerations of family, community, and sociocultural influences.
- It is important to understand the migration history of an immigrant child (or the history of their family), which provides context for infectious disease screening and exposure risk (including trauma).
- Discussions about child development should occur within a cultural context after building rapport and establishing trust with immigrant parents.
- Immigrant families benefit from support in understanding and navigating complex social, educational, and health care systems.

INTRODUCTION

Imagine you are a child. Imagine being forced to flee your home in the middle of night, bringing with you only what you can carry. Imagine spending your entire life in a large US city, seamlessly navigating between the languages

Disclosure Statement: Dr. Dawson-Hahn is the recipient of the Seattle Children's Center for Diversity and Health Equity Mentored Scholars Award.

*Corresponding author. *E-mail address:* abigail_kroening@urmc.rochester.edu

https://doi.org/10.1016/j.yapd.2019.04.003

and cultures of your home and the greater community. Imagine traveling with strangers, thousands of exhausting miles, on a journey to seek safety. Imagine growing up in a metropolitan suburb, offered opportunities unavailable to your parents in their childhoods.

The experiences of immigrant and refugee children are as individual and diverse as the children themselves. These experiences and these children, however, are not uncommon. One in 4 children in the United States–nearly 18 million children and youth–lives in a family with at least 1 immigrant parent and approximately 90% of these children were born in and are citizens of the United States [1].

The US population includes more immigrants than any other nation worldwide, and there are many reasons why individuals emigrate to this country. Most immigrants live legally within the United States [2]. Many individuals come voluntarily as international migrants, seeking educational or employment opportunities. Due to escalating global conflicts, many come as asylees or refugees, seeking protection after forceful displacement from their countries of origin. Box 1 provides clarifying definitions of migration status. Refugee children are 1 subgroup of immigrant children. As such, this article refers to immigrant and refugee children as "immigrant children" unless distinctly highlighting children of refugee status.

The health considerations of immigrant children are diverse in scope and applicability, depending on a child's specific needs and circumstances. This document offers a broad understanding of these considerations through an ecological framework that places an individual immigrant child's health within the context of family, community, and sociocultural influences and provides a comprehensive overview of pediatric immigrant health, relevant for newly arrived and second-generation US children.

MIGRATION HISTORY

The experience of migration includes social and physical exposures and public health risk factors that can guide initial screening, management, and treatment of recently immigrated children and families. Therefore, it is imperative for providers to incorporate a migration history (Box 2) into the routine collection of a patient's historical data. For example, children may travel through areas that have different patterns of endemic infectious diseases than the country of origin; a family also may have experienced physical abuse or kidnapping during transit, which could influence their physical and psychological health. Other factors that may affect growth and development are the duration of transit time and access to public services, such as education [3]. Health care access preceding entry often has been for acute issues or hospitalization and not for routine preventive care [4].

The location of the child's birth provides information around available prenatal and postnatal health care services, including newborn screening. Globally, approximately one-third of children have a newborn screen [5]. Key conditions identified by newborn screening are congenital hypothyroidism, hemoglobinopathies, and metabolic acid disorders [5], for which early

Box 1: Definitions of migration status

Immigrants: individuals who have left their country of birth (country of origin) to establish residency in a new country (receiving country)

First-generation immigrants: parents and children all born in their country of origin

Second-generation immigrants: children who are born in the United States (US citizens) and have immigrant parents

Refugees: individuals outside of their country who are unable or unwilling to return home because they fear serious harm and are outside the United States when they seek protection

Secondary migration: voluntary movement of refugees to another state different from their initial state of resettlement (this movement may occur before or after public health screening)

Asylees: individuals who fit the definition of a refugee; however, they seek protection at a point of entry or once they are within the United States

Unaccompanied children: individuals under age 18 without legal status in the United States and without a legal guardian in the United States to provide care or physical custody

Unaccompanied refugee minors: refugee children under age 18 years old meeting previous definition of refugees, without a parent or guardian, and living with foster family under the protection of the Office of Refugee Resettlement

Undocumented immigrant children: children without lawful legal status in the United States with or without a guardian in the United States

Special immigrant visa: holders of this visa qualify for legal permanent residence under the US Citizenship and Immigration Services special immigrant program (most recently this includes Afghani and Iraqi families who worked for the US military)

Temporary visitors: children with permission from the government (a visa) to reside in the United States for a specified period of time due to their parents' work or education, visiting family, or tourism

Legal permanent residents: children with a green card; they qualify for many of the programs that children with US citizenship qualify for

Refugees, asylees, unaccompanied children, and unaccompanied refugee minors are required to have some form of public health screening and a civil surgeon examination to continue their lawful permanent resident eligibility process.

identification is critical to early treatment. Some US states allow children to have a newborn screen drawn even outside the traditional neonatal collection window, and providers can contact their state department of health for more information. Alternatively, providers can consider ordering relevant tests to evaluate for conditions routinely identified by newborn screen.

In the authors' experience, it is most helpful to ask about migration history at the first encounter because it guides initial management, it builds rapport in having a shared understanding of the patient's story (path to migration), and it is more challenging to ask later. The questions of the migration history

Box 2: Migration history question guide

Preferred language
Number of years in the United States
Location of birth
Path to the United States
Location lived in during migration
Number of years in migration
Members of the family who traveled during migration
School attendance before and during migration
Health access before and during migration
Overseas presumptive treatment receipt (if refugee, see details in text)
Location of first residence in the United States

can be readily developed into a dot phrase or template within an electronic health record and can serve as a provider prompt for discussion [6].

Eliciting a migration history also clarifies a patient's migration status (see Box 1), which helps determine what screening, presumptive treatment, immunizations, or physical examination may have occurred prior to immigration. Although a patient's migration status category maybe inquired about verbally, it is not recommended to include this documentation in the medical record [7,8]. Exceptions to the recommendation of not documenting migration status in the medical record include conducting medical or psychological affidavits for an asylum case for an attorney [7].

As part of their immigration entry process, immigrants and refugees have a medical evaluation based on technical guidelines written by the Centers for Disease Control and Prevention (CDC) [9]. These technical guidelines focus on inadmissible health conditions–for example, active tuberculosis [9]. The contents of this medical evaluation may serve as 1 data point in piecing together the broader story of a family's migration history and the child's health and growth. The American Academy of Pediatrics (AAP) policy statement on *Providing Care for Immigrant, Migrant, and Border Children* and its accompanying *Immigrant Child Health Toolkit* build on applying the CDC domestic guidelines for caring for refugees [10] to immigrant children more broadly [11]. The AAP recommends that all immigrant children have a comprehensive medical evaluation after immigration and incorporation into a medical home [11]. There is notable heterogeneity in the migration history of immigrant children welcomed into practices. Ongoing research in migration health will inform and refine postimmigration recommendations.

PHYSICAL HEALTH

The recommendations for screening, presumptive treatment, and testing in this section primarily apply to newly immigrated children; however, the history is applicable to all generations of immigrant children.

The World Health Organization (WHO) Alma-Ata agreement was updated approximately 20 years ago to include the provision of primary health care as a human right [12]. Despite this, many individuals around the world remain without routine access to primary care [13]. For children, this may mean that they are under-immunized and that anatomic abnormalities or developmental disabilities go undiagnosed and routine surveillance of growth and development are incomplete. Education about routine preventive health care [4] may be unfamiliar and require explanation for new immigrant families.

Orientation of new immigrant families to a practice and the local health care system can be helpful, including topics, such as the primary care medical home, subspecialty care, urgent and emergent care, and the importance of and right to having professional interpretation (by phone, video, or in person) in a patient's preferred language for all medical encounters [14]. All members of the health care team should maintain awareness about the wide variation in preimmigration health care experiences and in cultural differences and expectations.

Chronic disease

Even though health providers encounter the usual range of chronic diseases in immigrant children, there are a few chronic diseases that are more prevalent and are highlighted in Table 1.

Nutrition

Refugee and immigrant children are affected by both undernutrition and overnutrition, both before and after immigration [15–19]. Undernutrition–including fetal growth restriction, micronutrient deficiencies, wasting, and stunting–contributes to 45% of all child deaths under age 5 [20]. Child overweight and obesity are rising in prevalence globally and are associated with an increased burden of noncommunicable diseases in adulthood [21].

The anthropometric definitions of undernutrition and overnutrition are based on WHO [22] and CDC [23] growth parameters (Table 2). The intergenerational cycle of malnutrition, in which a malnourished mother gives birth to an infant small for gestational age, can increase the likelihood of a child being stunted [24]. Families may not know their child's birth weight or growth trajectory. Applying anthropometric definitions from growth curves requires a clear understanding of a child's age, which may be unknown or inaccurate. An age assessment tool [25] was developed in Australia as a holistic approach to determining a child's age when it is unknown. The age assessment tool includes an oral narrative, developmental and pubertal assessments, and anthropometric measures. Children, regardless of ethnicity, have the potential to achieve similar growth parameters when their nutritional needs are met, according to the Multicentre Reference Growth Study from the WHO [26].

Immigrant and refugee children may experience comorbid micronutrient deficiencies, especially if they have experienced severe acute malnutrition or chronic malnutrition. Common micronutrient deficiencies are described in Table 3, and deficiencies in zinc, vitamin C, and other B vitamins should be considered in other rare scenarios. Based on elicited patient history, the authors

Table 1
Clinical pearls for selected chronic diseases

Chronic Disease	Clinical Pearls
Thyroid disease	• Contributes to abnormalities in child growth [75]. Congenital hypothyroidism leads to intellectual disability [76]. • May be undiagnosed in new immigrant children due to the lack of routine newborn screening in many settings globally [5]. • There is an uneven distribution of iodine throughout the world, which contributes to differences in etiologies in thyroid disease for children coming from different regions [77,78].
Cerebral palsy	• One of the most common causes of childhood physical disability. The overall prevalence of cerebral palsy globally is 2.11 per 1000 live births [79] and has been reported to be higher in some low-income countries (2.9 per 1000 live births) [80]. • Although preterm birth is a leading cause of cerebral palsy in many high-income countries [81], it is not a leading cause of cerebral palsy in low-income countries [80]. • Etiology of cerebral palsy includes brain injuries through the early childhood years and cerebral infections (including cerebral malaria) [80]. • When children establish care in their medical home after immigration with a diagnosis of cerebral palsy, it is prudent to assess whether they have characteristics of other neurologic disorders. In the authors' clinical practices, the authors have met children misdiagnosed with cerebral palsy who had spinal muscular atrophy and other conditions missed because of the limited opportunity for testing and lack of pediatric providers or specialists with familiarity with these conditions. • Children with cerebral palsy may not have had access to physical or occupational therapy or to adaptive equipment prior to immigration.
Sickle cell anemia	• Highly prevalent in global regions with a high burden of malaria. Nigeria, the Democratic Republic of Congo, and India are estimated to represent 57% of the annual cases of sickle cell anemia diagnosed in newborns [82]. • Routine universal screening for sickle cell anemia is not commonplace globally [5,83,84]. • Inquire about a history of multiple transfusions or need for pain medications (due to sickle cell pain crises). • A hemoglobin electrophoresis is a routine component of our tiered screening among children from countries with a high prevalence of sickle cell anemia or with a concerning history [32].
Thalassemias	• Highly prevalent genetic conditions. They are most prevalent in the Mediterranean, Middle East, Indian Peninsula, sub-Saharan Africa, and Southeast Asia [85,86]. • Not routinely screened for in settings without routine newborn screening [5,84]. • Varying degrees of anemia from thalassemia minor to transfusion-dependent and nontransfusion-dependent thalassemia; affected individuals also may experience growth impairment, bone disease, and endocrine abnormalities [85]. • Children with thalassemia are at risk for iron overload due to multiple transfusions, increased intestinal absorption of iron, and ineffective erythropoiesis [85]. • A hemoglobin electrophoresis is a routine component of our tiered screening [32].

(*continued on next page*)

Table 1
continued

Chronic Disease	Clinical Pearls
Glucose-6-phosphate dehydrogenase deficiency	• X-linked enzyme disorder that is more common in low-income countries near the equator [84]. It is more common in highly malaria endemic areas [87]. • May not be diagnosed in a community that does not have routine universal newborn screening [84,86], including in the United States, where it is not screened for in all states [88]. • Glucose-6-phosphate dehydrogenase deficiency places affected individuals at increased risk of hemolysis from insults, including febrile illnesses, fava beans, and certain oxidative drugs (including primaquine) [89,90]. • Immigrant children with a family history of jaundice, splenomegaly, cholelithiasis, anemia, or hemolytic anemia secondary to an infection should be tested for glucose-6-phosphate dehydrogenase with the rapid fluorescent spot test [87].
Rheumatic heart disease	• Found primarily in low-income and middle-income countries. • Sequelae of untreated streptococcal pharyngitis. • The global burden of rheumatic heart disease was found to be 10 per 1000 people in South Asia and central sub-Saharan Africa and 15 per 1000 people in Oceania [91]. • Clinical diagnosis of rheumatic heart disease is based on auscultating a pathologic valvular murmur on physical examination and is associated most often with mitral valve pathology confirmed by echocardiogram [92].

recommend optional and tiered screening for micronutrient deficiencies (other than iron, which should be screened routinely).

Oral health

Children of immigrant status, especially refugee children, may present with significant oral health care needs. Regional differences in dietary practices, natural sources of fluoride-containing drinking water, cultural beliefs/practices, and access to professional care influence a child's risk for dental decay [27]. African children have significantly lower dental caries and fewer untreated caries compared with similarly aged children from Eastern Europe, Asia, and the Middle East [27]. The prevalence of caries in African immigrant children is half that of either white or African American children, although their rate of untreated caries is comparable to that of African American children [28].

Immunizations and infectious diseases

The burden of infectious disease varies widely across geographic regions. Health Profiles [29,30] specific to regions of origin and transit can inform public-health grounded care. Ideally, recommendations for infectious disease screening for immigrant children correlates with a child's countries of origin,

Table 2
Anthropometric definitions of nutritional status categories

Nutritional Status Category	Age <2 Years (World Health Organization Definitions)	Age 2 Years to 18 Years (Centers for Disease Control and Prevention Definitions)
Severe acute malnutrition (severe wasting)	Weight-for-length ≤1st percentile	BMI 1st percentile
Moderate acute malnutrition (moderate wasting)	Weight-for-length ≤2.3rd and >1st percentile	BMI ≤5th percentile and >1st percentile
Healthy	Weight-for-length >2.3rd percentile and <97.7th percentile	BMI >5th percentile and ≤85th percentile
Overweight/obese	Weight-for-length ≥97.7th percentile	BMI >85th percentile
Chronic malnutrition[a] (stunting)	Length-for-age ≤2.3rd percentile	Height-for-age <5th percentile

Abbreviation: BMI, body mass index.

The <1st percentile is equal to a *z* score of −3.00, 2.3rd percentile is equal to *z* score of −2.00, 5th percentile is equal to *z* score of −1.65, 85th percentile is equal to a *z* score of 1.04, 95th percentile is equal to a *z* score of 1.65, and 97.7th percentile is equal to a *z* score of 2.00.

[a]Children classified into the wasting, healthy weight, or overweight/obese categories also could be classified into the height/length-for-age category of stunting.

through transit and departure. In the absence of this information, it is helpful to utilize the best existing evidence (Table 4) [31,32].

Immigrant children applying for a visa overseas or an adjustment of their status to become legal permanent residents are required to provide proof of vaccinations as part of their related medical examination [33]. Those lacking the necessary vaccinations have to receive immunizations based on the Advisory Committee on Immunization Practices (ACIP) recommendations [34]. Immigrant children who do not apply for a visa before entry to the United States may be unimmunized or under-immunized and should have an evaluation of their immunization status when they establish care in a primary care medical home. Refugee children are not required to have immunizations for US entry. The CDC, however, in partnership with the US State Department, began a vaccination program for US-bound refugees in 2013 that starts their ACIP-recommended immunizations prior to US resettlement [34]. Variations in cultural beliefs and immunization requirements for immigration may partially explain different patterns of immunizations across countries of origin [34].

Exposures

War/conflict

Children growing up in settings of war/conflict are at risk for physical and mental health consequences. Physical injuries may include burns, loss of limbs, traumatic brain injury (TBI), and other blast injuries [35]. Depending on regional resources, children may not have access to imaging for injuries,

Table 3
Clinical pearls for selected micronutrient deficiencies

Micronutrient	Clinical pearls
Iron	• Iron deficiency accounts for 50% of anemia globally [93]. • Increased risk of iron deficiency due to food scarcity, parasitic disease, prematurity, and exclusive breastfeeding without intake or iron-fortified foods. • Iron deficiency is associated with impaired neurodevelopmental outcomes [94]. • The authors recommend routine screening with a complete blood cell count and zinc protoporphyrin/heme ratio [95].
Iodine	• Most common preventable cause of cognitive disability globally [78] • Differential access to iodine globally [78] • Iodine deficiency can lead to hypothyroidism or hyperthyroidism [77].
Vitamin A	• Leading cause worldwide of preventable childhood blindness [96] • Associated with an increased risk of mortality from measles and diarrhea • Clinical features include poor night vision, impaired bone growth, impaired immunity. • Most common in southern Asia and sub-Saharan Africa
Vitamin B_{12}	• Causes megaloblastic anemia, peripheral neuropathy, and other neurologic signs • Individuals most at risk are those who consume diet without meat, eggs, and dairy products (the major dietary sources) [97]
Vitamin D	• Increased risk may be due to poor diet quality, prolonged periods of time inside due to concern for safety, higher melanin in the skin, and decreased skin exposure to sunlight due to clothing [98] • Disturbance in vitamin D production, absorption, or metabolism can cause the development of rickets [99]

appropriate assessment for mild-to-moderate TBI, or recommended therapy, such as that to prevent burn-related contractures [36]. The long-term sequelae of TBI include neurocognitive impairment and mood disorders and are particularly important to consider.

Despite the strong stance of the United Nations against chemical weapons [37], their use has been reported most recently in Syria [38]. Exposure to sarin, a nerve toxin, can cause seizures and cholinergic crisis in the short-term or long-term morbidity due to organophosphorus ester-induced delayed neurotoxicity in those who survive [39]. Tear gas, used for crowd and riot control globally and domestically, is associated with lung, cutaneous, and ocular complications in adults [40]. Although the acute and chronic impact on children is unknown, it is reasonable to anticipate that children experience the same or more serious physical health effects, along with potential mental health problems.

Lead

Immigrant children (refugee children, in particular) are at increased risk for elevated blood lead levels due to acute and chronic exposures. Lead absorption also is increased with anemia and malnutrition. Conduits for exposure include

Table 4
Infectious diseases to consider in the care of immigrant children

Infectious Diseases	Clinical Pearls	Routine Screening vs Optional Screening Vs Presumptive Treatment (Screening Test)	Presumptive Treatment[a,c] from Region of Origin or Transit
Soil-transmitted helminths (ascariasis, hookworm, whipworm)	• Infection may be asymptomatic or may have abdominal pain, vomiting, diarrhea, or anemia and fatigue.	Presumptive treatment with albendazole (3 stool ova and parasites)	Asia, Middle East, North Africa, Latin American, Caribbean, sub-Saharan Africa
Strongyloidiasis	• Can persist asymptomatically for decades because it can replicate in a human host. • Patient may have eosinophilia; however, it is neither sensitive nor specific for *Strongyloides* [100] • Hyperinfection syndrome can occur unexpectedly and many years after parasite acquisition in the setting of immunosuppression, including from steroids.	Presumptive treatment with ivermectin (*Strongyloides* IgG)	Asia, Middle East, North Africa, Latin American, Caribbean, sub-Saharan Africa[c]
Schistosomiasis	• Latent disease may persist for up to 25 y [101]. • Patient may have eosinophilia; however, it is neither sensitive nor specific for schistosomiasis [100].	Presumptive treatment with raziquantel[b] (schistosomiasis IgG)	Sub-Saharan Africa
Malaria	• Young children are at greatest risk in highly endemic areas to poor health outcomes. • Immigrants and refugees have arrived with malaria [102].	Presumptive treatment with atovaquone-proguanil or artemether-lumefantrine (rapid diagnostic test or thick and thin smears)	Sub-Saharan Africa
Giardia	• May be asymptomatic or lead to acute symptoms of diarrhea and abdominal pain or chronic symptoms of failure-to thrive, malabsorption, anorexia [32]	Optional (giardia stool antigen)	

Helicobacter pylori	• More than half of the world's population is infected. Prevalence estimates are highest in Central and Western Africa, Central Asia, and South America [103]. • Multigenerational colonization is common [104]. • Presenting symptoms in children may include nausea, regurgitation, vomiting, abdominal pain. • Consider in children with poor appetite or poor growth.	Optional (*H pylori* stool antigen)
Tuberculosis	• Children are more likely to convert latent tuberculosis infection to active disease, particularly in the first year of life [105]. • Children experience higher rates of extrapulmonary disease than adults [106].	Routine (QuantiFERON (if >2 y old) or tuberculin skin test
HIV	• Not universally screened for during pregnancy globally • Children whose mothers have immigrated may be at higher risk [107].	Routine (HIV ELISA [HIV-1 and HIV-2]); if child <18 mo, order HIV polymerase chain reaction)
Syphilis	• Commonly asymptomatic latent infection [108]	Routine if child >13 y old (syphilis enzyme immunoassay)
Hepatitis B	• Chronic disease is asymptomatic. • Testing is recommended even if vaccinated before immigration [109].	Routine (hepatitis B surface antigen)
Hepatitis C	• Screen individuals with concern for high risk: blood transfusion, surgery prior to immigration, tattoo, intravenous drug use, maternal history. • Treatable condition	Optional (hepatitis C antibody)

[a]Presumptive treatment will be done overseas for the majority of immigrant children with refugee status [110]; however, it is unlikely that children with other statuses will have had presumptive treatment. For children who have not had presumptive treatment overseas, their geographic region of origin or travel may warrant presumptive treatment paralleling the CDC guidelines for the care of refugees from similar regions [110]. Recommendations for presumptive treatment are listed by country of origin or residence in transit.

[b]Children coming from neurocystercicosis endemic areas should be ruled out for disease if they have seizures or neurologic deficits before presumptive treatment with praziquantel.

[c]Among children from areas in sub-Saharan Africa with endemicity of *Loa loa* (Angola, Cameroon, Central African Republic, Chad, Republic of Congo, Democratic Republic of Congo, Equatorial Guinea, Gabon, Nigeria, and South Sudan), it is not recommended that they be treated with ivermectin presumptively for *Strongyloides* because it has been associated with encephalopathy in individuals with a high microfilarial load [111]. Children arriving from this region should either have a daytime (10:00 AM to 2:00 PM) Giemsa-stained blood smear or be treated with high-dose albendazole if *Loa loa* cannot be ruled out [111].

traditional medicines, cosmetic products, cookware, in-home use of car batteries as power sources, and leaded gasoline [41,42]. Lead exposure also may occur from exposure to munitions being present in areas where children play. A child's risk for lead exposure is stratified by country of origin and pre-emigration locations [31]. Screening for lead exposure as per CDC guidelines [43] is important because elevated blood lead levels are associated with toxicity, including irreversible neurocognitive and behavioral sequelae.

Female genital cutting

WHO defines female genital cutting (also known as circumcision or mutilation) as a procedure that intentionally alters or causes injury to the female genitalia for nonmedical reasons [44]. At least 200 million children and women have been affected globally and 3 million girls are reported at risk [44]. Female genital cutting is most frequently reported in northern sub-Saharan Africa, the Middle East, and India. Due to the illegality of the procedure in the United States [45], girls sometimes are sent back to their country of origin for vacation cutting. Complications include infection, bleeding, and urinary retention. Longer-term complications include urinary, psychological, dermatologic, fertility, and sexual function–related problems [45].

Violence/exploitation/trafficking

Violence toward immigrant children comes in many forms and risks are pervasive throughout the migration process. Forms of violence include state action (such as migration enforcement or detention), employer (forced child labor), peer-to-peer (bullying and school abuse), familial (domestic violence), the general public (xenophobia), and child smuggling or trafficking [46]. Available data indicate that trafficking affects children worldwide, and 1 in 3 detected victims is a child [47]. Exposure to violence is one of the most predictive risk factors for adverse mental health outcomes in immigrant children.

Xenophobia

Immigrant families experience xenophobia and racism on their path to migration and after immigration. Both xenophobia and racism are social determinants of health, with long-term implications for mental and physical health as well as access to health services [48]. Changes in politics, policy, or global events may increase bullying or harassment [49] and should be considered in supporting an immigrant child's health over the long term.

DEVELOPMENTAL HEALTH

One in 6 children in the United States is reported to have 1 or more developmental delays or disabilities [50]. Although there are no reliable and representative data on the global prevalence of childhood developmental disabilities, research indicates that hundreds of millions of children worldwide are not meeting their developmental potential and may not have access to interventions that could positively alter their developmental trajectories [51,52].

Although they come from widely varying backgrounds, children of immigrant status are at increased risk for developmental delays and disabilities. This risk is influenced by many factors preimmigration and postimmigration (Box 3). Acknowledging a child's migration history (or the migration history of the family) is particularly important. Many children have experienced significant, cumulative stressors and adverse experiences during critical periods of cognitive, language, and social-emotional development. Such toxic stress and trauma increase a child's risk for poor developmental outcomes [53].

It often is challenging to assess the developmental status of an immigrant child. Many cultural communities do not monitor a child's developmental progress or track developmental milestones, as in the United States. The word, *development*, does not even exist in all languages, sometimes making communication of this concept difficult [54].

The AAP highlights the importance of early childhood developmental screening through the use of standardized developmental assessments [55]. Various cultural considerations have an impact on the feasibility and effectiveness of standardized developmental screening for immigrant children. Such considerations include use of translated tools and interpreters, cultural connection/relevance to the questions being asked, a caregiver's foundational literacy or educational status (in their preferred language), and a caregiver's rapport with a child's health care provider. The AAP does not endorse any specific standardized developmental screening tool but does provide a comprehensive database for provider use [56]. Despite the limitations of standardized screening for children of immigrant status, these assessments provide opportunities for structured attention and discussion of developmental status. Increasing conversations around typical and atypical child development may promote increased awareness and identification of developmental concerns within diverse cultural communities.

Although parents/caregivers of immigrant children may not specifically track their child's acquisition of developmental milestones, most are aware of their child's developmental path and whether this path adheres to cultural expectations and is consistent with that of peers or older siblings. Parents of immigrant children, however, may not spontaneously disclose developmental concerns. In

Box 3: Influences on child development

Heredity and genetic considerations (including family history of consanguinity)
Nutritional status
Physical health
Exposures (infections, toxins, trauma)
Family safety and stability
Early childhood learning environment
Educational opportunities
Opportunities for community integration

many cultural communities, having a child with a developmental disability is viewed as a curse on the family, leading to the child and family being ostracized from the larger community. A family thus may choose to withhold concerns because of fear of isolation or of how such disclosure may have an impact on their family's security within the United States, given the increased scrutiny of immigration status.

Many families emigrate from resource-poor settings, believing there is nothing to be done for their child or worrying that identification and disclosure of their child's disability will prevent their child from going to school, as was the custom in their countries of origin and transit. Although some parents understand that they have greater access to developmental or educational interventions in the United States, others may not realize the breadth of supports that their child is now entitled to receive.

Given the increased challenges associated with eliciting and assessing an immigrant child's developmental status, clinical pearls guiding surveillance and screening may be helpful (Table 5). As concerns are identified, a child should be referred to a subspecialist trained in developmental and behavioral pediatrics, neurodevelopmental disabilities, or pediatric physical medicine and rehabilitation for further evaluation. A child under age 3 years can access early intervention services in their state, whereas the home school district is a resource for children over age 3 years.

BEHAVIORAL/MENTAL HEALTH

An immigrant child's behavioral/mental health is also strongly influenced by experiences and exposures. Behaviors provide valuable insight into an immigrant child's overall well-being and family functioning. In younger children, close attention to eating, sleeping, and toileting patterns may reveal underlying psychological stressors. In older children, it often is helpful to elicit additional information about school engagement/performance and peer interactions.

Overall, immigrant children are well adjusted and their behavioral/mental health care should reflect the care provided to all children in the pediatric medical home [32]. The AAP highlights 4 key elements of special consideration in the pediatric immigrant mental health assessment [57]:

1. Screening for trauma and adversities
2. Influence of acculturation
3. Consideration of changing social support structure
4. Resilience

Screening for trauma

Immigrant children may experience trauma at any point in their journey from country of origin to living in the United States. Children of refugee status and children who have been separated from their families (including unaccompanied minors and immigrant children in foster care) are at particular risk for traumatic exposures, as are children who are detained in Department of

Table 5
Clinical pearls for developmental surveillance and screening of refugee children

Build rapport/establish trust.	Maintain continuity of care over several visits. Express empathy.
Ask questions about child development at every visit.	Do not assume that parents will spontaneously disclose concerns; use examples and visual supports when possible.
Appreciate a cultural context.	Offer explanation for the term, development, such as, "the way your child moves, speaks, learns, or behaves." Ask questions about how child development is understood within a parents' community. Ask questions to appreciate parental expectations. Recognize potential societal implication of having a child with a developmental concern.
Designate specific clinical time for screening.	Results are likely to be more informative if providers directly administer screening tools (versus a parent completing independently).
Use an interpreter (in person, when possible).	Translations of screening tools may be helpful if available in preferred languages AND if parents are literate in preferred language.
Explain the roles of early intervention or educational service providers	Many families do not have a cultural context for therapists and special educators. They benefit from support in understanding and navigating early intervention and educational systems.

Homeland Security facilities [57,58]. Immigrant children may face increased risk for targeted discrimination, microaggressions, and bullying within their receiving country (Table 6). Additional complexity arises with multiple identities–such as being an immigrant youth with a disability or an immigrant youth who identifies as lesbian, gay, bisexual, or transgender–and, depending on cultural and community contexts, the intersection of multiple identities may increase a child's or adolescent's risk for adverse experiences. Pediatric providers must remain attentive to this increased risk and offer routine and ongoing surveillance for trauma, with further assessment as necessary. Taking time to establish trust with parents and youth is critical to supporting those with trauma histories. Standardized mental health screening instruments may be useful but only some instruments offer translations, whereas others are available only in English [57]. Skilled medical interpreters can be helpful, but parents or youth may be hesitant to disclose information, especially if the interpreter is a member of their local cultural community.

Influence of acculturation

Understanding the influence of acculturation on a child's mental health requires an appreciation for multigenerational experiences. The mental health stressors of first-generation immigrants are not identical to stressors experienced by second-generation or third-generation immigrants. First-generation immigrants may have more recent trauma related to their migration journeys but be reluctant to disclose experiences due to cultural expectations or fear of deportation. Second-generation children may experience distress associated with persistent poverty, intergenerational conflicts, parental legal status, and societal discrimination. Research indicates that second-generation children demonstrate increased mental health service utilization compared with first-generation immigrant children [57].

Considerations of changing social support structure

The process of migration often leads to loss of familiar support networks, including extended family and community [57]. Within the receiving country, families may experience shifts in traditional roles and expectations, because children often acculturate more quickly than adults to their new home.

Resilience

Several studies have examined risk and protective factors influencing the mental health and resiliency of immigrant children, in particular displaced and refugee children (see Table 6) [59,60]. Healthy families with positive interpersonal connectedness are key to mitigating mental health difficulties. Adaptive responses promote biculturalism and bilingualism with the integration of values from the culture of origin and the receiving culture [57].

Table 6
Risk and protective factors for immigrant child mental health[a]

Risk factors	Protective factors
Individual • Exposure to premigration violence • Exposure to postmigration violence • Female gender	Individual[b] • Temperament (eg, easy going, stress-reactive) • Intellectual functioning/academic achievement • Executive functioning skills (in particular, self-regulation/inhibitory control skills) • Sense of self-efficacy and positive self-concept • Belief in higher power/religiosity or belief that life has meaning
Family • Parental exposure to violence • Parental mental health concerns • Poor financial support • Single-parent household • Unaccompanied by caregiver	Family • High parental support and family cohesion • Positive school experience (self-reported) • Same ethnic origin foster care
Community • Perceived discrimination • Multiple relocations/changes in residence in host country	Community • Support from friends (self-reported)

[a]Specific to displaced refugee children [59].
[b]Children with variety of adverse life experiences [60].

Vicarious trauma/secondary traumatic stress

Providers who work closely with immigrant children and their families, and have opportunities to hear their narratives, are at elevated risk for vicarious trauma. Mindful attention to this risk allows providers to engage in resilience-building strategies, including

1. Psychoeducation: learning the signs and symptoms of secondary traumatic stress
2. Skills training: learning specific tools to prevent or target the signs and symptoms
3. Supervision: connecting with other professionals to share and discuss experiences [61]

EDUCATION

Early childhood education

Research highlights the immediate and long-term benefits of high-quality early childhood education programs (ECEPs) for all children [62]. These programs are particularly valuable for children of immigrant status, given their increased developmental and behavioral risks. ECEPs establish a solid foundation for school readiness through promotion of healthy physical, cognitive, socioemotional, and language development [63,64]. ECEPs also build literacy skills by providing language instruction in the receiving country's majority language. Evidence shows that young immigrant children may benefit even more than their native-born peers from participation in high-quality ECEPs [65] and that participation reduces future disparities (academic, employment, income, and overall health) between these 2 groups [66].

High-quality ECEPs are additionally valuable for their role in supporting integration and inclusion of entire immigrant families. Parents/caregivers are able to build meaningful relationships with community partners who facilitate immigrant parents' understanding and navigation of complex health, social, and educational systems [67].

Given the clear benefits of ECEPs for immigrant children, pediatric providers should remain thoughtful of the barriers that interfere with program access and participation. These barriers are strikingly common to the overall immigrant experience and include lack of awareness of service options, cultural and linguistic barriers, difficulties in finding reliable/affordable transportation, conflicting schedules (with parents' work hours), cost of services/difficulty accessing financial assistance, distrust of providers, and concerns connected to legal status [63]. Addressing these barriers with immigrant families will benefit children and their families through improved care coordination, social cohesion, and self-efficacy.

Elementary and secondary education

All children, regardless of immigration status, have the right to receive a free public education under the US Constitution [68]. The US Department of Education provides clear mandates in support of the successful civic, linguistic, and economic integration of immigrant children and their families [68]. The Department of Education Office of English Language Acquisition guides state policies in supporting English learners (ELs) through dedicated curricula that incorporate languages and cultures of origin, because research does not support a "1 child, 1 language" approach to learning [69]. Even with this focus, however, states and local school districts may struggle to effectively teach Els, and, consequently, immigrant children often lag behind peers in academic achievement [70]. ELs have a national graduation rate of 63% compared with an overall national graduation rate of 82% [70].

As discussed previously, school-aged immigrant children, especially refugee children, commonly experience significant educational disruption prior to emigration. More than 4 million refugee children worldwide currently are not in school, with 500,000 children added to this group in the past year [71]. Educational disruption places immigrant children at an academic disadvantage compared with US peers and creates challenges for educators in understanding the complex interplay of factors contributing to a child's learning differences. Differences may result from limited English proficiency, absent or interrupted educational exposure, developmental disabilities, effects of past traumatic experiences, inadequate EL programs, or any combination of these influences.

Assessing immigrant ELs for language or learning disabilities is challenging. Recommendations from the Individuals with Disabilities Education Act and the American Speech-Language-Hearing Association describe the importance of conducting assessments in a child's preferred language using interpreters and translations, gathering information from a variety of sources, and using alternative assessment procedures–such as dynamic assessment (test-teach-retest) [72]. Evaluation by a developmental subspecialist also can be helpful.

Parents of immigrant children are likely to benefit from support in navigating US educational systems and expectations, particularly if their child receives special education. Parents may need reassurance of their child's school enrollment, because children with disabilities are not uniformly educated worldwide. Parents also are likely to benefit from guidance and support regarding the role they play in their child's education, especially as an advocate, an unfamiliar role for many immigrant families.

SUMMARY

Health considerations for immigrant and refugee children are vast, diverse, and complex. Thoughtful attention to the physical, developmental, educational, and behavioral health of immigrant children demands a broader appreciation for their experiences, exposures, and roles within their families, communities, and society. Supporting immigrant and refugee children requires intentional, interdisciplinary partnerships across social, educational, legal, political, and health care systems [73], with an emphasis on a

2-generation approach: addressing the needs of children is key to the success of their parents and vice versa [74]. Immigrant and refugee children require attention and advocacy.

References

[1] Migration Policy Institute. Children in US immigrant families 2016. Available at: https://www.migrationpolicy.org/programs/data-hub/charts/children-immigrant-families. Accessed December 31, 2018.

[2] Lopez G, Bialik K, Radford J. Key findings about US immigrants 2018. Available at: http://www.pewresearch.org/fact-tank/2018/11/30/key-findings-about-u-s-immigrants/. Accessed December 30, 2018.

[3] Dryden-Peterson S. The educational experiences of children in a country of first asylum. Washington, DC: Migration Policy Institute; 2015.

[4] Hagan JF Jr, Shaw JS, Duncan PM. Bright futures: guidelines for health supervision of infants, children, and adolescents. Elk Grove Village (IL): American Academy of Pediatrics; 2017.

[5] Therrell BL Jr, Padilla CD. Newborn screening in the developing countries. Curr Opin Pediatr 2018;30(6):734–9.

[6] Dawson-Hahn E, Pidaparti V, Ibrahim A, et al. WCAAP: immigrant health toolkit 2018. Available at: http://wcaap.org/wp-content/uploads/2018/09/WCAAP-Immigrant-Health-Toolkit-2.pdf. Accessed December 28, 2018.

[7] Kim G, Sanchez Molina U, Saadi A. Should immigration status information be included in a patient's health record? AMA J Ethics 2019;21(1):8–16.

[8] National Immigration Law Center. Health care providers and immigration enforcement: know your rights, know your patients' rights. 2017. Available at: https://www.nilc.org/issues/immigration-enforcement/healthcare-provider-and-patients-rights-imm-enf/. Accessed January 6, 2019.

[9] The Division of Global Migration and Quaratine, The Centers for Disease Control and Prevention. Medical examination of immigrants and refugees 2014. Available at: https://www.cdc.gov/immigrantrefugeehealth/exams/medical-examination.html. Accessed January 1, 2019.

[10] Division of Global Migration and Quarantine, The Centers for Disease Control and Prevention. Guidelines for the U.S. Domestic medical examination for newly arriving refugees. 2014. Available at: https://www.cdc.gov/immigrantrefugeehealth/guidelines/domestic/domestic-guidelines.html. Accessed January 5, 2019.

[11] Council on Community Pediatrics. Providing care for immigrant, migrant, and border children. Pediatrics 2013;131(6):e2028–34.

[12] World Health Organization. Declaration of Alma Ata 2000. Available at: http://www.who.int/publications/almaata_declaration_en.pdf. Accessed January 5, 2019.

[13] Rao M, Pilot E. The missing link–the role of primary care in global health. Glob Health Action 2014;7:23693.

[14] Chen AH, Youdelman MK, Brooks J. The legal framework for language access in healthcare settings: title VI and beyond. J Gen Intern Med 2007;22(Suppl 2):362–7.

[15] Dawson-Hahn E, Pak-Gorstein S, Matheson J, et al. Growth trajectories of refugee and nonrefugee children in the United States. Pediatrics 2016;6:e20160953.

[16] Dawson-Hahn EE, Pak-Gorstein S, Hoopes AJ, et al. Comparison of the nutritional status of overseas refugee children with low income children in Washington State. PLoS One 2016;11(1):e0147854.

[17] Creighton MJ, Goldman N, Pebley AR, et al. Durational and generational differences in Mexican immigrant obesity: is acculturation the explanation? Soc Sci Med 2012;75(2):300–10.

[18] Oza-Frank R, Cunningham SA. The weight of US residence among immigrants: a systematic review. Obes Rev 2010;11(4):271–80.

[19] Smock L, Nguyen T, Metallinos-Katsaras E, et al. Refugee children's participation in the women, infants, and children supplemental nutrition (WIC) program in Massachusetts, 1998-2010. J Public Health Manag Pract 2019;25(1):69–77.
[20] Black RE, Victora CG, Walker SP, et al. Maternal and child undernutrition and overweight in low-income and middle-income countries. Lancet 2013;382(9890):427–51.
[21] International Food Policy Research Institute. Global nutrition report 2015: actions and accountability to advance nutrition and sustainable development. Washington, DC: International Food Policy Research Institute; 2015.
[22] World Health Organization. WHO child growth standards: length/height-for-age, weight-for-age, weight-for-length, weight-for-height and body mass index-for-age: methods and development. Geneva (Switzerland): World Health Organization; 2006.
[23] Kuczmarski RJ, Ogden CL, Grummer-Strawn LM, et al. CDC growth charts: United States. Adv Data 2000;(314):1–27.
[24] Mosites E, Dawson-Hahn E, Walson J, et al. Piecing together the stunting puzzle: a framework for attributable factors of child stunting. Paediatr Int Child Health 2017;37(3): 158–65.
[25] Sypek SA, Benson J, Spanner KA, et al. A holistic approach to age estimation in refugee children. J Paediatr Child Health 2016;52(6):614–20.
[26] de Onis M, Garza C, Victora CG, et al. The WHO multicentre growth reference study: planning, study design, and methodology. Food Nutr Bull 2004;25(1 Suppl):S15–26.
[27] Quach A, Laemmle-Ruff IL, Polizzi T, et al. Gaps in smiles and services: a cross-sectional study of dental caries in refugee-background children. BMC Oral Health 2015;15:10.
[28] Cote S, Geltman P, Nunn M, et al. Dental caries of refugee children compared with US children. Pediatrics 2004;114(6):e733–40.
[29] The Division of Global Migration and Quarantine, The Centers for Disease Control and Prevention. Refugee health profiles 2018. Available at: https://www.cdc.gov/immigrantrefugeehealth/profiles/index.html. Accessed January 1, 2019.
[30] Ethnomed. Cultures. 2019. Available at: http://ethnomed.org/culture. Accessed January 1, 2019.
[31] Yun K, Matheson J, Payton C, et al. Health profiles of newly arrived refugee children in the United States, 2006-2012. Am J Public Health 2016;106(1):128–35.
[32] The American Academy of Pediatrics, Meneses C, Chilton L, et al. AAP policy statement: providing care for immigrant, migrant, and border children. Pediatrics 2013;131(6): e2028–34.
[33] National Center for Immunization and Respiratory Disease. Vaccines for immigrants and refugees 2018. Available at: https://www.cdc.gov/vaccines/adults/rec-vac/immigrants-refugees.html. Accessed January 7, 2019.
[34] National Center for Immunization and Respiratory Disease. Recommended immunization schedule for children and adolescents aged 18 years or younger, United States, 2018. 2018. Available at: https://www.cdc.gov/vaccines/schedules/hcp/child-adolescent.html#catchup. Accessed January 7, 2019.
[35] Kadir A, Shenoda S, Goldhagen J, et al, Section On International Child Health. The Effects of Armed Conflict on Children. Pediatrics 2018;142(6) [pii:e20182586].
[36] Sarmiento K, Waltzman D, Lumba-Brown A, et al. CDC guideline on mild traumatic brain injury in children: important practice takeaways for sports medicine providers. Clin J Sport Med 2018. [Epub ahead of print].
[37] United Nations Office of Disarmament Affairs. Chemical weapons 2013. Available at: https://www.un.org/disarmament/wmd/chemical/. Accessed January 7, 2019.
[38] Stellström Å. Report of United Nations mission to investigate allegations of the use of chemical weapons in the Syrian Arab Republic on the alleged use of chemical weapons in the Ghouta Area of Damascus on 21 August 2013. 2018. Available at: https://undocs.org/A/67/997. Accessed January 4, 2019.

[39] Abou-Donia MB, Siracuse B, Gupta N, et al. Sarin (GB, O-isopropyl methylphosphonofluoridate) neurotoxicity: critical review. Crit Rev Toxicol 2016;46(10):845–75.
[40] Rothenberg C, Achanta S, Svendsen ER, et al. Tear gas: an epidemiological and mechanistic reassessment. Ann N Y Acad Sci 2016;1378(1):96–107.
[41] Geltman PL, Brown MJ, Cochran J. Lead poisoning among refugee children resettled in Massachusetts, 1995 to 1999. Pediatrics 2001;108(1):158–62.
[42] Mitchell T, Jentes E, Ortega L, et al. Lead poisoning in United States-bound refugee children: Thailand-Burma border, 2009. Pediatrics 2012;129(2):e392–9.
[43] Division of Global Migration and Quarantine, Centers for Disease Control and Prevention. Screening for lead during the domestic medical examination for newly arrived refugees 2013. Available at: https://www.cdc.gov/immigrantrefugeehealth/guidelines/lead-guidelines.html. Accessed January 8, 2019.
[44] World Health Organization. Female genital mutilation 2018. Available at: https://www.who.int/news-room/fact-sheets/detail/female-genital-mutilation. Accessed January 7, 2019.
[45] Hearst AA, Molnar AM. Female genital cutting: an evidence-based approach to clinical management for the primary care physician. Mayo Clin Proc 2013;88(6):618–29.
[46] UNICEF. Uprooted: the growing crisis for refugee and migrant children. New York: UNICEF; 2016.
[47] United Nations Office on Drugs and Crime. Global report on trafficking in persons. New York: United Nations; 2014.
[48] Suleman S, Garber KD, Rutkow L. Xenophobia as a determinant of health: an integrative review. J Public Health Policy 2018;39(4):407–23.
[49] Sirin S, Fine M. Hyphenated selves: muslim american youth negotiating identities on the fault lines of global conflict. Appl Dev Sci 2007;11(3):151–63.
[50] Boyle CA, Boulet S, Schieve LA, et al. Trends in the prevalence of developmental disabilities in US children, 1997-2008. Pediatrics 2011;127(6):1034–42.
[51] Black MM, Walker SP, Fernald LCH, et al. Early childhood development coming of age: science through the life course. Lancet 2017;389(10064):77–90.
[52] World Health Organization. Early childhood development and disability: a discussion paper 2012. Available at: http://apps.who.int/iris/bitstream/handle/10665/75355/9789241504065_eng.pdf;jsessionid=8DE1C1B573E0341F3DD5B226E85DA039?sequence=1. Accessed January 7, 2019.
[53] Shonkoff JP, Garner AS, Committee on Psychosocial Aspects of Child and Family Health, et al. The lifelong effects of early childhood adversity and toxic stress. Pediatrics 2012;129(1):e232–46.
[54] Kroening AL, Moore JA, Welch TR, et al. Developmental screening of refugees: a qualitative study. Pediatrics 2016;138(3):1–11.
[55] Council on Children With Disabilities, Section on Developmental Behavioral Pediatrics, Bright Futures Steering Committee, Medical Home Initiatives for Children With Special Needs Project Advisory Committee. Identifying infants and young children with developmental disorders in the medical home: an algorithm for developmental surveillance and screening. Pediatrics 2006;118(1):405–20.
[56] American Academy of Pediatrics STAR (Screening Technical Assistance and Resource) Center. Screening Time: tuning in to the needs of families 2018. Available at: https://screeningtime.org/star-center/#/screening-tools#top. Accessed December 15, 2018.
[57] American Academy of Pediatrics. Immigrant and child health toolkit, section on mental and emotional health 2013. Available at: https://www.aap.org/en-us/advocacy-and-policy/aap-health-initiatives/Immigrant-Child-Health-Toolkit/Pages/Mental-and-Emotional-Health.aspx. Accessed December 31, 2018.
[58] Linton JM, Griffin M, Shapiro AJ, Council on Community Pediatrics. Detention of Immigrant Children. Pediatrics 2017;139(5) [pii:e20170483].

[59] Fazel M, Reed R, Panter-Brick C, et al. Mental health of displaced and refugee children resettled in high-income countries: risk and protective factors. Lancet 2012;379: 266–82.
[60] Masten AS. Resilience in children threatened by extreme adversity: frameworks for research, practice, and translational synergy. Dev Psychopathol 2011;23(2): 493–506.
[61] National Child Traumatic Stress Network. Secondary traumatic stress 2018. Available at: https://www.nctsn.org/trauma-informed-care/secondary-traumatic-stress/. Accessed January 1, 2019.
[62] Garcia JL, Heckman JJ, Leaf DE, et al. The life-cycle benefits of an influential early childhood program. 2016. Available at: https://heckmanequation.org/www/assets/2017/01/F_Heckman_CBAOnePager_120516.pdf. Accessed December 20, 2018.
[63] Park M, Katsiaficas C, McHugh M. Responding to the ECEC needs of children of refugee and asylum seekers in Europe and North America 2018. Available at: https://www.migrationpolicy.org/research/responding-ecec-needs-children-refugees-asylum-seekers-europe-north-america. Accessed December 27, 2018.
[64] Crosnoe R. Preparing the children of immigrants for early academic success 2013. Available at: www.migrationpolicy.org/research/preparing-children-immigrants-early-academic-success. Accessed December 27, 2018.
[65] Park M. Accessibility of early childhood education and care services in the United States for children of immigrants or diverse origin background paper: transatlantic forum on, inclusive early years meeting. 2013. Available at: www.europe-kbf.eu/~/media/Europe/TFIEY/TFIEY-1_InputPaper/Accessibility-of-ECEC-in-US.pdf. Accessed January 2, 2019.
[66] US Department of Health and Human Services and US Department of Education. Policy Statement on supporting the development of children who are dual language learners in early childhood education programs 2016. Available at: www.acf.hhs.gov/sites/default/files/ecd/dll_policy_statement_final.pdf. Accessed January 1, 2019.
[67] Park M, McHugh M. Immigrant parents and early childhood education programs: addressing barriers of literacy, culture, and systems knowledge 2014. Available at: www.migrationpolicy.org/research/immigrant-parents-early-childhood-programs-barriers. Accessed January 5, 2019.
[68] US Department of Education and US Department of Justice. Educational resources for immigrants, refugees, asylees, and other new Americans 2014. Available at: https://www2.ed.gov/about/overview/focus/immigration-resources.html. Accessed January 6, 2019.
[69] Byers-Heinlein K, Lew-Williams C. Bilingualism in the early years: what the science says. Learn Landsc 2013;7(1):95–112.
[70] Sanchez C. English language learners: how your state is doing 2017. Available at: https://www.npr.org/sections/ed/2017/02/23/512451228/5-million-english-language-learners-a-vast-pool-of-talent-at-risk. Accessed January 8, 2019.
[71] United Nations High Commissioner for Refugees (UNHCR). Turn the tide: refugee education in crisis 2018. Available at: https://www.unhcr.org/news/latest/2018/8/5b86342b4/four-million-refugee-children-schooling-unhcr-report.html. Accessed December 18, 2018.
[72] Caesar LG, Kohler PD. The state of school-based bilingual assessment: actual practice versus recommended guidelines. Lang Speech Hear Serv Sch 2007;38(3):190–200.
[73] McNeely CA, Morland L. The Health of the Newest Americans: How US public health systems can support Syrian refugees. Am J Public Health 2016;106(1):13–5.
[74] Greenberg M, Gelatt J, Bolter J, et al. Promoting Refugee Integration in Challenging Times: the potential of two-generation strategies. 2018. Available at: https://www.migrationpolicy.org/research/refugee-integration-two-generation-strategies. Accessed January 6, 2019.
[75] Homan GJ. Failure to thrive: a practical guide. Am Fam Physician 2016;94(4):295–9.

[76] New England Congenital Hypothyroidism Collaborative. Effects of neonatal screening for hypothyroidism: prevention of mental retardation by treatment before clinical manifestations. Lancet 1981;381(8255):1095–8.
[77] Taylor PN, Albrecht D, Scholz A, et al. Global epidemiology of hyperthyroidism and hypothyroidism. Nat Rev Endocrinol 2018;14(5):301–16.
[78] Iodine Global Network. Iodine global network - annual report 2017. Seattle (WA): Iodine Global Network; 2017.
[79] Oskoui M, Coutinho F, Dykeman J, et al. An update on the prevalence of cerebral palsy: a systematic review and meta-analysis. Dev Med Child Neurol 2013;55(6):509–19.
[80] Kakooza-Mwesige A, Andrews C, Peterson S, et al. Prevalence of cerebral palsy in Uganda: a population-based study. Lancet Glob Health 2017;5(12):e1275–82.
[81] Van Naarden Braun K, Doernberg N, Schieve L, et al. Birth prevalence of cerebral palsy: a population-based study. Pediatrics 2016;137(1):1–9.
[82] Piel FB, Hay SI, Gupta S, et al. Global burden of sickle cell anaemia in children under five, 2010-2050: modelling based on demographics, excess mortality, and interventions. PLoS Med 2013;10(7):e1001484.
[83] Odame I. Developing a global agenda for sickle cell disease: report of an international symposium and workshop in Cotonou, Republic of Benin. Am J Prev Med 2010;38(4 Suppl):S571–5.
[84] Verma IC, Puri RD. Global burden of genetic disease and the role of genetic screening. Semin Fetal Neonatal Med 2015;20(5):354–63.
[85] Amid A, Saliba AN, Taher AT, et al. Thalassaemia in children: from quality of care to quality of life. Arch Dis Child 2015;100(11):1051–7.
[86] Suchdev PS, Ruth LJ, Earley M, et al. The burden and consequences of inherited blood disorders among young children in western Kenya. Matern Child Nutr 2014;10(1):135–44.
[87] Frank JE. Diagnosis and management of G6PD deficiency. Am Fam Physician 2005;72(7): 1277–82.
[88] Watchko JF, Kaplan M, Stark AR, et al. Should we screen newborns for glucose-6-phosphate dehydrogenase deficiency in the United States? J Perinatol 2013;33(7): 499–504.
[89] Spring R, Schlaack H, Rice M, et al. Glucose-6-phosphate dehydrogenase deficiency in internationally adopted children. Pediatr Blood Cancer 2018;65(5):e26990.
[90] Beutler E. G6PD deficiency. Blood 1994;84(11):3613–36.
[91] Watkins DA, Johnson CO, Colquhoun SM, et al. Global, Regional, and National Burden of Rheumatic Heart Disease, 1990-2015. N Engl J Med 2017;377(8):713–22.
[92] Marijon E, Mirabel M, Celermajer DS, et al. Rheumatic heart disease. Lancet 2012;379(9819):953–64.
[93] Lopez A, Cacoub P, Macdougall IC, et al. Iron deficiency anaemia. Lancet 2016;387(10021):907–16.
[94] Siu AL, US Preventive Services Task Force. Screening for iron deficiency anemia in young children: USPSTF recommendation statement. Pediatrics 2015;136(4):746–52.
[95] Rettmer RL, Carlson TH, Origenes ML, et al. Zinc protoporphyrin/heme ratio for diagnosis of preanemic iron deficiency. Pediatrics 1999;104(3):e37.
[96] Stevens GA, Bennett JE, Hennocq Q, et al. Trends and mortality effects of vitamin A deficiency in children in 138 low-income and middle-income countries between 1991 and 2013: a pooled analysis of population-based surveys. Lancet Glob Health 2015;3(9): e528–36.
[97] The Centers for Disease Control and Prevention. Vitamin B12 deficiency in resettled Bhutanese refugees, United States 2008–2011. MMWR Morb Mortal Wkly Rep 2011;60: 343–6.
[98] Hintzpeter B, Scheidt-Nave C, Muller MJ, et al. Higher prevalence of vitamin D deficiency is associated with immigrant background among children and adolescents in Germany. J Nutr 2008;138(8):1482–90.

[99] Nield LS, Mahajan P, Joshi A, et al. Rickets: not a disease of the past. Am Fam Physician 2006;74(4):619–26.
[100] Dawson-Hahn EE, Greenberg SL, Domachowske JB, et al. Eosinophilia and the seroprevalence of schistosomiasis and strongyloidiasis in newly arrived pediatric refugees: an examination of Centers for Disease Control and Prevention screening guidelines. J Pediatr 2010;156(6):1016–8.e1.
[101] Division of Global Migration and Quarantine, Centers for Disease Control and Prevention. Presumptive treatment and screening for strongyloidiasis, schistosomiasis and infections caused by soil-transmitted helminths for refugees. 2013. Available at: https://www.cdc.gov/immigrantrefugeehealth/guidelines/domestic/intestinal-parasites-domestic.html. Accessed January 6, 2019.
[102] Division of Global Migration and Quarantine, The Centers for Disease Control and Prevention. Malaria: domestic guidelines. 2012. Available at: https://www.cdc.gov/immigrantrefugeehealth/guidelines/domestic/malaria-guidelines-domestic.html. Accessed January 6, 2019.
[103] Hooi JKY, Lai WY, Ng WK, et al. Global prevalence of helicobacter pylori infection: systematic review and meta-analysis. Gastroenterology 2017;153(2):420–9.
[104] Iwanczak BM, Buchner AM, Iwanczak F. Clinical differences of Helicobacter pylori infection in children. Adv Clin Exp Med 2017;26(7):1131–6.
[105] Cruz AT, Stark JR. Pediatric tuberculosis. Pediatr Rev 2010;31(1).
[106] Division of Global Migration and Quarantine, The Centers for Disease Control and Prevention. Guidelines for screening for tuberculosis infection and disease during the domestic medical examination for newly arrived refugees. 2010. Available at: https://www.cdc.gov/immigrantrefugeehealth/guidelines/domestic/tuberculosis-guidelines.html. Accessed January 6, 2019.
[107] MacPherson DW, Zencovich M, Gushulak BD. Emerging pediatric HIV epidemic related to migration. Emerg Infect Dis 2006;12(4):612–7.
[108] Division of Global Migration and Quarantine, The Centers for Disease Control and Prevention. Clinical presentations and diagnostic testing for specific STDs. 2017. Available at: https://www.cdc.gov/immigrantrefugeehealth/guidelines/domestic/sexually-transmitted-diseases/syphilis.html. Accessed January 6, 2019.
[109] Division of Global Migration and Quarantine, The Centers for Disease Control and Prevention. Screening for hepatitis during the domestic medical examination. 2014. Available at: https://www.cdc.gov/immigrantrefugeehealth/guidelines/domestic/hepatitis-screening-guidelines.html. Accessed January 6, 2019.
[110] Division of Global Migration and Quarantine, Centers for Disease Control and Prevention. Treatment schedules for presumptive treatment of infections. 2017. Available at: https://www.cdc.gov/immigrantrefugeehealth/guidelines/overseas/interventions/interventions.html. Accessed January 2, 2019.
[111] Division of Global Migration and Quarantine, The Centers for Disease Control and Prevention. Guidelines for overseas presumptive treatment of strongyloidiasis, schistosomiasis, and soil-transmitted helminth infections. 2018. Available at: https://www.cdc.gov/immigrantrefugeehealth/guidelines/overseas/intestinal-parasites-overseas.html. Accessed January 6, 2019.

Advances in Pediatrics 66 (2019) 111–122

ADVANCES IN PEDIATRICS

The Essentials of Essential Oils

Rebecca M. Plant, MD*, Lisa Dinh, MD,
Shaara Argo, MD, Monica Shah, MD

University of South Florida, 2 Tampa General Circle, 5th Floor, Tampa, FL 33606, USA

Keywords

• Essential oils • Aromatics • Pediatrics • Aromatherapy • Peppermint • Neonate

Key points

- Essential oils have been used for centuries as medicine and are now much more readily available and inappropriately advertised for the treatment of specific diseases.
- There is very little reliable evidence in favor of using essential oils in pediatrics, except for peppermint in the treatment of irritable bowel syndrome and a combination of tea tree oil and iodine for molluscum contagiosum.
- With the increased access to essential oils, there have been more cases of toxic exposures to children.

INTRODUCTION

Essential oils (EOs) are the basic components of aromatherapy, with records of their use in the practice of herbal medicine dating from 4500 BC. The composition and potency of each EO can vary depending on the part of the plant from which they are extracted. EOs are a mixture of hydrocarbons, terpenes, phenols, and aldehydes; 1 oil can contain 80 to 300 different hydrocarbons [1]. Historically, EOs have been used in a variety of applications including perfumes, food flavorings, aromatics, paints, cleaners, and medications. Many studies have reported mechanisms of action with clinical effects of specific EOs described herein. However, data are limited and most evidence is not high quality.

MANUFACTURING AND MARKETING

Manufacturers of EOs distill the hydrocarbon components from the desired part of the plant. Thus, the word "essential" refers to the essence of the plant

Disclosure Statement: The authors have nothing to disclose.

*Corresponding author. *E-mail address:* rplant@health.usf.edu

https://doi.org/10.1016/j.yapd.2019.03.005

that is distilled, instead of an invaluable active ingredient. Manufacturers describe their products as ranging from cosmetic grade C, food grade B, to therapeutic grade A. However, there is no regulatory body that determines these quality standards; the determinations are made by each manufacturer [1]. Although many companies conduct testing, safety, and treatment studies on their EOs, the studies are designed and funded by the companies themselves, which introduces bias and questions regarding validity.

Numerous brands are available for consumer purchase including doTERRA, Plant Therapy, Young Living, and Rocky Mountain Oils. Most of these companies function with a multilevel marketing system with no store, and products only available through an approved member. Although multilevel marketing is a legitimate sales model, multilevel marketing sales people are motivated by commissions, which can lead to overzealous marketing.

THE LAW

EOs are covered by the Dietary Supplement Health and Education Act of 1994. Thus, they are not regulated by the US Food and Drug Administration and do not have any other government agency oversight. Although the act specified that companies cannot "claim to treat, prevent, cure, mitigate, or diagnose disease," many EO manufacturers violate this act with claims on their websites. Manufacturers are allowed to make claims of "structure or functional help," such as their product "improves prostate health" or "maintains a healthy immune system."

Critically, they are not required to show safety or to report adverse events. It is the responsibility of the by the US Food and Drug Administration to prove the product is unsafe, thereby enabling the removal of products from market. With companies growing at a remarkable rate, this task is challenging.

OILS MOST COMMONLY USED (BOX 1)

Clove oil

Historically, clove oil has been combined with zinc for use as a tooth sealant and an analgesic; 60% to 90% of the content is eugenol, which is the active ingredient [1,2]. Eugenol works by blocking certain ion channels and inhibiting prostaglandin synthetase, which contributes to its antiinflammatory effects. Its

Box 1: Most commonly used EOs

Clove
Eucalyptus
Lavender
Nutmeg
Peppermint
Tea Tree

effects are similar to benzocaine. For these reasons, it is used as a skin anesthetic [1].

Thomassen and colleagues [3] reported in 1991 that clove oil can deplete glutathione, resulting in hepatotoxicity in rats. Toxic effects from human ingestion are altered mental status, increased anion gap resulting in a metabolic acidosis, coagulopathy, and hypoglycemia. Common reactions include contact dermatitis, skin irritation, and allergic reaction [1].

Eucalyptus oil

Eucalyptus oil is historically and currently used to treat the common cold. It reduces mucous secretions by inhibiting tumor necrosis factor-α and IL-1β and it decreases tracheal muscle contractions by potentiating acetylcholine. The oil inhibits potassium-induced contraction of airway smooth muscle, thereby enabling it to act as a myorelaxant [1]. These actions could be beneficial to patients with asthma or chronic obstructive pulmonary disease.

There are case reports of altered mental status, slurring of speech, nausea, vomiting, and seizures or coma when the oil is used topically in excess or ingested owing to its rapid absorption through the gastrointestinal (GI) tract. One teaspoon is toxic in children when ingested; however, inhaled or topical exposure is rarely toxic [1].

Lavender oil

Lavender oil has multiple uses: as a mood enhancer, anxiolytic, pain control, insect repellant, and for its antimicrobial effects. In vitro and in vivo studies in rats found that lavender oil inhibits mast cell degranulation and histamine release. One of the added benefits includes the ability to inhibit prostaglandins and leukotrienes. These analgesic and antiinflammatory properties support lavender oil as a possible therapeutic agent [4]. There is also evidence that it has antimicrobial activity against methicillin-resistant *Staphylococcus aureus*, vancomycin-resistant enterococcus, and other bacteria [1].

However, lavender oil is rapidly absorbed through the skin and commonly causes a contact dermatitis [5]. It also has dose-dependent estrogenic and antiandrogenic effects. A well-documented side effect is gynecomastia [6].

Nutmeg oil

During the Middle Ages, nutmeg was used as a digestive aid and to treat cholera and rheumatic disease. However, the scarlet-colored aril around the seed was used as an abortifacient. Unfortunately, it was often toxic to the mother as well as her unborn infant. Historically it has also been used as a natural high, providing the feeling of giddiness, detachment, or impending doom. Currently, mace spray is made from the aril [1].

Myristicin is currently being investigated as the possible psychoactive component of the oil; otherwise, the pathophysiology of nutmeg is largely unknown [1]. Side effects include tachycardia, reflexive bradycardia, nausea, vomiting, delirium, and dry mouth [1,7].

Peppermint oil

Peppermint oil is used for oral care, candy, cosmetics, and beverages. It is also used to treat upper respiratory infections, itching, inflammatory bowel syndrome, and as an anesthetic. Menthol is the main component, making up 29% to 48% of the oil [8].

Menthol acts as a smooth muscle relaxant through its actions on ion channels. At temperatures of 46° to 82°F, peppermint oil stimulates the calcium channels providing a warming sensation. Its action on sodium channels causes analgesia. By these mechanisms, it decreases peristalsis within the GI tract and alleviates symptoms of rhinitis. However, prolonged use can cause a reflexive increase in congestion [1]. Other properties of menthol include stimulating bile flow and helping relieve gas through burping or flatulence [8].

Although this oil is rapidly absorbed through the skin and GI tract, it is rarely toxic. Side effects include abdominal pain, hypersensitivity, rash, muscle tremor, and bradycardia. Menthol relaxes the lower esophageal sphincter, which worsens gastroesophageal reflux [8]. The dermatitis and hypersensitivity primarily result from topical use. It is speculated that neonates with glucose-6-phosphate deficiency cannot conjugate menthol, resulting in worsened jaundice [9].

Tea tree oil

Australian Aborigines inhaled crushed tea tree leaves in their hands to treat colds and applied tea tree poultices to wounds for its antimicrobial effects. There are also stories of "healing lakes," where tea tree leaves had fallen and steeped [1].

Investigations in the 1920s found the oil to be bactericidal and antiinflammatory. Later studies showed its specific lipophilic hydrocarbon disrupts lysosomal membranes, resulting in lysis in a hypertonic medium. It also inhibits tumor necrosis factor-α, IL-1α, IL-10, and prostaglandin E. There is speculation that it may function as a topical antiseptic and an in vitro bactericidal agent for staphylococcal and *Escherichia coli* species [1].

Tea tree oil is very allergenic, and its adverse effects include skin irritation. Repeated exposure can cause gynecomastia, and ingestion can cause altered mental status, ataxia, and slurred speech within 30 minutes [1].

OILS THAT ARE HIGHLY DANGEROUS TO CHILDREN (BOX 2)

Camphor Oil

Camphor oil is an abortifacient, a contraceptive, and a lactation suppressant. It has also been used as a cold remedy, antidiarrheal agent, and antiseptic. In the

Box 2: Most dangerous EOs

Camphor

Oil of wintergreen

19th and 20th centuries, this oil was used as a cardiac stimulant in patients with chronic heart failure during flu epidemics [1].

It is rapidly absorbed through the GI tract, skin, and mucous membranes, and can also cross the placenta and blood–brain barrier [1]. The name is similar to castor oil, which is purported to help induce labor; camphor and castor oil have been confused before with the mother accidently ingesting camphor oil causing serious injury to her and her unborn child. Toxicity occurs 5 to 90 minutes after ingestion, with nausea, vomiting, vertigo, headache, altered mental status, seizures, and hepatotoxicity. Symptoms can also occur from other exposures such as inhalation and dermal application [1,10]. One tablespoon can be fatal in children if ingested [1].

Oil of Wintergreen

Touted to help with rheumatism, inflammation, myalgias, and upper respiratory infections, wintergreen oil is another highly dangerous EO. With its minty smell and taste, it carries a high risk of accidental ingestion by children. It is rapidly absorbed by the GI tract and skin with 12% to 20% transdermal absorption within 10 hours. Quicker absorption occurs if heat is applied or if the skin is inflamed, broken, or an occlusive dressing is applied.

Wintergreen oil is metabolized by CYP450 which converts it to salicylic acid. This conversion can cause aspirin toxicity, with 1 teaspoon of ingested oil being the equivalent of 7 g of aspirin. Transdermal application has caused deaths in children [11]. Signs of toxicity with this oil are similar to salicylate toxicity: nausea, vomiting, tinnitus, fever, hyperpnea, and tachypnea [1].

TREATMENT AND LABORATORY TESTS

Measurement of EO levels in the blood of patients with suspected toxicity is generally not available or useful. Blood samples are sent to outside laboratories that take a long time to return results, so they are not generally used to guide treatment. Treatment usually is supportive, with laboratory measurements made as needed. Local poison control centers should be contacted immediately for specific treatments and if any further specific monitoring for the patient is needed.

THE EVIDENCE OF EFFICACY

As described elsewhere in this article, limited data exist on the pharmacology and therapeutic effects of EOs. The few extant randomized, controlled studies are described.

Evidence for anxiolysis

A double-blind, placebo-controlled, randomized study was done by Ndao and colleagues [12] in 2012 to evaluate the effects of inhalation of bergamot EO on the anxiety, nausea, and pain of 37 patients ages 5 to 21 years old undergoing stem cell transfusion; the parents were also included [13,14]. The placebo was a scented shampoo that did not contain EOs.

Children were assessed before infusion, at infusion completion, and 1 hour after infusion using validated anxiety, pain, and nausea scales (Spielberger State-Trait Anxiety Inventory, Children's Behavioral Style Scale, visual analogue scale, and the Emotionality Activity Sociability and Impulsivity instrument). Parents were assessed with the Spielberger State-Trait Anxiety Inventory for parents before, during, and after the infusion as well. The children were randomized into 2 groups: 20 into the placebo group and 17 into the experimental group controlling for age, transplant type, and amount of dimethyl sulfoxide in grafts. Dimethyl sulfoxide is added to stem cells as a cryoprotectant and has been associated with nausea and vomiting owing to its unpleasant odor [15].

The investigators concluded that bergamot EO did not significantly reduce transitory anxiety and may have contributed to persistent anxiety after transfusion, with children in the treatment group experiencing greater anxiety 1 hour after the transfusion ($P = .05$). In the treatment group, reported pain was higher at baseline ($P = .04$), but it decreased in both groups and was not significantly different 1 hour after the infusion.

Nausea was significantly greater in patients in the treatment group upon completion of transfusion ($P \leq .01$) and 1 hour after the transfusion ($P = .03$). Parental anxiety declined in both groups; however, the difference between groups was not significant. This study indicates that there is no benefit of aromatherapy with bergamot EO for decreasing anxiety, nausea, or pain in children receiving stem cell infusions, and in their parents.

Nord and Belew (2009) [7] conducted a single-blinded, randomized, controlled, prospective clinical trial to determine the effectiveness of combined aromatherapy with lavender and ginger EOs in lessening postoperative distress in children. Forty-eight children (from <1 to 21 years old) were assigned to aromatherapy with lavender and ginger EOs, and 46 were assigned to placebo, which was aromatherapy with jojoba EO, which has no known effects and a light scent.

All children received standard care in addition to EO inhalation (EO on cotton ball taped on the subject's hospital gown) and topical administration (EO placed over a pulse point and covered with a nonocclusive adhesive bandage). Parents completed the Faces, Legs, Activity, Cry, Consolability tool as a measure of pain and distress before anesthesia was administered and after surgery when they were reunited with their children. Parent satisfaction was assessed by asking, "In your opinion, do you think the aromatherapy enhanced the patient's overall comfort?", "Would you choose to use aromatherapy for future health care comfort measures?", and additional open-ended comments were encouraged.

The distress scales after surgery were lower for the children in the lavender/ginger EO group, although the difference was not statistically significant. There were no differences between the 2 groups in parental responses to questions. However, more than 78% of the parents in both groups stated that they would choose to use aromatherapy interventions in the future.

Nord and Belew (2009) [7] identified several limitations: parents who agreed to participate were likely biased in their beliefs about EOs and were more accepting of the treatment than the general population; parental bias may have influenced the Legs, Activity, Cry, Consolability scores; and variations in length of surgery case (and therefore length of EO exposure) was not controlled for; and jojoba oil was not a valid placebo because its effects have not been well-investigated.

Evidence for pain control

Soltani and colleagues (2013) [16] evaluated the effect of aromatherapy on pain in children in a single-blinded, randomized, controlled, prospective clinical trial. The investigators measured the effect of lavender EO on posttonsillectomy pain [5].

Forty-eight posttonsillectomy patients (ages 6–12 years old) were randomly assigned to a treatment or a control group. After surgery, all patients received acetaminophen as needed to relieve pain. The treatment group also inhaled lavender EO every 6 hours (4 droplets were rubbed on their palms and patients were instructed to inhale it for 3 minutes). The frequencies of acetaminophen use, nocturnal awakening owing to pain, and pain intensity (measured via visual analogue scale) were documented for 3 days after surgery. The control group received the acetaminophen only.

The treatment group required significantly less acetaminophen on all 3 postoperative days ($P < .05$), but there were no significant differences between groups in pain intensity and frequency of nocturnal awakening. The investigators concluded that aromatherapy with lavender EO can decrease analgesics usage after tonsillectomy in children. However, the study had major limitations, including the small sample size, the lack of a placebo in the control group, the lack of double-blinding, and the lack of control for the size of drop used.

Evidence for molluscum contagiosum

Markum and Baillie (2012) [17] conducted a double-blinded, randomized, controlled, prospective trial to compare the effectiveness of topical application of EOs: (1) tea tree oil, (2) a combination of tea tree oil and organically bound iodine, and (3) iodine alone (as the control) for the treatment of molluscum contagiosum in children. Tea tree oil and iodine are both known as topical antiseptics [18,19].

Fifty-three children (mean age, 6.3 ± 5.1 years) diagnosed with molluscum contagiosum were randomized to receive 1 of the 3 treatments. Children or their parents were instructed to apply their assigned treatment topically to the affected area twice daily and the results were documented after 30 days of treatment. Successful treatment was defined as more than a 90% decrease in the number of lesions. Forty-eight children completed the study.

The treatment was successful in 16 of 19 children treated with a combination of tea tree oil and iodine, 3 of 16 children treated with tea tree oil alone, and 1 of 18 treated with iodine alone. Two children treated with iodine only had worsening of lesions. Side effects were limited and included 4 cases of a mild, noninfectious erythema around the base of lesions, and included children from all 3 therapy groups.

The investigators concluded that the combination of tea tree oil and organically bound iodine is a safe and effective treatment for molluscum contagiosum in children. The response within 30 days is a therapeutic improvement given that molluscum contagiosum typically requires 12 to 30 months to resolve spontaneously, and can require tissue destruction for treatment (curettage, cryotherapy, laser, topical caustics, etc).

The mechanism by which tea tree oil and iodine worked synergistically is unclear, but the authors proposed that it could be due to the lipophilic properties of tea tree oil allowing further penetration of the iodine into skin. A major limitation of the study is that the length of infection before treatment was not specified.

Evidence for treatment of lice

Greive and Barnes (2017) [19] conducted an assessor-blinded, randomized, multicenter, controlled, prospective clinical trial in Australia to compare the safety and efficacy of a head lice treatment containing Australian eucalyptus oil and *Leptospermum petersonii* (lemon-scented tea tree) oil versus pyrethrins and piperonyl butoxide in children [19]. Ninety-seven children (ages 6 months to 11 years old) were randomized to have 1 of the 2 treatments applied per manufacturer instructions: MOOV Head Lice Solution (eucalyptus oil and *L petersonii*) which was applied 3 times with 1 week between applications (at days 0, 7, and 14); Banlice Mousse (pyrethrins and piperonyl butoxide), which was applied twice with 1 week between applications (at days 0 and 7). Banlice Mousse is a leading product for treating head lice in Australia, but contains a neurotoxin. Effective treatment was defined as the absence of live lice, adults, or nymphs identified by wet combing 1 week after the final treatment.

The results were statistically significant with 83% versus 36% cure rates in the eucalyptus oil and *L petersonii* group and pyrethrins and piperonyl butoxide group, respectively. As a secondary measure, the investigators immersed eggs for 10 seconds in the eucalyptus oil and *L petersonii* solution or water and monitored hatch rates. No body louse eggs hatched after 10 days immersion in the eucalyptus oil and *L petersonii* solution, whereas 24%, 76%, 92% and 92% of eggs hatched after 7, 8, 9 and 10 days, respectively, after immersion in water.

The investigators concluded that the eucalyptus oil and *L petersonii* solution was safe, effective, and superior to the pyrethrins and piperonyl butoxide. A major limitation was that the eucalyptus oil and *L petersonii* solution was applied 3 times, whereas the pyrethrins and piperonyl butoxide was only applied 2 times.

Evidence for apnea in premature infants

Edraki and colleagues (2013) [20] conducted a randomized, controlled, prospective clinical trial to study the efficacy of olfactory stimulation by vanillin in preventing apnea in premature newborns, a concept first proposed by Marlier and colleagues [21]). The proposed mechanism is passage of vanillin through the nasal mucosa and into the brain, where it reportedly affects the respiratory center [21]. Thirty-six newborns were randomized into experimental and control groups. The experimental group received olfactory stimulation by saturated vanillin solution, which was placed on a cotton ball in the newborn's incubator, with no skin contact. The control group received no interventions. Apnea, arterial blood oxygen saturation, and heart rate were continuously monitored for 5 days.

The experimental group had a statistically significant decrease in the number of apnea episodes ($P = .001$) and a 3.1-fold decrease in apnea compared with the control group. The authors suggested that the vanillin decreased newborn distress, which subsequently prevented apnea related to stress, and they recommended its use. A major limitation of the study was the lack of controls to determine if the vanillin or olfactory stimulation alone produced the results.

Evidence for irritable bowel syndrome

Peppermint oil is used to treat a variety of ailments, including headaches, muscle pain, and abdominal distress. Most studies regarding the efficacy of peppermint oil in alleviating abdominal symptoms have been done in adults. Pittler and Ernst (1998) [22] conducted a critical review and metaanalysis on adult studies that used peppermint oil to treat irritable bowel syndrome; of the 8 studies that met criteria, 5 were double-blind, placebo-controlled, randomized clinical trials. Their analyses revealed "a significant ($P < .001$) global improvement of irritable bowel syndrome symptoms in patients treated with peppermint oil compared with placebo." However, the authors identified many limitations, including a lack of consistent diagnostic criteria, publication bias, length of treatment, and carry-over effects (only 1 trial had a washout period). Because of these limitations, the authors concluded that it is still not clear if peppermint oil alleviates symptoms of irritable bowel syndrome in adults [8].

A randomized, double-blind study by Kline and colleagues [23] indicated the efficacy of peppermint oil in children with irritable bowel syndrome. The investigators used enteric-coated peppermint oil capsules, which release the oil in the small bowel versus the stomach owing to the pH-dependent coating. The placebo was a capsule of arachis oil. Fifty children (ages 8–17 years) recruited from the University of Missouri, Georgetown University, and a private practice in Charleston, South Carolina, had previously been diagnosed with irritable bowel syndrome using the 2 most accepted criteria for diagnosis, either Manning or Rome. Forty-two children who met the criteria and who had symptoms and pain the prior 2 weeks were randomized to the treatment or placebo group, with weight-based dosing. Children maintained a journal of symptoms and clinicians ranked the severity of pain and the improvement in symptoms from day 1 to day 14.

Significantly more children in the peppermint oil versus placebo group reported a change in the severity of symptoms (76% vs 19%, respectively; $P < .001$) and improvements in symptoms (71% vs 43%; $P < .002$). There was no improvement in other symptoms, including gas, urgency, or features of stool, and children reported no side effects from the peppermint oil [23].

In summary, the studies of EOs being used to treat various ailments are generally limited owing to small sample sizes and many have inadequate control groups. However, the studies provide much-needed data that can help to guide recommendations on this growing and controversial topic.

NATIONAL POISON CONTROL DATA

The increasing popularity and availability of EOs have resulted in increasing numbers of exposures and toxicities. The American Association of Poison Control Centers annual report reveals 20,109 case mentions of EO exposures in 2016, of which 18,997 were single exposures (Table 1) [24]. A majority of the exposures were listed as miscellaneous EO, with the other most commonly listed oils being tea tree (22%), followed by eucalyptus (6%), and then cinnamon (3%) and clove oils (2.7%). In 2016, 70% of all calls to poison control for an exposure to an EO were for a child less than 6 years old. For all ages, 93.6% of calls were for an unintentional exposure and 9.6% needed treatment in a health care facility.

Of all exposures, 20% had minor effects that were "minimally bothersome . . . usually resolve[d] rapidly" [24] and had no permanent effects. One out of every 100 people exposed had moderate to major effects (Table 2). All of these exposures had similar side effect profiles listed under the individual oil information described elsewhere in this article. Moderate effects were "more pronounced, more prolonged or more of a systemic nature than minor symptoms. Usually some form of treatment is or would have been indicated." Again, the symptoms left no permanent effects and were not life-threatening. Major effects were "life-threatening or resulted in significant residual disability or disfigurement" [21]. There were no reported deaths owing to an EO exposure.

Table 1
American Association of Poison Control Centers 2016 and 2017 annual report from clinical toxicology

Age, y	Total exposures in 2016, n (%)	Total exposures in 2017, n (%)
<6	13,264 (69.8)	15,249 (69.1)
6–12	756 (3.9)	853 (3.9)
12–19	420 (2.2)	553 (2.5)
>20	3722 (19.5)	4403 (20.0)
Unknown age[a]/adult of unknown age[b]	835/716 (4.4%/3.7)	1010/891 (4.6%/4)

[a]Unknown age of patient involved in exposure (child or adult).
[b]Adult of unknown age: listed as an adult but their exact age was not listed. A majority of the calls that did not have an exact age listed were adults.
Data from Gummin DD, Mowry JB, Spyker DA, et al. 2017 Annual report of the American Association of Poison Control Centers' National Poison Data System (NPDS): 35th Annual Report. Clin Toxicol (Phila), 2018 in press.

Table 2
Examples of side effects associated with EO exposures, American Association of Poison Control Centers Annual Report, 2017

Minor	Moderate	Major
Mild GI symptoms	Acid–base disturbance	Repeated seizures or status
Drowsiness	High fever	Cardiovascular instability
Skin irritation	Disorientation	Cardiac or respiratory arrest
Transient cough	Isolated brief seizures	Esophageal stricture
	Minor creatinine elevations	Renal failure
	Hypoglycemia with confusion	Rhabdomyolysis

Data from Gummin DD, Mowry JB, Spyker DA, et al. 2017 Annual Report of the American Association of Poison Control Centers' National Poison Data System (NPDS): 35th Annual Report. Clin Toxicol (Phila), 2018 in press.

There was a 16% increase in single exposure calls from 2016 to 2017 (an increased from 18,997 to 22,068, respectively); the types of oils in the exposures were similar between years. Between 2016 and 2017, there was a 15% increase in children less than 6 years old being exposed (see Table 1). Ninety-four percent of exposures were unintentional with 9.3% of people needing treatment at a health care facility. Minor effects were reported in 15.2% of all cases and moderate to major outcomes were reported in 0.8% of cases. There were no deaths reported in 2017.

In summary, EOs have a long history of usage for their possible medicinal effects. Although the pharmacology and potential treatments applications are being studied, large, blinded, randomized studies are needed to clarify their efficacy and safety.

Potentially effective EOs are peppermint in the treatment of irritable bowel syndrome and a combination of tea tree oil and iodine in the treatment of molluscum contagiosum. The other studies with significant positive effects have too many limitations to draw reliable conclusions or there are already available effective and safe treatments. However, there needs to be better defined regulations of the EOs before true testing can occur if the results are to be reliably reproduced. Safety is a particularly important issue with children given their high risk of unintentional exposures and toxicities. Most importantly, EOs must be handled as potential poisons and stored out of a child's reach.

Acknowledgments

I would like to express my deep gratitude to Dr.s Jane Carver, PhD MS, Tamas Peredy, MD, Jemima Desir MD MBA, and Alfred Aleguas Jr, Pharm D D. ABAT FCAAT for their valuable and constructive input during the planning and development of this chapter. Their willingness to give so much of their time so generously has been very much appreciated.

References

[1] Hoffman RS, Howland MA, Lewin NA, et al. Essential oils, Goldfrank's toxicologic emergencies. 10th edition. Hong Kong, China: McGraw-Hill Education; 2015. p. 575–85.

[2] Barkin ME, Boyd JP, Cohen S. Acute allergic reaction to eugenol. Oral surgery, oral medicine. Oral Pathol 1984;57(4):441–2.
[3] Thomassen D, Pearsin PG, Slattery JT, et al. Partial characterization of biliary metabolites of pulegone by tandem mass spectrometry. Detection of glucuronide, glutathione, and glutathinyl glucuronide conjugates. Drug Metab Dispos 1991;19:997–1003.
[4] Kim HM, Cho SH. Lavender oil inhibits immediate-type allergic reaction in mice and rats. J Pharm Pharmacol 1999;51(2):221–6.
[5] Jager W, Buchbauer G, Jirovetz L, et al. Percutaneous absorption of lavender oil from a massage oil. J Soc Cosmet Chem 1992;43:49–54.
[6] Henley DV, Lipson N, Korach KS, et al. Prepubertal gynecomastia linked to lavender and tea tree oils. N Engl J Med 2007;356(5):479–85.
[7] Nord DA, Belew J. Effectiveness of the essential oils lavender and ginger in promoting children's comfort in a perianesthesia setting. J Perianesth Nurs 2009;24(5):307–12.
[8] Charrios TL, Hrudey J, Gardiner P, et al. Peppermint oil. Pediatr Rev 2006;27:e49–51.
[9] Olowe SA. The risk of jaundice in glucose-6-phosphate dehydrogenase deficient babies exposed to menthol. Acta Paediatr Scand 1980;69(3):341–5.
[10] Craig JO. Poisoning by the volatile oils in childhood. Arch Dis Child 1953;28:475–83.
[11] Gross M, Greenberg L. Salicylates: a critical bibliographic view. New Haven (CT): Hillhouse Press; 1948. p. 380.
[12] Ndao DH, Ladas EJ, Cheng B, et al. Inhalation aromatherapy in children and adolescents undergoing stem cell infusion: results of a placebo-controlled double-blind trial. Psychooncology 2012;21(3):247–54.
[13] Wildwood C. The encyclopedia of aromatherapy. Rochester (NY): Healing Arts Press; 1996.
[14] Payne RB. Nutmeg intoxication. N Engl J Med 1963;269:36–8.
[15] Zambelli A, Poggi G, Da Prada G, et al. Clinical toxicity of cryopreserved circulating progenitor cells infusion. Anticancer Res 1998;18:4705–8.
[16] Soltani R, Soheilipour S, Hajhashemi V, et al. Evaluation of the effect of aromatherapy with lavender essential oil on post-tonsillectomy pain in pediatric patients: a randomized controlled trial. Int J Pediatr Otorhinolaryngol 2013;77(9):1579–81.
[17] Markum E, Baillie J. Combination of essential oil of Melaleuca alternifolia and iodine in the treatment of molluscum contagiosum in children. J Drugs Dermatol 2012;11(3):349–54.
[18] Wutzler P, Sauerbrei A, Klocking R, et al. Virucidal activity and cytotoxicity of the liposomal formulation of povidone-iodine. Antiviral Res 2002;54:89–97.
[19] Greive KA, Barnes TM. The efficacy of Australian essential oils for the treatment of head lice infestation in children: a randomised controlled trial. Australas J Dermatol 2018;59(2): e99–105.
[20] Edraki M, Pourpulad H, Kargar M, et al. Olfactory stimulation by vanillin prevents apnea in premature newborn infants. Iran J Pediatr 2013;23(3):261–8.
[21] Marlier L, Gaugler C, Messer J. Olfactory stimulation prevents apnea in premature newborns. Pediatrics 2005;115(1):83–8.
[22] Pittler M, Ernst E. Peppermint oil for irritable bowel syndrome: a critical review and metaanalysis. Am J Gastroenterol 1998;93:1131–5.
[23] Kline RM, Kline JJ, Di Palma J, et al. Enteric-coated, pH-dependent peppermint oil capsules for the treatment of irritable bowel syndrome in children. J Pediatr 2001;138:125–8.
[24] Gummin DD, Mowry JB, Spyker DA, et al. 2017 annual report of the American Association of Poison Control Centers' National Poison Data System (NPDS): 35th annual report. Clin Toxicol (Phila) 2018;56(12):1213–415.

Advances in Pediatrics 66 (2019) 123–145

ADVANCES IN PEDIATRICS

Feeding Issues in Young Children

Melissa Harada, MD[a], Nelly Amariglio, PhD[b],
Hope Wills, MA, RD, CSP, IBCLC[c],
Irene Koolwijk, MD, MPH[a,*]

[a]Department of Pediatrics, UCLA David Geffen School of Medicine, 300 UCLA Medical Plaza, Suite 3300, Los Angeles, CA 90095, USA; [b]Department of General Pediatrics, Children's Hospital of Los Angeles, 4650 Sunset Boulevard, MS #53, Los Angeles, CA 90027, USA; [c]Department of Clinical Nutrition Services, Children's Hospital of Los Angeles, 4650 Sunset Boulevard, MS #53, Los Angeles, CA 90027, USA

Keywords

• Feeding • Mealtime • Picky • Oral-motor

Key points

- Feeding experiences are influenced by developmental level, age, family relationships, and additional systems in children's lives (eg, culture, health, and childcare).
- A biopsychosocial lens is essential when assessing and treating a child's feeding challenges.
- After challenging feeding experiences, it is important to support the restoration of a sense of safety, predictability, and agency around feeding and to support the caregiver–child feeding relationship.

INTRODUCTION

Feeding challenges are one of the most common caregiver concerns discussed with primary care providers for infants, toddlers, and preschool-aged children [1,2]. Approximately 20% to 45% of caregivers of typically developing young children have expressed an eating behavior or feeding concern, and this number increases to approximately 40% to 80% for caregivers of children with chronic medical conditions and children with developmental disabilities [2–4]. To address these concerns, a comprehensive

Disclosure Statement: The authors have nothing to disclose.

*Corresponding author. *E-mail address:* ikoolwijk@mednet.ucla.edu

https://doi.org/10.1016/j.yapd.2019.03.004
0065-3101/19/Published by Elsevier Inc.

approach which considers several factors involved in feeding is required, including [5–7]:

- The broad environment of the child (culture, community, childcare setting);
- Caregiver–child interactions (temperament, behavior, caregiver feeding style); and
- The health status of the child (oral–motor skills, medical and dental factors).

Several classifications of feeding challenges and feeding disorders have been published over time. Feeding disorders have most recently been described in the *Diagnostic and Statistical Manual of Mental Disorders*, 5th edition, with the diagnostic category of avoidant/restrictive food intake disorder, which now covers all ages and a heterogeneous group of patients with avoidant and/or restrictive food intake, without fear of weight gain or body image disturbance [8]. To warrant an avoidant/restrictive food intake disorder diagnosis, the avoidant and restrictive eating must lead to significant medical or psychosocial problems that require independent clinical attention [9]. The *Diagnostic and Statistical Manual of Mental Disorders*, 5th edition, provides 3 example presentations of avoidant/restrictive food intake disorder, which can occur independently or in combination:

- Those with sensory sensitivity who avoid eating specific foods (owing to tastes, textures, smells);
- Those who restrict the amount they eat owing to a lack of interest in eating or low appetite; and,
- Those who avoid specific foods or stop eating after a traumatic experience with eating.

In 2015, Kerzner and colleagues [5] provided a more practical classification for the broader area of feeding difficulties, describing 4 categories: those not eating enough, those eating an inadequate variety, those afraid to eat, and difficulties owing to parental feeding styles. In this article, we chose to describe 3 of the most common feeding challenges that occur in young children (oral motor delay, picky eating, and fear of feeding), and how they can be approached in the primary care setting. Additionally, we added the topic of caregiver feeding relationship and style, and started with this topic, because this dynamic in the child's most proximal relationship is an important determinant of child feeding behaviors.

FEEDING RELATIONSHIP AND FEEDING STYLES

Case 1: *A 15-month-old girl with history of being small for gestational age, presents for evaluation of "not eating enough." The child was hospitalized in the neonatal intensive care unit at birth for hypoglycemia and her mother was initially instructed to feed her child every 2 hours. She was discharged after 2 days. The child has always fed small amounts, but progressed nicely from purees to chopped table foods. Her mother now worries that her daughter only wants to eat every 6 to 8 hours. She therefore supplements every 3 hours with whole milk. Although the child can feed independently, she will not finish her plate so her mother spoon feeds her. During spoon feeding, the child tends to close her mouth and turn away or get up and leave. She currently only accepts food while watching television. A review of the child's growth chart reveals weight less than the 5th percentile until 5 months of age, with a steady increase to the 25th percentile and weight for length of 30th percentile at the clinic visit today.*

Case 1 illustrates a feeding relationship disrupted by a prior history of medical intervention for hypoglycemia. The mother's authoritarian feeding practice is likely rooted in this initial problem and is her response to her perception that the child's intake is insufficient. Consequently, the child has developed an aversion to her mother's assertive feeding approaches. This feeding relationship would benefit from reassuring the parent about the child's growth and sharing of information about how to recognize feeding cues and support child independence during meals.

Early child development and behavior, including feeding, are heavily influenced by parent–child interactions. The relationships that caregivers develop with their children during feeding exist on a spectrum, from positive and supportive behaviors at one end to controlling or neglectful behaviors at the other [10]. Ellen Satter has long proposed that a division of responsibility during feeding in which caregivers determine what, where, and when their child eats and the child decides how much and whether they eat [11] is the ideal. In some instances, when these characteristics are atypical, aberrant feeding relationships develop. As demonstrated in case 1, the feeding relationship may be at risk when there is a mismatch between parental feeding behaviors and beliefs and the child's eating characteristics and abilities [11]. These disruptions can result from a prior history of difficult feeding interactions, attributes of the caregiver or child, or a poor fit between caregiver and child [12].

Children with a history of prematurity, failure to thrive, or complex medical and/or developmental conditions may have experienced intensive medical or nutritional interventions in the past. Although the child's medical condition improves or resolves, the caregiver's perception of the child as medically fragile may persist. This feeling can contribute to a mismatch between the child's nutritional needs and the caregiver's feeding practices [12]. Caregivers may be more controlling, less organized, or aloof. The child may have medical or developmental challenges that interfere with feeding. The child may exhibit behaviors or have a temperament that does not match the caregiver's expectations [12]. Further, other psychosocial stressors can also negatively influence the parent's interaction with the child. These challenging dynamics around feeding can create an ongoing cycle of distress that further contributes to disrupted feeding relationships.

Screening and Assessment Strategies

Evaluation of the feeding relationship and anticipatory guidance regarding feeding should be included for every child with feeding challenges. The guiding principle in Satter's feeding relationship is that children have an innate desire to learn and grow and that the role of caregivers is to support their child. As such, the primary goal in assessing the feeding relationship is to identify environmental factors that do not support a child's capacity to learn to feed and grow [12]. Providers can ask the following questions to assess the feeding relationship and caregiver feeding style [5]:

- How worried are you about your child's eating?
- What happens during mealtimes?
- What happens if your child doesn't eat?

Additionally, providers can request a video of a mealtime to observe the parent–child interactions. Responses to these questions or review of the video may reveal red flags (Table 1) that could be suggestive of a disrupted feeding relationship. The responses can be categorized into 1 of 4 caregiver feeding styles, based on parenting styles originally developed by Baumrind [13,14]: authoritative, authoritarian, permissive, and uninvolved. The 4 caregiver feeding styles are classified according to the level of caregiver demandingness (degree of caregiver control and encouragement of their child to eat during feeding) and responsiveness (level of caregiver sensitivity to and recognition of their child's feeding cues and needs; Table 2). Parent feeding style can be further characterized by 6 feeding practices: responsibility, monitoring, modeling, encouraging, restriction, and pressure to eat [15,16]. These caregiver feeding styles are important for the feeding relationship, because they help to capture caregiver–child interactions and feeding dynamics during meals [17–20].

Authoritative

An authoritative style is preferred for feeding and appropriately follows Satter's division of responsibility during feeding. Authoritative feeders guide and support, rather than control, their child's feeding [5]. They set limits and establish

Table 1
Red flags for caregiver feeding style [5,7]

Characteristic	Potential undesired outcome
Forceful feeding	Child develops aversion to feeding or develops inappropriate behaviors at meals
Disruptive, chaotic, or stressful mealtimes	Lack of appropriate food, structure, or meal-related social patterns for the child
Lack of appropriate independent feeding	Child does not have the opportunity to learn appropriate feeding skills
Distractions during mealtime	Child/parent relies on distractions (television, electronics) during feeding
Positive reinforcement	Caregiver bribes child who turns head away and cries; child's behavior is reinforced
Negative reinforcement	Caregiver ends a meal when the child acts out; child's behavior is reinforced

Table 2
Caregiver feeding styles

		DEMANDINGNESS: Caregiver control and encouragement to eat during feeding	
		HIGH	LOW
RESPONSIVENESS: Caregiver sensitivity to child's needs during feeding	HIGH	AUTHORITATIVE *High Demand/High Response* Reasonable demands Responsive to needs	INDULGENT *Low Demand/High Response* Reduced Structure Highly sensitive to needs
	LOW	AUTHORITARIAN *High Demand/Low Response* Highly controlling Less sensitive to needs	UNINVOLVED *Low Demand/Low Response* Reduced control Reduced involvement

clear expectations, while being sensitive to their child's needs [21]. Authoritative feeding has been associated with increased child intake of dairy, fruit, and vegetables and lower intake of junk foods [22–24].

Authoritarian

Authoritarian feeders may use force, punishment, or rewards to pressure their child to eat, with disregard for their child's feeding cues [17]. They may demand that their child eat their vegetables to leave the table or may restrict access to desirable/unhealthy foods and use these foods as rewards [21]. Authoritarian feeding can be associated with overeating and poorer self-regulation of energy intake in preschool-aged children [25], lower fruit and vegetable intake [26], higher intake of dietary fat [27] among young girls, and an increased risk for overweight [28].

Indulgent

Indulgent feeders give in more to their child's demands and cater to their child's every need. They might ignore the child's hunger cues and provide less structural guidance and limit setting [17]. They may prepare special or multiple foods for their child [5]. Indulgent feeding can be associated with lower consumption of nutrient-rich foods and higher consumption of dietary fat [17].

Uninvolved

Uninvolved feeders may not offer food on a predictable basis. They provide less guidance, structure, or limit setting. They might not pick up on their child's feeding cues or other emotional and physical needs [5]. Uninvolved feeding has been associated with increased weight status [17,28] and risk for adult obesity [29].

When considering how to address an atypical feeding relationship, a cornerstone of intervention is to support and develop a caregiver's sensitivity and responsiveness to their child's feeding cues. If the caregiver does not recognize or respond appropriately to their child's cues, the child is less able to learn how to interpret or address their own cues [10]. Ideal feeding relationships should provide developmentally appropriate support, while teaching feeding skills in a manner that is sensitive to a child's needs. The focus during feeding is shifted from getting food into the child to the feeding relationship and allowing a child to gain confidence and acquire new skills [11].

Feeding Approach

The following strategies can be used to support the parent–child feeding relationship in general [10,11,30]:

- Appropriate food selection: Provide information on developmentally appropriate food selection and the developmental progression of eating skills and food acceptance. Teaching caregivers to base food selection on developmental readiness reinforces responsiveness to their child's feeding cues.
- Teach positive feeding skills: Teach caregivers how to recognize and respond to their child's feeding cues, such as hunger, satiety, and food preferences. Avoid distractions during meals, such as television and cell phones. Model appropriate eating behaviors and maintain a pleasant, neutral attitude during meals. Once a caregiver offers their child appropriate food in a positive way, their job is done. Their child ultimately decides how much and whether they eat.
- Avoid intrusion: Children have an innate desire to learn feeding skills and to regulate food intake. The caregiver's role is to support their child so that their feeding cues are disrupted as little as possible by outside forces. Encourage self-feeding and tolerate age appropriate mess.

The following strategies can be used to support the parent–child feeding relationship per specific feeding styles.

- Authoritarian: Maintain a relaxed and pleasant mealtime. Focus on conversation and time together rather than on eating. Meals will be more fun, with less conflict. Allow children to select foods for their plate and decide how much to eat from the healthy food choices you offer. Your child will gain confidence and learn to sense when they are hungry and full.
- Indulgent: Be a positive example. Set limits and offer the same foods to everyone at meal times. Your child learns from watching you eat. It is alright if the child does not like what is offered. Let the child decide how much and if they will eat the foods offered to everyone. Avoid preparing special food for your child. Trust your child to eat enough over time. It is normal for a child's appetite to vary through the day and week. Continue to offer a variety of food options throughout the day.
- Uninvolved: Work on setting a regular schedule for meal times and snacks. A daily routine helps a child to develop good eating habits and teaches a child that there are more opportunities during the day to eat. Make mealtime family time. Sit together to eat and talk. Avoid distractions, such as electronics and television, during meals. This allows your child to focus on meal time and socializing.

With the educational guidance and behavior changes described herein, most disrupted feeding relationships that result from a lack of information will improve [10]. However, should significant challenges remain despite these measures, providers should consider referral to a mental health provider or to an interdisciplinary feeding team for evaluation and treatment (Fig. 1). If a feeding team is unavailable, providers have to refer to each relevant provider individually.

Online resources for support with caregiver–child feeding relationship

- https://www.ellynsatterinstitute.org/resources-and-links-professionals/.
- https://www.fns.usda.gov/core-nutrition/child-feeding.

SELECTIVE INTAKE BASED ON ORAL–MOTOR DELAY

Case 2: *An 18-month-old girl is seen in clinic for difficulty with eating "regular food." As an infant, she had difficulty latching on, and when drinking from a bottle she was a slow feeder. When offered smooth baby cereal at 6 months of age she turned her head away; cereal was discontinued owing to repeated gagging on small amounts. She gagged on smooth purees offered at 7 months but started eating these in small amounts at 10 months of age. Currently, she mainly eats smooth puree and meltable crackers and consumes infant formula from a bottle. She is quiet in the examination room, has excellent eye contact, and gestures nicely to express what she wants. Although as an infant she had failure to thrive, she caught up at 9 months of age and her weight for length has since been at the 55th percentile, with her height at the 60th percentile.*

This case illustrates a child who presents with delays in oral–motor skills, which have led to delays in feeding skills, and in speech–language

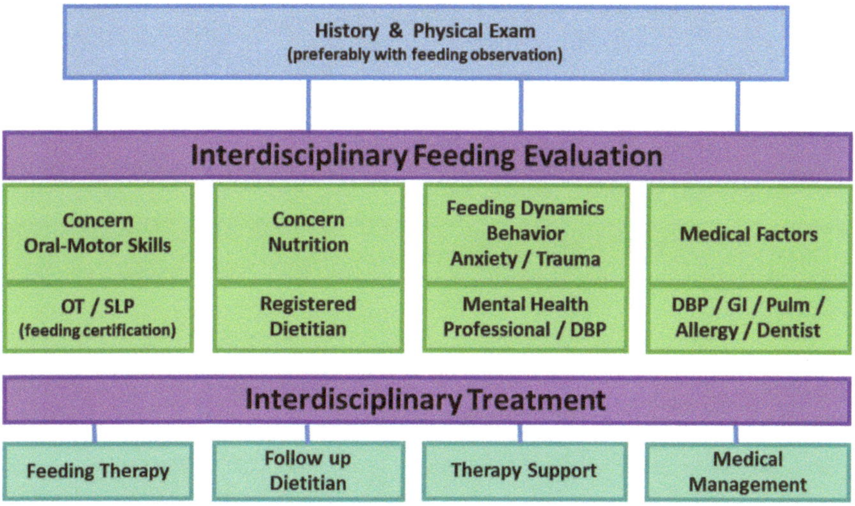

Fig. 1. General evaluation and management of feeding concerns. Allergy, allergy-immunologist; DBP, developmental-behavioral pediatrician; GI, gastro-enterologist; OT, occupational therapist; Pulm, pulmonologist; SLP, speech-language pathologist.

development. There is no concern about overall caloric intake, although the child's nutritional intake is likely affected by a higher than recommended milk and formula intake. However, the child's limited ability to manage a range of textures can be a challenge for caregivers, who report spending increased time on planning, meal preparation, and supporting the child during mealtimes [31]. Moreover, the child's limited diet can create social isolation because menus offered at childcare, restaurants, and birthday parties may not be congruent with what she can manage.

In the first 5 years of life, children are expected to make rapid gains in terms of feeding skills from safely sucking and swallowing, to chewing, drinking from a cup, to eating table food and serving themselves [32–34]. An infant's ability to efficiently coordinate suck and swallow with respiration is essential for safe oral feeding [35]. When feeding challenges are reported, the safety of oral intake is an important question, especially in populations at greater risk for aspiration, such as children who are born prematurely or have complex medical conditions (cardiac or respiratory problems or neurodevelopmental challenges, like cerebral palsy) [36–39]. Table 3 indicates red flags for possible overt or silent (no cough) aspiration, and in these cases an evaluation for dysphagia should be initiated.

Infants born prematurely, especially those less than 30 weeks gestational age, are much more likely to experience feeding–swallowing difficulties. Difficulty with lip and jaw movement and swallowing can persist up to 12 months corrected age or beyond [40]. At 18 months adjusted age, premature infants with a history of feeding difficulties are also more likely to have language delay. Neuromotor impairment and the number of days of mechanical ventilation are both important risk factors associated with these outcomes [41].

The American Academy of Pediatrics and the World Health Organization recommend breastfeeding as the sole source of nutrition for the first 6 months of life, with the introduction of complementary foods around 6 months of age if

Table 3
Red flags indicating risk for aspiration during oral feedings

During feeding	Gagging Choking Food refusal Apnea Cyanosis Taking >30 min/feeding

Directly after feeding	Difference in respiratory quality
	  Sounding "wet/congested"
	  Wheezing
	  Coughing

Over time	Recurrent pneumonias Failure to thrive

the infant seems to be developmentally ready for this [42,43]. In terms of motor skills, sitting with some stability, having good head control, reaching for items, and bringing foods to the mouth are prerequisites for complementary and self-feeding [32]. A gradual transition from a liquid diet to smooth and then courser purees, and eventually to table food has been recommended by the American Academy of Pediatrics and the World Health Organization, with the introduction of finger foods around 8 months. However, an alternative approach called baby-led weaning (BLW), a term coined by Gill Rapley, has gained popularity in recent years [44–46]. In BLW, infants self-feed family foods that are deemed safe to manage from the very start of weaning around 6 months of age, with an emphasis on being part of family mealtimes and child choice of what and how much they eat (without the use of purees or caregiver spoon feeding). Proponents of BLW note that this approach promotes child exploration and a responsive parental feeding style. However, most studies are limited by a reliance on self-report and caregivers mostly self-selecting into the BLW approach. Concerns were raised about a possible increased choking risk with BLW; however, a randomized trial, the BLISS study, showed no significant difference in choking risk between the BLW and the traditional group. However, there was a high frequency of choking events in both groups, with a total of 35% of children between 6 and 8 months of age having at least 1 reported choking event, most commonly on a hard cracker or a raw vegetable [47]. No difference was noted in body mass index scores of BLISS participants at 12 and 24 months of age, but caregivers self-reported less food fussiness in the BLW group [48].

After children learn to coordinate suck–swallow–and–breathe [35], the next critical period generally affected by oral–motor delay is between 6 and 12 months, when a rapid progression of skills should occur from a liquid diet to managing a variety of textures and table foods at 12 months of age. Spoon-feeding capabilities in typically developing infants occurs between 6 to 8 months and takes 5.7 weeks on average [49]. A longer time to develop this skill could indicate a feeding problem. Additional symptoms of oral–motor delay affecting feeding include poor lip closure, decreased awareness of quantity and location of food in the mouth, difficulty with chewing, and feeding times of greater than 30 minutes per meal. A child's diet texture needs to match their oral–motor skill level. When a mismatch occurs with food textures being too challenging for a child, food refusal tends to occur. This refusal might be misinterpreted as disruptive behavior, although a deficit in skills is the actual cause. Additionally, prolonged holding of food in the mouth and gagging or choking events can occur. Table 4 provides an overview of developmental feeding milestones from 0 to 5 years of age.

Assessment Strategies

A basic feeding assessment includes a history of the child's past and current feeding patterns; a developmental, medical, and family history; and a physical examination. Additionally, a large amount of information can be gathered by

Table 4
Developmental feeding milestones

Age (mo)	Motor/social	Feeding skill	Food/consistency
Birth to 3	Many reflexes to protect the airway	Suck–swallow	Liquid
4–5	Sits with some support	Suck–swallow	Liquid
6–8	Sits without support Reaches for food	Gag response declines Starts munching (6 mo) Clearing spoon with top lip (7 mo)	Pureed food
9–12	First teeth erupted Points to food they like	Begins to chew Interest in self-feeding	Ground and lumpy purees Mashed table food Soft/dissolvable solids
13–24	Rejection of new food peaks at 20 mo Sits in booster chair	Most can spoon feed themselves by 15 mo Most can drink from open cup by 19 mo Moves food from one side to other side of mouth while chewing (immature rotary chew)	Table food Chews juicy foods
24–36	Total self-feeding Imitates adult eating preferences	Chews with more mature rotary chew Drinks from open cup without spilling	Table food Tougher solids
36–60	Imitates peers eating preferences	Starts using fork to stab food Progresses with chewing and swallowing of advanced textures under close supervision of caregiver	Table food Better manages advanced textures (meats, whole fruits, fried food)

a feeding observation if feeding is considered safe, even if the feeding is 5 minutes or less. Alternatively a video of feeding can be requested [50]. Because of its danger, a high index of suspicion should be maintained about silent aspiration, especially in children at higher risk, such as those with multisystem diagnoses [38].

When a child's history of past and current feeding challenges is suggestive of oral–motor delay, it is important to determine if their feeding skills match their current diet and if caregiver feeding expectations match the child's ability to manage different textures. If a clinician has a concern about a risk of aspiration, a referral should be placed for a dysphagia evaluation to assess the safety of oral intake. Referral for an interdisciplinary feeding team assessment, if available, is ideal [38], because the team can simultaneously assess different aspects of feeding, including oral–motor skills, nutritional, medical, developmental, and mental health needs (see Fig. 1). If such a team is not available, then individual providers with feeding experience need to be found for evaluation and treatment of feeding challenges. Because oral–motor delays affecting feeding often strain the caregiver–child feeding relationship, assessing this is an important component of any feeding evaluation [31].

Online resources for feeding difficulties

- https://www.infantandtoddlerforum.org/health-childcare-professionals/fact sheets.
- www.healthychildren.org/English/ages-stages/baby/feeding-nutrition/Pages/Signs-of-Feeding-Difficulties.aspx.

PICKY EATING

Case 3: *A 3-year-old boy presents in clinic for well child care. His mother expresses concern that her son will barely eat anything compared with his 5-year-old cousin. The child was exclusively breastfed for the first 6 months of life. He easily made the transition to oral solids. His mother provides 3 meals and 2 snacks per day. She reports that he refuses most vegetables. She has tried to hide them in his preferred foods, but he finds them and picks them out. The child will sit at the table, eat for approximately 10 to 15 minutes, and then get up from the table, saying, "All done." A review of the growth chart indicates that the child has maintained a steady rate of weight gain and linear growth, with a body mass index at the 25th percentile. His mother reports that she will often make the child return to the table to eat more. This sometimes results in the child crying or gagging on his food.*

Case 3 illustrates a caregiver's frustration with a child who is a picky eater. Parental anxiety around the child "not eating enough" despite evidence that he is growing well could bring more pressure into the mealtime environment. Brown and colleagues [51] found that 33% of mothers expressed concern about their child being a picky eater despite evidence of adequate growth. This concern was associated with greater use of pressure and coercive strategies at mealtime to encourage intake. This often contributes to battles that disrupt family mealtimes.

Children with picky eating frequently demonstrate an unwillingness to eat either familiar or new foods (neophobia) and consume a limited variety of foods (selective eating). Parental concern about picky eating correlates with perceived or actual low weight status and with concerns about nutritional adequacy [51]. Children are often identified as being picky based on parent report as opposed to formal screening tools [51,52]. Despite a lack of a singular definition of picky eating there are several recurring themes that appear in the literature. These challenging eating behaviors interfere with daily routines and can be problematic for the caregiver, the child, and the caregiver–child relationship. Parents feel pressured to prepare alternative meals to ensure adequate intake. Picky eating contributes to stress in the household and impacts meal preparation and even food purchases [53].

A recent systematic review estimated the prevalence of picky eating in young children at 22% [54]. Data from the Feeding in Infant and Toddlers study reports prevalence rates of 34.4% for somewhat picky eating and 10.2% for very picky eating [55]. Although picky eating is typically transient in nature, it can be amplified by other behavioral concerns. A secondary data analysis of the Duke Preschool Anxiety study examined selective/picky eating and its relationship with anxiety or depression [56]. The authors reported that 20.3% of children were identified with selective eating, 17.7% with moderate selective eating, and 3% with severe selective eating. Children identified with severely selective eating were 2 times more likely to have comorbid social anxiety or depression. The prevalence rates of picky eating can be influenced by who is observing the behavior. An observational study assessed the agreement between childcare providers and parents in identifying picky eaters. Although the sample was limited, parents were more likely to identify a child as a picky eater compared with a childcare provider, regardless of whether childcare was home based or center based [54,57].

Picky eating is a common concern among parents of young children. However, it tends to be transient in nature with no lasting impact on growth and development [58]. The major risk factor associated with the development of persistent picky eating is the late introduction of lumpy foods [59]. The Generation R study [56,60] reported that breastfeeding for fewer than 2 months correlated with a higher rate of food fussiness at age 4 years compared with children who were breastfed more than 6 months. Later introduction of solids (beyond 6 months of age) is also associated with greater food fussiness. Preterm infants have a higher prevalence of food refusals and picky eating than term infants [61]. Genetic influences on selective or picky eating have long been reported in the literature. A recent study reinforced the heritability of selective eating behaviors, noting a positive association in these behaviors between middle-aged parents and their adult children [62].

Screening and assessment strategies

The Children's Eating Behavior Questionnaire is a validated instrument to identify picky eating [63], although its length (35 items) precludes routine use in a general pediatric office. However, researchers have identified 3 questions that correlate with picky eating.

- Is your child a picky eater?
- Does your child have strong likes?
- Does your child accept new foods?

Further questions that support the identification of picky eaters would assess variety and frequency of disruptive behaviors like tantrums at meal times. Children identified as picky eaters at 3 years of age were noted to be picky eaters as early as 15 months of age, a time when most children have made the transition to table foods [59]. Thus, well-child visits occurring between 12 and 24 months are opportune times to screen for feeding behaviors that can become more problematic in the future.

Feeding approach

Challenges around feeding typically focus on child noncompliance. However, children's eating habits are also influenced by parent behavior. A study of parents of children with picky eating reported a higher use of inappropriate behaviors, such as threats using foods or activities as awards and offering extra snacks to encourage eating [64]. Parents using such approaches can become frustrated when the child no longer responds to threats or promised rewards. This refusal amplifies tension at mealtimes. To ameliorate the tension, providers can advise parents to reduce the emphasis on specific foods or food groups while focusing on variety and positive mealtime behaviors. See Table 5 for strategies to reduce picky eating. The mnemonic TASTE is another way to frame this for parents:

Time	Choosing the best time of day to explore a challenging food, such as after a nap.
Activity	Engage the child in age-appropriate activities in the kitchen, such as tearing lettuce.
Senses	Use all the child's senses to explore a new food by looking at, smelling, and touching it.
Taste	Choose the right taste approach for your child such as kissing, licking, or biting.
Experience	Talk about the experience, not just the taste (eg, "What sound did it make?").

Online resources for picky eating

- https://www.healthychildren.org/English/healthy-living/nutrition/Pages/Picky-Eaters.aspx.
- https://healthychildren.org/English/ages-stages/toddler/nutrition/Pages/default.aspx.
- https://www.superkidsnutrition.com/nutrition-articles/nutrition-concerns/picky-eaters/.

FEAR OF FEEDING: MEDICAL TRAUMA AND FEEDING CHALLENGES

Case 4: *A 3-year-old boy with Tetralogy of Fallot who had undergone several surgeries was born premature and spent 3 weeks in the neonatal intensive care unit. His developmental trajectory has been mainly within normal limits, despite a mild speech–language delay. Several months ago, the child underwent another medical procedure, for which he was hospitalized for a week. Since discharge, he has been irritable and displays diminished interest in playing with his peers. He started having daily nightmares and is now sleeping in his parents' room. His mother reports that he cries and is aggressive any time he has an appointment with a physician. He recently started refusing to eat solids and to participate in family mealtime. On examination, the child seems to be fearful and teary, and his parents express worry over his poor growth and lack of interest in eating.*

Table 5
Strategies to reduce picky eating

Strategies		Examples
Using all the senses	Looking at the food Smelling the food Touching the food	"What does this look like?" "What does this smell like?" "How does it feel?"
Focusing on positive interaction	Give verbal (not tangible) praise	"You took a brave bite."
Respecting no after tasting	Allowing expression of dislikes Trying it again at another meal	"Thank you for trying."
BEING A ROLE MODEL	Eat *with* your child Let child *watch you try new foods*	"It's my turn to take a bite."
Including your child in	Grocery shopping Meal planning Cooking	"Can you find the apples?" Choose a new food based on: Color (eg yellow squash) Shape (eg round melon) Letter (eg M for mango) "Nice job adding raisins to your oatmeal." "Mix blueberries to the pancake batter."

Case 4 illustrates a child who presents with fear of feeding that began after a recent intrusive medical procedure and disruption of his daily routines. Although the child's complex medical history reportedly has not significantly impacted his overall cognitive and psychosocial development, his feeding experiences have been shaped by early tube feeding in the neonatal intensive care unit and repeated surgeries requiring intubation. The child's mild speech–language delay impacts his ability to verbalize his needs and experiences. In addition to the parental concerns about the child's medical care, the recent changes in his feeding behaviors add an additional layer of parental stress because his parents are concerned about his caloric intake and growth. This concern has strained their interactions with the child during mealtime.

A fear of feeding can be understood as a phobia [65], where the child who has experienced an event perceived as traumatic (choking, allergic reaction, pain during mealtime) is highly activated when reminded of the event and makes ongoing attempts to avoid further insults. The avoidance of a specific food item may not be detrimental to a child's development. However, avoidance of multiple food items and to multiple aspects of the mealtime indicate a larger scale problem. Children who experience ongoing uncomfortable experiences related to feeding or to their mealtime experiences, who have organic and structural abnormalities resulting in painful feeding, and/or who undergo medical and dental procedures related to their oral structures or to the gastrointestinal tract [5,66] may present with more pervasive avoidant behaviors and overall fearfulness, which goes beyond mealtime and feeding, and resembles symptoms of posttraumatic stress. In these instances, the fear of feeding can be understood and treated as posttraumatic stress, which develops among children whose sense of safety, predictability, and agency, and ability to explore their environment and thrive [12,66] are hindered by painful and uncomfortable daily feeding experiences.

A certain degree of fear of feeding is common among children who have gastroesophageal reflux [67], craniofacial disorders, neurologic and neuromuscular disorders, and/or undergo intrusive procedures to their oropharynx or esophagus [68]. Additionally, children who have experienced a single traumatic episode related to feeding (choking) [69] or had a food allergy reaction [70,71] can also present with fear of feeding. Additional risk factors for fear of feeding include prematurity, young age and developmental level [72,73], child's premorbid symptoms of anxiety [74] or depression [75], characteristics of parent–child feeding interactions where there is a controlling, indulgent or neglectful parenting style, incompatibility between parent feeding style and the child's temperament, and poor relationship quality [11,12]. Parental anxiety, depression, and trauma symptoms [76] also increase risk for difficulties around the feeding interactions. The degree of symptomatology vastly varies from 1% to 5% in the general population to approximately 80% among young children who present with comorbid complex medical conditions and medical histories and with neurodevelopmental conditions [77–79].

Screening and assessment strategies

The development of aversive feeding behaviors and fear of feeding occurs within the context of a child's feeding experiences, which are influenced by their developmental level and age, family relationships, and additional systems in their lives, such as their educational status, health care, and culture. A biopsychosocial lens is, therefore, essential when assessing for a child's feeding behaviors [79].

A thorough medical, psychosocial, and feeding history is needed to conceptualize the context in which the fear of feeding developed and is maintained and to acquire detailed information clarifying the caregiver's perception regarding the possible antecedents leading to the reported changes in feeding behaviors. It is beneficial to explore any strategies caregivers might have implemented to address a child's feeding behaviors and to obtain information regarding the child's responses. Objective information such as a feeding observation can be very helpful. A child with fear of feeding may present as vigilant around mealtimes and may cry or refuse to eat [80], become distressed or aggressive if pressured to eat, or present with physiologic responses like gagging or vomiting [66].

Specific questions to ask caregivers

- What events occurred before the change in the child's feeding behaviors?
- What are some of the child's behaviors during mealtime?
- What are some of the child's behaviors when presented with certain food items?
- What strategies were implemented in response to the child's feeding behaviors?
- What are the child's responses to the caregiver's strategies?
- How do these changes impact the family mealtime dynamics?

Further questions about general symptoms of posttraumatic stress beyond feeding [8,81]

- Presence of notable distress and/or dysregulation (eg, fears, defeated/depressed, tantrums)
- Changes in child's sleeping/toileting habits
- Reduced interest in previously enjoyed activities
- More aggressive or thematic play
- Presence of hypervigilance
- Developmental regression
- Avoidant behaviors
- Nightmares

Finally, it has been shown that parental distress and symptoms of posttraumatic stress increase the child's risk of development and maintenance of posttraumatic stress symptoms [82,83]. Screening for caregiver stress symptoms can also inform family functioning.

Feeding approach

Table 6 provides an overview of the signs, symptoms, and strategies to address fear of feeding. It is essential to support the development or restoration of a sense of safety around feeding and around the parent–child feeding relationship as the foundation for regulation and for food exploration. Validate,

Table 6
Fear of feeding: signs, symptoms, and strategies

Scenario	Observed behaviors	Strategies
Anticipation of mealtime (bottle, food items)	Vigilance and tension Shallow/fast breathing Crying Signs of nausea Gagging Vomiting	Identify behaviors as signs of fear Reassure the child Implement predictability (duration of mealtime, expectations) Promote regulation for child (deep pressure, Yoga, breathing) Promote regulation for caregiver (breathing, mindfulness)

During mealtime	Crying
	Arching backward
	Closing their mouth
	Pushing food away
	Aggression (eg, hitting)
		Help the child understand their fear
		Create a positive mealtime environment
		Restore safety and trust
		  Attunement to the child's cues
		  Communication between child and caregiver
		Provide the child with a sense of control
		  Infant holding their bottle
		  Toddler helps to set the table
		Promote regulation for child and caregiver

While feeding	Refusing to swallow
	Spitting out food
	Pocketing food
		Avoid force feeding
		Follow the child's lead
		  Whether and how much they choose to eat
		Promote independence
		  Serve themselves, serve others, self-feed

reassure, and provide the family with information about the impact of the child's medical condition, medical interventions, and the event(s) that was experienced as traumatic on their feeding behaviors, regulation, interpersonal relations, and communication. Teach the parent that healing from these traumas will require some specific steps. Goals are to:

- Address any medical and/or organic issues impacting mealtime experiences;
- Develop a sense of trust and restoration of safety;
- Strengthen the parent–child feeding interactions and overall communication;
- Provide the child with predictability, a sense of control and mastery;
- Promote developmentally appropriate food exploration; and
- Promote a positive mealtime experience.

A systemic approach is warranted to address the multiple biopsychosocial factors influencing the development and maintenance of the fear of feeding. This is best done through an interdisciplinary team evaluation staffed by a physician, dietitian, mental health clinician, occupational or speech–language pathologist (see Fig. 1) [50,84,85]. Once medically cleared to participate in oral feeding activities, a cotreatment model between mental health and an oral–motor specialist such as an occupational therapist or speech–language therapist ensues. Dyadic or family trauma-informed mental health therapy is aimed at promoting systemic change and symptom reduction [65,86–93].

- Address symptoms of anxious or/and depressed mood and of posttraumatic stress disorder.
- Address symptoms of trauma in both the child and the caregiver.
- Promote structural change in the family system.
- Enhance communication between family members.
- Promote emotional and behavioral regulation.
- Implement parent education and training.

Nutritional consultation and guidance are often required to ensure sufficient caloric and nutrient intake [50,84].

Ongoing collaboration and consultation with medical teams is ideal. Trauma-informed evidence-based models, such child–parent psychotherapy (CPP), are particularly effective in addressing fear of feeding symptoms that develop and are maintained within the context of traumatic relational, medical, and/or feeding experiences. CPP is an attachment-based treatment model that promotes the parent–child relationship as a foundation for regulation and safe exploration. CPP has been shown to positively ameliorate a myriad of trauma symptoms in young children and their caregivers. CPP strategies have also been effectively used as part of feeding interventions in medical and clinical settings, despite the lack of specific studies on CPP and its effects on feeding interaction. Table 7 provides an overview of mental health–related treatment options and their goals.

Online resources for medical trauma related feeding challenges

- http://drchatoor.com/ptfd/

Table 7
Overview mental health treatment options

Type of intervention	Strategies	Targeted symptoms and outcome
Cognitive therapy and behavioral therapy [65,91,94–96]	Stimulus control Extinction Gradual exposure Shaping Cognitive restructuring Relaxation strategies	Promote food exploration Reduce avoidance Reduce anxiety Reduce fear response Reduced caregiver distress
Parent support and training [84,97,98]	Reassurance Validation Information Skill acquisition and practice	Improve caregiver–child interaction Promote developmentally appropriate caregiver strategies Reduce caregiver distress
Trauma-informed family/dyadic therapy [87,88,99,100]	CPP Culturally sensitive attachment-focused intervention Play therapy, and cognitive and behavioral strategies Trauma narrative	Promote secure child–caregiver attachment bond Promote communication Promote regulation Reduce anxious/depressed mood Reduce traumatic stress symptoms
Trauma-informed child therapy (ages 3–21) with co-joint caregiver support https://paperpile.com/c/3kopwd/OpkR [101]	Trauma-focused cognitive–behavioral therapy Psychoeducation and parenting skills Relaxation and affect regulation Cognitive strategies Trauma narrative Safety maintenance	Reduce anxious mood Reduce traumatic stress symptoms Promote communication Promote regulation Promote effective parenting Reduce relapse
Medication referral https://paperpile.com/c/3kopwd/aSyB [65,102]	Medication treatment (selective serotonin reuptake inhibitor, guanfacine)	Reduce anxious mood Reduced symptoms of posttraumatic stress disorder

- The National Child Traumatic Stress Network: https://www.nctsn.org/
- https://www.nctsn.org/sites/default/files/resources//pediatric_toolkit_for_health_care_providers.pdf.

SUMMARY

Feeding experiences are influenced by developmental level, age, family relationships, and additional systems in children's lives (eg, culture, health, childcare/preschool). A biopsychosocial lens is thus essential when assessing and treating a child's feeding challenges. With the educational guidance and behavior changes described in this article, most disrupted feeding relationships that result from a lack of information will improve. However, should significant challenges remain despite these measures, providers should consider referral to a mental health provider or to an interdisciplinary feeding team for evaluation and treatment. If a feeding team is unavailable, providers have to refer to each relevant provider individually.

References

[1] Field D, Garland M, Williams K. Correlates of specific childhood feeding problems. J Paediatr Child Health 2003;39:299–304.

[2] Carruth BR, Ziegler PJ, Gordon A, et al. Prevalence of picky eaters among infants and toddlers and their caregivers' decisions about offering a new food. J Am Diet Assoc 2004;104:s57–64.

[3] Bryant-Waugh R, Markham L, Kreipe RE, et al. Feeding and eating disorders in childhood. Int J Eat Disord 2010;43:98–111.

[4] Reau NR, Senturia YD, Lebailly SA, et al. Infant and toddler feeding patterns and problems: normative data and a new direction. Pediatric Practice Research Group. J Dev Behav Pediatr 1996;17:149–53.

[5] Kerzner B, Milano K, MacLean WC Jr, et al. A practical approach to classifying and managing feeding difficulties. Pediatrics 2015;135:344–53.

[6] Rybak A. Organic and nonorganic feeding disorders. Ann Nutr Metab 2015;66(Suppl 5): 16–22.

[7] Phalen JA. Managing feeding problems and feeding disorders. Pediatr Rev 2013;34: 549–57.

[8] American Psychiatric Association. Diagnostic and statistical manual of mental disorders (DSM-5®). Arlington (VA): American Psychiatric Pub; 2013.

[9] Thomas JJ, Lawson EA, Micali N, et al. Avoidant/restrictive food intake disorder: a three-dimensional model of neurobiology with implications for etiology and treatment. Curr Psychiatry Rep 2017;19:54.

[10] Satter EM. The feeding relationship. J Am Diet Assoc 1986;86:352–6.

[11] Satter E. The feeding relationship: problems and interventions. J Pediatr 1990;117:S181–9.

[12] Davies WH, Hobart Davies W, Satter E, et al. Reconceptualizing feeding and feeding disorders in interpersonal context: the case for a relational disorder. J Fam Psychol 2006;20: 409–17.

[13] Baumrind D. Current patterns of parental authority. Dev Psychol 1971;4:1.

[14] Damon W. Child development today and tomorrow. San Francisco (CA): Jossey-Bass Incorporated Pub; 1989.

[15] Hubbs-Tait L, Kennedy TS, Page MC, et al. Parental feeding practices predict authoritative, authoritarian, and permissive parenting styles. J Am Diet Assoc 2008;108:1154–61 [discussion: 1161–2].

[16] Arlinghaus KR, Vollrath K, Hernandez DC, et al. Authoritative parent feeding style is associated with better child dietary quality at dinner among low-income minority families. Am J Clin Nutr 2018;108:730–6.

[17] Hughes SO, Power TG, Orlet Fisher J, et al. Revisiting a neglected construct: parenting styles in a child-feeding context. Appetite 2005;44:83–92.

[18] Hughes SO, Power TG, O'Connor TM, et al. Maternal feeding styles and food parenting practices as predictors of longitudinal changes in weight status in Hispanic preschoolers from low-income families. J Obes 2016;2016:7201082.

[19] Hughes SO, Power TG, Papaioannou MA, et al. Emotional climate, feeding practices, and feeding styles: an observational analysis of the dinner meal in Head Start families. Int J Behav Nutr Phys Act 2011;8:60.

[20] Hughes SO, Shewchuk RM, Baskin ML, et al. Indulgent feeding style and children's weight status in preschool. J Dev Behav Pediatr 2008;29:403.

[21] Savage JS, Fisher JO, Birch LL. Parental influence on eating behavior: conception to adolescence. J Law Med Ethics 2007;35:22–34.

[22] Cullen KW, Baranowski T, Rittenberry L, et al. Social–environmental influences on children's diets: results from focus groups with African-, Euro- and Mexican-American children and their parents. Health Educ Res 2000;15:581–90.
[23] Patrick H, Nicklas TA, Hughes SO, et al. The benefits of authoritative feeding style: caregiver feeding styles and children's food consumption patterns. Appetite 2005;44:243–9.
[24] Nicklas TA, Baranowski T, Baranowski JC, et al. Family and child-care provider influences on preschool children's fruit, juice, and vegetable consumption. Nutr Rev 2001;59: 224–35.
[25] Faith MS, Scanlon KS, Birch LL, et al. Parent-child feeding strategies and their relationships to child eating and weight status. Obes Res 2004;12:1711–22.
[26] Fisher JO, Mitchell DC, Smiciklas-Wright H, et al. Parental influences on young girls' fruit and vegetable, micronutrient, and fat intakes. J Am Diet Assoc 2002;102:58–64.
[27] Lee Y, Birch LL. Diet quality, nutrient intake, weight status, and feeding environments of girls meeting or exceeding the American Academy of Pediatrics recommendations for total dietary fat. Minerva Pediatr 2002;54:179–86.
[28] Rhee KE, Lumeng JC, Appugliese DP, et al. Parenting styles and overweight status in first grade. Pediatrics 2006;117:2047–54.
[29] Lissau I, Sørensen TI. Parental neglect during childhood and increased risk of obesity in young adulthood. Lancet 1994;343:324–7.
[30] Kerzner B. Clinical investigation of feeding difficulties in young children: a practical approach. Clin Pediatr 2009;48:960–5.
[31] Estrem HH, Thoyre SM, Knafl KA, et al. 'It's a long-term process': description of daily family life when a child has a feeding disorder. J Pediatr Health Care 2018;32:340–7.
[32] Carruth BR, Ziegler PJ, Gordon A, et al. Developmental milestones and self-feeding behaviors in infants and toddlers. J Am Diet Assoc 2004;104:s51–6.
[33] Miles G, Siega-Riz AM. Trends in food and beverage consumption among infants and toddlers: 2005–2012. Pediatrics 2017;139:e20163290.
[34] Birch LL. Learning to eat: behavioral and psychological aspects. Nestle Nutr Inst Workshop Ser 2016;85:125–34.
[35] Lau C. Development of infant oral feeding skills: what do we know? Am J Clin Nutr 2016;103:616S–21S.
[36] Lefton-Greif MA, Arvedson JC. Pediatric feeding and swallowing disorders: state of health, population trends, and application of the international classification of functioning, disability, and health. Semin Speech Lang 2007;28:161–5.
[37] Gisel E. Interventions and outcomes for children with dysphagia. Dev Disabil Res Rev 2008;14:165–73.
[38] Dodrill P, Gosa MM. Pediatric dysphagia: physiology, assessment, and management. Ann Nutr Metab 2015;66(Suppl 5):24–31.
[39] Kuperminc MN, Gottrand F, Samson-Fang L, et al. Nutritional management of children with cerebral palsy: a practical guide. Eur J Clin Nutr 2013;67(Suppl 2):S21–3.
[40] Sanchez K, Spittle AJ, Slattery JM, et al. Oromotor Feeding in children born before 30 weeks' gestation and term-born peers at 12 months' corrected age. J Pediatr 2016;178: 113–8.e1.
[41] Adams-Chapman I, Bann CM, Vaucher YE, et al. Association between feeding difficulties and language delay in preterm infants using Bayley Scales of Infant Development-Third Edition. J Pediatr 2013;163:680–5.e1–3.
[42] World Health Organization. Global strategy for infant and young child feeding. Geneva, Switzerland: World Health Organization; 2003.
[43] Schwarzenberg SJ, Georgieff MK, Committee on Nutrition. Advocacy for improving nutrition in the first 1000 Days to support childhood development and adult health. Pediatrics 2018;141; https://doi.org/10.1542/peds.2017-3716.
[44] Cameron SL, Heath A-LM, Taylor RW. How feasible is Baby-led Weaning as an approach to infant feeding? A review of the evidence. Nutrients 2012;4:1575–609.

[45] Rapley G, Murkett T. Baby-led weaning: the essential guide to introducing solid foods—and helping your baby to grow up a Happy and confident eater. New York: The Experiment; 2010.
[46] Brown A, Jones SW, Rowan H. Baby-led weaning: the evidence to date. Curr Nutr Rep 2017;6:148–56.
[47] Fangupo LJ, Heath A-LM, Williams SM, et al. A baby-led approach to eating solids and risk of choking. Pediatrics 2016;138; https://doi.org/10.1542/peds.2016-0772.
[48] Taylor RW, Williams SM, Fangupo LJ, et al. Effect of a baby-led approach to complementary feeding on infant growth and overweight: a randomized clinical trial. JAMA Pediatr 2017;171:838–46.
[49] van den Engel-Hoek L, van Hulst KCM, van Gerven MHJC, et al. Development of oral motor behavior related to the skill assisted spoon feeding. Infant Behav Dev 2014;37:187–91.
[50] Arvedson JC. Assessment of pediatric dysphagia and feeding disorders: clinical and instrumental approaches. Dev Disabil Res Rev 2008;14:118–27.
[51] Brown CL, Pesch MH, Perrin EM, et al. Maternal concern for child undereating. Acad Pediatr 2016;16:777–82.
[52] Taylor CM, Wernimont SM, Northstone K, et al. Picky/fussy eating in children: review of definitions, assessment, prevalence and dietary intakes. Appetite 2015;95:349–59.
[53] Trofholz AC, Schulte AK, Berge JM. How parents describe picky eating and its impact on family meals: a qualitative analysis. Appetite 2017;110:36–43.
[54] Cole NC, An R, Lee S-Y, et al. Correlates of picky eating and food neophobia in young children: a systematic review and meta-analysis. Nutr Rev 2017;75:516–32.
[55] van der Horst K, Deming DM, Lesniauskas R, et al. Picky eating: associations with child eating characteristics and food intake. Appetite 2016;103:286–93.
[56] Zucker N, Copeland W, Franz L, et al. Psychological and psychosocial impairment in preschoolers with selective eating. Pediatrics 2015;136:e582–90.
[57] Luchini V, Musaad SM, Donovan SM, et al. Differences and agreement in perception of child picky eating among center- and home-based childcare providers and parents and its impact on utilized mealtime strategies. Nutr Metab Insights 2017;10:1178638816684830.
[58] Taylor CM, Steer CD, Hays NP, et al. Growth and body composition in children who are picky eaters: a longitudinal view. Eur J Clin Nutr 2018; https://doi.org/10.1038/s41430-018-0250-7.
[59] Emmett PM, Hays NP, Taylor CM. Antecedents of picky eating behaviour in young children. Appetite 2018;130:163–73.
[60] de Barse LM, Jansen PW, Edelson-Fries LR, et al. Infant feeding and child fussy eating: the Generation R Study. Appetite 2017;114:374–81.
[61] Johnson S, Matthews R, Draper ES, et al. Eating difficulties in children born late and moderately preterm at 2 y of age: a prospective population-based cohort study. Am J Clin Nutr 2016;103:406–14.
[62] Elkins A, Zickgraf HF. Picky eating and food neophobia: resemblance and agreement in parent/young adult dyads. Appetite 2018;126:36–42.
[63] Steinsbekk S, Sveen TH, Fildes A, et al. Screening for pickiness - a validation study. Int J Behav Nutr Phys Act 2017;14:2.
[64] Chao H-C, Chang H-L. Picky eating behaviors linked to inappropriate caregiver–child interaction, caregiver intervention, and impaired general development in children. Pediatr Neonatol 2017;58:22–8.
[65] Chatoor I, Conley C, Dickson L. Food refusal after an incident of choking: a posttraumatic eating disorder. J Am Acad Child Adolesc Psychiatry 1988;27:105–10.
[66] Chatoor I, Ganiban J, Harrison J, et al. Observation of feeding in the diagnosis of posttraumatic feeding disorder of infancy. J Am Acad Child Adolesc Psychiatry 2001;40:595–602.
[67] Dellert SF, Hyams JS, Treem WR, et al. Feeding resistance and gastroesophageal reflux in infancy. J Pediatr Gastroenterol Nutr 1993;17:66–71.

[68] Di Scipio WJ, Kaslon K, Ruben RJ. Traumatically acquired conditioned dysphagia in children. Ann Otol Rhinol Laryngol 1978;87:509–14.
[69] McNally RJ. Choking phobia: a review of the literature. Compr Psychiatry 1994;35:83–9.
[70] Haas AM. Feeding disorders in food allergic children. Curr Allergy Asthma Rep 2010;10: 258–64.
[71] Christie L. Food fears in children with food allergies. J Allergy Clin Immunol 2004;113: S154.
[72] Wilken M, Bartmann P, Dovey TM, et al. Characteristics of feeding tube dependency with respect to food aversive behaviour and growth. Appetite 2018;123:1–6.
[73] Kassam-Adams N, Butler L. What do clinicians caring for children need to know about pediatric medical traumatic stress and the ethics of trauma-informed approaches? AMA J Ethics 2017;19:793–801.
[74] Norris ML, Robinson A, Obeid N, et al. Exploring avoidant/restrictive food intake disorder in eating disordered patients: a descriptive study. Int J Eat Disord 2014;47:495–9.
[75] Psychological and psychosocial impairment in preschoolers with selective eating. Pediatrics 2015;136:X19.
[76] Ammaniti M, Ambruzzi AM, Lucarelli L, et al. Malnutrition and dysfunctional mother-child feeding interactions: clinical assessment and research implications. J Am Coll Nutr 2004;23:259–71.
[77] Chatoor I. Diagnosis and treatment of feeding disorders in infants, toddlers, and young children. Washington, DC: Zero to Three; 2009.
[78] Aldridge VK, Dovey TM, Martin CI, et al. Identifying clinically relevant feeding problems and disorders. J Child Health Care 2010;14:261–70.
[79] Manikam R, Perman JA. Pediatric feeding disorders. J Clin Gastroenterol 2000;30: 34–46.
[80] Benoit D, Coolbear J. Post-traumatic feeding disorders in infancy: behaviors predicting treatment outcome. Infant Ment Health J 1998;19:409–21.
[81] Kazak AE, Kassam-Adams N, Schneider S, et al. An integrative model of pediatric medical traumatic stress. J Pediatr Psychol 2005;31:343–55.
[82] Price J, Kassam-Adams N, Alderfer MA, et al. Systematic review: a reevaluation and update of the integrative (trajectory) model of pediatric medical traumatic stress. J Pediatr Psychol 2016;41:86–97.
[83] De Young AC, Hendrikz J, Kenardy JA, et al. Prospective evaluation of parent distress following pediatric burns and identification of risk factors for young child and parent posttraumatic stress disorder. J Child Adolesc Psychopharmacol 2014;24:9–17.
[84] Silverman AH. Interdisciplinary care for feeding problems in children. Nutr Clin Pract 2010;25:160–5.
[85] Sharp WG, Volkert VM, Scahill L, et al. A systematic review and meta-analysis of intensive multidisciplinary intervention for pediatric feeding disorders: how standard is the standard of care? J Pediatr 2017;181:116–24.e4.
[86] Reyes V, Stone BJ, Dimmler MH, et al. Child-parent psychotherapy: an evidence-based treatment for infants and young children. In: Landolt MA, Cloitre M, Schnyder U, editors. Evidence-based treatments for trauma related disorders in children and adolescents. Cham, Switzerland: Springer International Publishing; 2017. p. 321–40.
[87] U.S. Department of Health and Human Services, Administration for Children and Families, Administration on Children, Youth and Families, Children's Bureau. Child maltreatment 2013. 2015.
[88] Lieberman AF, Van Horn P. Psychotherapy with infants and young children: repairing the effects of stress and trauma on early attachment. New York: Guilford Press; 2011.
[89] Williams KE. Childhood feeding disorders, J. H. Kedesdy and K. S. Budd, 1998, Brookes, Baltimore, 416 pp. Behav Interv 2001;16:140–1.

[90] Bryant-Waugh RJ, Piepenstock EHC. Childhood disorders: feeding and related disorders of infancy or early childhood. In: Tasman A, Kay J, Lieberman JA, et al, editors. Psychiatry. Hoboken (NJ): John Wiley & Sons, Ltd; 2008. p. 830–46.
[91] Lukens CT, Silverman AH. Systematic review of psychological interventions for pediatric feeding problems. J Pediatr Psychol 2014;39:903–17.
[92] Seiverling L, Burns J, Rodriguez J, et al. The effects of a brief behavioral intervention on food refusal in a child with a fear of choking. Clin Case Stud 2015;15:117–25.
[93] Duncan LG, Coatsworth JD, Greenberg MT. A model of mindful parenting: implications for parent-child relationships and prevention research. Clin Child Fam Psychol Rev 2009;12: 255–70.
[94] Sharp WG, Jaquess DL, Morton JF, et al. Pediatric feeding disorders: a quantitative synthesis of treatment outcomes. Clin Child Fam Psychol Rev 2010;13:348–65.
[95] Kerwin ME. Pediatric feeding problems: a behavior analytic approach to assessment and treatment. Behav Anal Today 2003;4:162–76.
[96] Okada A, Tsukamoto C, Hosogi M, et al. A study of psycho-pathology and treatment of children with phagophobia. Acta Med Okayama 2007;61:261–9.
[97] Kaminski JW, Valle LA, Filene JH, et al. A meta-analytic review of components associated with parent training program effectiveness. J Abnorm Child Psychol 2008;36:567–89.
[98] Babbitt RL, Hoch TA, Coe DA, et al. Behavioral assessment and treatment of pediatric feeding disorders. J Dev Behav Pediatr 1994;15:278–91.
[99] Ghosh Ippen C, Harris WW, Van Horn P, et al. Traumatic and stressful events in early childhood: can treatment help those at highest risk? Child Abuse Negl 2011;35:504–13.
[100] Paul HA. Treating trauma and traumatic grief in children and adolescents (2nd Ed.) by J. A. Cohen, A. P. Mannarino, & E. Deblinger. Child Fam Behav Ther 2017;39:318–24.
[101] Cohen JA, Deblinger E, Mannarino AP. Trauma-focused cognitive behavioral therapy for children and families. Psychother Res 2018;28:47–57.
[102] Banerjee SP, Preeya Banerjee S, Bhandari RP, et al. Use of low-dose selective serotonin reuptake inhibitors for severe, refractory choking phobia in childhood. J Dev Behav Pediatr 2005;26:123–7.

Advances in Pediatrics 66 (2019) 147–159

ADVANCES IN PEDIATRICS

Review of Narcolepsy and Other Common Sleep Disorders in Children

Sagarika Nallu, MD[a,*], Giselle Y. Guerrero, MD[b], Jaclyn Lewis-Croswell, PsyD[c], Lara M. Wittine, MD[d]

[a]Department of Pediatrics, University of South Florida, Morsani College of Medicine, 17 Davis Blvd. Suite#200, Tampa, FL 33606, USA; [b]University of South Florida, 17 Davis Blvd. Suite#200, Tampa, FL 33606, USA; [c]Tampa General Hospital, 1 Tampa General Center, Tampa, FL 33606, USA; [d]University of South Florida, Morsani Center for Advanced Healthcare, 13330 USF Laurel Drive, Tampa, FL 33612-4799, USA

Keywords

• Narcolepsy • Sleep-related breathing disorders • Circadian rhythms disorders • Parasomnias • Restless leg syndrome

Key points

- Common sleep disorders in children include narcolepsy, sleep disordered breathing, circadian rhythm disorders, parasomnias, restless leg syndrome, periodic limb movements in sleep, and periodic limb movement disorder.
- These disorders can have a wide range of effects in children, including severe daytime sleepiness, abnormal behaviors, hyperactivity, lack of concentration, and difficulties in school.
- Ongoing research is helping to clarify the pathophysiology and clinical features of these disorders.
- Early diagnosis can significantly improve quality of life, and there are increasing options for management.

INTRODUCTION

The identification of sleep problems in children and adolescents is increasingly important given the growing evidence indicating that disrupted sleep in children can impair cognitive, emotional, neurobehavioral, and social development

Disclosure: The authors have no conflict of interests or relevant disclosures to declare.

*Corresponding author. *E-mail address:* snallu@health.usf.edu

https://doi.org/10.1016/j.yapd.2019.03.008

[1,2]. Sleep is essential in children's learning, memory processes, school performance, and general well-being [3]. The prevalence of sleep problems in children is at least 25% [2,3]. A misdiagnosis of narcolepsy or other sleep disorders has resulted in delayed treatment, causing increased symptom burden. We provide an overview of the common sleep disorders that are seen in children and adolescents.

NARCOLEPSY

Narcolepsy is a complex sleep disorder that can manifest in childhood or adolescence. It is the most common cause of excessive daytime sleepiness and can occur in isolation or in combination with other symptoms such as cataplexy, hypnogogic/hypnopompic hallucinations, disturbed nocturnal sleep, and sleep paralysis [3,4]. Cataplexy distinguishes type 1 (narcolepsy with cataplexy) from type 2 narcolepsy (narcolepsy without cataplexy) [4]. Cataplexy is reported by 60% to 75% of patients with narcolepsy and is defined as a transient, sudden-onset loss of skeletal muscle tone with retained consciousness. It is often in seen in response to a strong emotion (eg, laughter, startle, or anger) [4,5]. Narcolepsy is rare, occurring in 0.025% to 0.050% of the population, with a peak incidence between the ages of 10 and 19 years. The exact prevalence of narcolepsy in children is unknown, but studies indicate that symptoms began during childhood in more than one-half of adult narcolepsy patients [6]. Delays in diagnosis have been reported with a mean delay of up to 15 years [6,7]. Diagnosis in children can be difficult owing to a lack of general awareness of this disorder, atypical presentations of cataplexy, and the associated medical, sleep, and behavioral comorbidities that often lead to misdiagnosis [8]. Narcolepsy can impair social and academic performance in otherwise intellectually normal children [5,7,9], and its implications are often misunderstood by patients, parents, teachers, and health care professionals.

Genetic and environmental factors reportedly play a role in the etiology of narcolepsy [7,10]. Evidence suggests that the loss of hypocretin is highly associated with its development [10]. Hypocretin, a neuropeptide found in the lateral and posterior hypothalamus, targets monoaminergic and cholinergic areas. The loss of hypocretin neurons results in the characteristic symptoms of narcolepsy, including the inability to sustain long periods of wakefulness and frequent lapses into sleep [7,10]. Evidence suggests a link between HLA DQB1*06:02 and narcolepsy, indicating an autoimmune basis for narcolepsy that is mediated by hypocretin neurons [10].

Sleepiness is a normal, cyclic experience that invariably occurs after prolonged wakefulness. In healthy persons, mild sleepiness during the daytime is apparent only during boring, sedentary situations (eg, watching television). Children often lapse into sleep when not stimulated (eg, being driven in a car or during school). The majority of children stop requiring daytime naps by the age of 5 years [11]. Hypnagogic or hypnopompic hallucinations are vivid, dreamlike sensations that an individual feel, hears, or sees and that occur near the onset of sleep (hypnogogic) or upon waking up from sleep (hypnopompic). Sleep paralysis is defined as the temporary inability to move or speak while being conscious and that occurs when a person is falling asleep or waking up from sleep. These hallucinations and sleep paralysis are less common in children than adults, but can be confused with seizures in children. A lack of stereotypical features distinguishes these events from seizures, and the relationship of sleep with these hallucinations distinguishes them from hallucinations of psychosis. Cataplexy in children with narcolepsy may present as a wide range of motor disturbances that do not meet the classic definition of cataplexy, and can include more complex active movements (eg, perioral movements, dyskinetic–dystonic movements, or stereotypic movements) [8]. These motor disturbances may resolve later in the course of the disorder. Other predominating features of narcolepsy in children are restlessness and motor overactivity. Academic deterioration, inattentiveness, and emotional lability are common in affected children. Patients with narcolepsy tend to take short and refreshing naps (ie, REM-type naps) during the day. Their daytime naps may be accompanied by dreams [5–7].

Many patients with narcolepsy also have trouble sleeping at night, and children with narcolepsy have difficulty with morning arousal, which can be associated with aggressive behavior. Over the past several years, various common comorbidities have been described in children with narcolepsy [9,12], including obesity, accelerated pubertal development, and attention deficit hyperactivity disorder symptoms [3,9,12,13]. These children often were misdiagnosed as having attention deficit hyperactivity disorder, learning disability, depression, or another neurologic disorder.

Diagnosis

The diagnosis of narcolepsy requires a detailed clinical history and diagnostic studies such as an overnight polysomnography (PSG) followed by a multiple sleep latency test (MSLT) [5,7,14,15]. An MSLT includes 4 or 5 nap periods of 20 minutes, each with a 2-hour break between naps. An MSLT with sleep latency of 8 minutes of less and 2 or more sleep-onset REM periods and the exclusion of other sleep disorders on PSG provide a definitive diagnosis of narcolepsy [14,16]. The PSG performed the night before MSLT is important for excluding other primary sleep disorders such as sleep apnea and periodic limb movement disorder. Abnormal MSLT findings are not specific for narcolepsy and may be produced by other sleep disorders, such as sleep apnea, circadian misalignment, other mental or medical conditions, medications or substance use, or sleep deprivation [16]. An alternative criterion for diagnosis is a cerebrospinal fluid hypocretin level of 110 pg/mL or less [4,17].

Treatment

Narcolepsy is treatable; however, a multimodal approach with both nonpharmacologic and pharmacologic components is required for the most favorable outcome. Currently, no US Food and Drug Administration (FDA)-approved pharmacotherapy is available for children; however, the medications used to treat adults have been used off-label in children with positive results.

The primary treatment is stimulant therapy, which aims to improve alertness and functioning. Wake-promoting medications such as modafinil and armodafinil are considered first line therapy for excessive daytime sleepiness and are FDA approved for patients older than17 years. Both methylphenidate and modafinil have been used off label for patients 6- to 15-year-old children and are effective [18]. Stimulants such as methylphenidate and amphetamines such as dextroamphetamine and methamphetamine are commonly prescribed in younger children. The undesirable side effects of stimulant medications include headache, irritability, nervousness, and gastrointestinal complaints. Nocturnal sleep may be impaired, resulting in decreased total sleep time. Sleep hygiene is important. Most patients improve if they maintain a regular sleep schedule, usually 7.5 to 8.0 hours of sleep per night.

Sodium oxybate, a precursor for GABA, is the only treatment for cataplexy that has been approved by the FDA. Although sodium oxybate was approved by the FDA for narcolepsy in patients 18 years old or older, off-label use in younger children reportedly controls the cataplexy and severe hypersomnia [19]. Tricyclic antidepressants (eg, clomipramine), selective serotonin reuptake inhibitors (eg, fluoxetine), serotonin, and norepinephrine reuptake inhibitors (eg, venlafaxine) have all been used to treat cataplexy [20].

Although pharmacologic management is at the forefront, behavioral and lifestyle modifications can play a crucial role in decreasing the impact of the disease. Nonpharmacologic treatments include scheduled brief naps, practicing good sleep hygiene, and regular exercise during the day to improve alertness. People with narcolepsy should also be cautious around moving equipment/machinery and heights. Children should be encouraged to participate in afterschool activities and sports. School personnel should have narcoleptic children refrain from unsupervised activities if they seem to be drowsy. Avoiding foods high in refined sugars may improve daytime sleepiness. Providing emotional and educational support to children with narcolepsy, counseling regarding high-risk behaviors such as drug and alcohol use, and inquiring about depression, family conflict, and other psychosocial problems are important.

Regular follow-up with a sleep physician is recommended for children with narcolepsy to monitor response to treatment, to assess for the presence of comorbid sleep disorders such as obstructive sleep apnea or periodic limb movement disorder, and to assess for other psychosocial issues that often arise. Research into future treatments is focusing on preventing the loss of hypocretin (orexin)-producing neurons by targeting the proposed autoimmune-driven mechanism of narcolepsy [20].

SLEEP DISORDERED BREATHING IN CHILDREN

Sleep disordered breathing (SDB) refers to several different disorders that affect the quality of oxygenation and ventilation during sleep. About 1% to 5% of children have SDB, and some may have more than 1 disorder simultaneously [1,21]. SDB prevalence is much higher in children with certain risk factors, especially those with underlying genetic syndromes (eg, Down syndrome), craniofacial abnormalities, and neuromuscular disease.

Obstructive sleep apnea syndrome

Obstructive sleep apnea syndrome (OSAS) is characterized by recurrent partial or complete upper airway obstruction that causes fluctuations in oxygenation and sleep fragmentation. OSAS is accompanied by frequent snoring (>3 nights/wk), labored breathing during sleep, gasping for air, observed apneas, restless sleep, enuresis, morning headaches, daytime sleepiness, hyperactivity, and/or concentration/learning problems [4,22]. The children at greatest risk for OSAS are those with adenotonsillar hypertrophy, obesity, craniofacial anomalies (eg, Pierre Robin sequence, Crouzon and Treacher Collins syndrome), disorders resulting in hypotonia (eg, Down syndrome, Prader-Willi syndrome, cerebral palsy, neuromuscular disorders), metabolic diseases, and laryngomalacia [21].

Polysomnography with oximetry and end-tidal carbon dioxide monitoring are used to diagnose OSAS and other SDB disorders in children. The severity of upper airway obstruction is determined by the apnea-hypopnea index, which is the mean number of apneas and hypopneas that occurred per hour of total sleep time. In children, OSAS is present when the apnea-hypopnea index is 1 or greater, and AHIs of 1 to 4, 5 to 9, and 10 or greater are considered mild, moderate, and severe, respectively.

Untreated childhood OSAS can contribute to neurocognitive, behavioral, cardiovascular, and metabolic comorbidities. Children may suffer from attention problems, hyperactivity, aggression, as well as poor social, communication, and adaptive skills [22]. Metabolic abnormalities have also been reported, including increased low-density lipoprotein cholesterol, reduced high-density lipoprotein cholesterol, reduced insulin sensitivity, and elevated liver enzymes, especially in obese children [23]. Children with underlying congenital heart disease, chronic lung disease, or sickle cell anemia may be more vulnerable to the effects of intermittent nocturnal hypoxia.

Fortunately, the treatment of OSAS improves behavior, learning, OSA symptoms, quality of life, and health indices. The first-line treatment of OSAS in children is adenotonsillectomy. Risk factors for residual OSAS after surgery include obesity, severe OSAS before surgery with an apnea-hypopnea index of greater than 20 per hour, age greater than 7 years, high Mallampati score, African American ethnicity, and underlying asthma, craniofacial abnormalities, and neuromuscular disease [24,25].

For children who are not surgical candidates or whose surgery did not fully resolve their OSA, there are additional treatment options. Nasal corticosteroids and/or oral montelukast can be used in children with mild to moderate OSA [26]. Continuous positive airway pressure or bilevel positive airway pressure can treat OSA of any severity. Positive airway pressure therapy should be titrated to the correct pressure for the child by a repeat in-laboratory PSG [24]. Mandibular distraction osteogenesis and mandibular advancement surgeries have also been shown to improve OSA in children with mandibular insufficiency [27]. Tracheostomy is an option in severe cases when all other treatment options have failed.

Central sleep apnea

Central sleep apnea (CSA) is the lack of airflow owing to the absence of any respiratory effort. There are 2 main physiologic mechanisms by which CSA occurs [28]. There is either instability in the autonomic nervous system that senses and responds to O_2 and CO_2 levels (ie, the input pathway to the central respiratory control center in the medulla) or there is dysfunction in the phrenic nerve output and/or respiratory apparatus that does not allow the respiratory system to correctly respond to systemic O_2 and CO_2 levels (ie, the output pathway from the central respiratory control center to the lungs). The latter usually results in hypoventilation.

CSA can be seen in newborns, especially those born preterm. In fact, most preterm infants have central apneas within the first week of life owing to the immaturity of their central respiratory drive and chemoreceptor responses to O_2 and CO_2, as well as abnormal upper airway reflexes [29]. The incidence and severity of CSA in preterm infants is inversely related to gestational age and is diagnosed by recurrent, prolonged apneas lasting more than 20 seconds and periodic breathing with cyanosis, oxygen desaturations, and bradycardia [29]. Apnea of prematurity does not require a PSG for diagnosis [29].

The initial intervention is physical stimulation of the infant to induce spontaneous breathing. Oxygen and caffeine therapies are supportive while the infant matures to term gestational age [29]. Significant prematurity may require early mechanical ventilation or continuous positive airway pressure support. The persistence of CSA after 43 weeks gestational age indicates the presence of another disorder and CSA should be classified accordingly (ie, CSA owing to a medical or neurologic condition) [4]. Additional comorbidities need to be considered, including abnormal neurodevelopment or intracranial pathology (eg, Chiari malformation), anemia, infection/sepsis, metabolic derangements, gastric reflux, toxic substance exposure, and respiratory depressant medications/anesthesia. Treatment is aimed at correcting the underlying condition.

CIRCADIAN RHYTHM DISORDERS

Circadian rhythm, a biological process that has an endogenous and entrainable oscillation of about 24 hours, is controlled by the suprachiasmatic nucleus located in the anterior hypothalamus. Circadian rhythm disorders (CRSDs) occur when there is a desynchrony between the biological and environmental clocks and can occur when the person's natural circadian timing differs from the sleep–wake times required by work or school [4,30]. *Zeitgebers*, German for "time givers," are cues or entraining forces that keep most people synchronized to the 24-hour clock. Zeitgebers include light, social interactions, timing of food and drink, activity, and temperature. CRSDs can lead to significant daytime sleepiness, which can cause difficulty for schoolchildren. Inconsistent or late bedtimes contribute to insufficient sleep and 25% of children get less than the recommended amount of sleep [11]. Daytime naps can worsen sleep hygiene by decreasing sleep drive and worsening the child's ability to fall asleep, contributing to insomnia.

Children's nighttime sleep needs vary, from infants who require 6 to 13 hours to teenagers who require 6 to 10 hours [11]. Beginning in infancy, a child may have a tendency for a delayed or advanced circadian rhythm and begin to show a preference of rising early or sleeping late [11].

Delayed sleep phase disorder (DSPD) is the most common CRSD with an estimated prevalence of 0.17% in the general population and 7% to 16% among adolescents and young adults [30]. It is estimated that 5% to 10% of patients with chronic insomnia in sleep clinics have DSPD. Several studies indicate a genetic predisposition for DSPD, with about 40% of patients having a positive family history [30]. DSPD is characterized by difficulty falling asleep before midnight and difficulty waking in the morning. People with DSPD often prefer to sleep until the late morning, and it is very common among high school and college/university students, who have later bedtimes and who wake later, especially on weekends. For many adolescents, school start times are too early for their circadian timing, which can lead to sleep deprivation. The deprivation can accumulate and lead to fatigue, poor cognitive functioning, and, if severe, growth delay. Insufficient sleep time decreases the amount of human growth hormone released and may alter the cortisol curve, which can further exacerbate sleep issues [30,31]. This sleep deprivation has public health implications, because teens are showing increasing signs of significant sleep deprivation owing to school starting much earlier than it did 20 years ago.

Irregular sleep–wake rhythm disorder (ISWRD) occurs when sleep timing is disorganized and must include a sleep wake pattern with multiple sleep and wake periods throughout the 24-hour cycle. The pattern is more common in children with developmental disabilities or the elderly with dementia, as well as patients with traumatic brain injury or other psychiatric problems. ISWRD may be caused by a weakened central circadian oscillation and temporal disorganization of circadian rhythms secondary to a decreased exposure to zeitgebers or degeneration of the suprachiasmatic nucleus neurons [30,32]. Treatment options include timed light and melatonin to improve daytime alertness, decrease napping, and consolidate nighttime sleep. Melatonin and light therapy are effective treatments for ISWRD. Combining melatonin, bright light, and behavioral interventions that engage the patient in a cognitively enriched environment with scheduled social and physical activities throughout the day, consistent bedtime routines, and good sleep hygiene are crucial in treating ISWRD [31,33–35].

Patients with advanced sleep phase disorder have difficulty staying awake from 6 PM to 9 PM, and they wake up between 2 AM and 5 AM. Advanced sleep phase disorder is less common in children than adults, and only occurs in 1% of the population. Advanced sleep phase disorder has a genetic component [32].

The treatment of CRSD includes lifestyle changes including improved sleep hygiene, bright light therapy, and melatonin supplementation given at precise times. Hypnotics can help to promote sleep and stimulants can promote wakefulness [30].

PARASOMNIAS IN CHILDREN

Parasomnias are classified by the *International Classification of Sleep Disorders* as non-REM (NREM) sleep arousal disorders and REM sleep behavior disorders. Parasomnias occur in 10% to 28% of children and differ in pathophysiology and management from sleep–wake disorders in adults. The NREM parasomnias are most common in children and adolescents but may persist into adulthood [36] (Table 1).

NREM-related parasomnias can be triggered by significant sleep deprivation, OSA, fever, psychological stress, or substances [4,36]. Parasomnias can be difficult to distinguish from nocturnal seizures and may require video-electroencephalogram PSG [4,37,38].

Treatment of NREM parasomnias includes ensuring a safe environment, especially for patients who sleep walk. NREM parasomnias often resolve by adulthood. Behavioral interventions include parental education, scheduled awakenings, resolution of sleep deprivation, hypnosis, treatment for medical causes, and minimizing the use of medications that contribute to the disorder [38,39]. Medications used to treat NREM parasomnias include clonazepam, temazepam, tricyclic antidepressants, and selective serotonin reuptake inhibitors.

Nightmares, which happen during REM sleep, occur in up to 50% of children between 3 and 6 years old, and in up to 80% of children with generalized and other anxiety disorders [38]. Most patients outgrow nightmares by adulthood [4,38,39]. Nightmare disorder includes recurrent episodes of awakenings from sleep, with the patient recalling intensely disturbing dreams that usually involve fear or anxiety; other emotions such as anger, sadness, disgust, and other dysphoric emotions can occur. The patient wakes to full alertness, has

Table 1
Parasomnias

NREM-related parasomnias	REM-related parasomnias
Disorders of arousal (from NREM sleep)	REM sleep behavior disorder
Confusional arousals	Recurrent isolated sleep paralysis
Sleepwalking	Nightmare disorder
Sleep terrors	
Sleep-related eating disorder	
Other parasomnias	Isolated symptoms and normal variants
Exploding head syndrome	Sleep talking
Sleep-related hallucinations	
Sleep enuresis	
Parasomnia owing to a medical disorder	
Parasomnia owing to a medication or substance	
Parasomnia, unspecified	

little confusion or disorientation, recalls being asleep and recalls the dream content. The presence of nightmare disorder can impair quality of life, resulting in sleep avoidance and sleep deprivation, with a consequent increase in the intensity of the nightmares. Other consequences such as insomnia and sleep avoidance, daytime sleepiness, and fatigue are also common. It can also cause or exacerbate underlying psychiatric distress and illness. Nightmare disorder is more prevalent in patients with comorbid psychiatric disorders or with trauma/posttraumatic stress disorder and requires trauma-focused intervention [38,39].

Effective behavioral treatment options include cognitive–behavioral therapy, image rehearsal therapy, eye movement desensitization reprocessing, exposure, relaxation, rescripting therapy, and desensitization. Clonazepam and venlafaxine are not recommended for the treatment of nightmare disorder. In some studies, prazosin was helpful for reducing nightmare frequency and intensity, increasing total sleep time and improving daytime symptoms of posttraumatic stress disorder [31,38,40].

RESTLESS LEGS SYNDROME, PERIODIC LIMB MOVEMENTS IN SLEEP, AND PERIODIC LIMB MOVEMENT DISORDER

Restless legs syndrome (RLS), also known as Willis-Ekbom disease, is a common neurologic sensorimotor disorder that manifests as an irresistible urge to move the body to relieve the uncomfortable sensations. These sensations always occur during resting, sitting or sleeping. Pediatric RLS, which occurs in about 2% of children [41], commonly worsens at night, causing difficulties with initiating sleep [42]. In adults, it is more prevalent in females, but there is no gender difference in pediatric RLS. A family history of RLS was detected in 90.9% of the patients with RLS, indicating high hereditability. RLS also has a significant association with circadian rhythm, with symptoms worsening in the evening and having a short remission in the morning after waking up [43]. Attention, sleep, mood, cognition, and quality of life are significantly affected in pediatric RLS patients [44], and attention deficit hyperactivity disorder, depressive symptoms, and anxiety are common comorbidities [45]. Pain is a common presentation in pediatric RLS, with 45% of patients using the terms "pain" and "hurting" to describe their symptoms; it is often misdiagnosed as growing pains [46]. A definitive diagnosis of RLS generally can be made in typically developing children by the age of 5 to 6 years, because they are able to accurately describe their symptoms [46,47]. The diagnosis of RLS in children is made using the criteria recommended by the International Restless Legs Syndrome Study Group. A definite diagnosis of RLS in children requires that the child meets all 4 essential adult criteria for RLS and is able to describe the leg discomfort in his or her own words, for example, "lot of energy in my legs," "my legs tickle," "feels like spiders crawling on my legs," and so on. Age-appropriate words to describe their symptoms are encouraged. If unable to describe these feelings, the child must meet all 4 essential adult criteria for RLS and 2 out of 3 supportive criteria. These criteria include the presence of a sleep disturbance for age, having a biologic parent or sibling with definite RLS, or a PSG-documented periodic limb movement index of 5 or more per hour of sleep [47,48].

RLS diagnostic criteria in adults include 4 core essential symptoms:

1. An urge to move the legs
2. The urge to move begins or worsens when sitting or lying down
3. The urge to move is partially or totally relieved by movement
4. The urge to move is worse in the evening or night than during the day or only occurs in the evening or night.

The diagnosis of RLS is more difficult in children who are developmentally delayed, and in preschool-aged children who have restless and fragmented sleep; PSG is recommended for these children. Periodic limb movements (PLMS) are polysomnographic findings and are characterized by stereotypical jerks lasting between 0.5 to 10.0 seconds and occurring at 15- to 40-second intervals. An index of 5 or more PLMS per hour is abnormal in pediatric patients [47,49]. PLMS are present in approximately 80% of patients with RLS, and a periodic limb movement index of 5 or greater, when associated with a sleep complaint not accountable by any other sleep disorder, may suggest a periodic limb movement disorder (PLMD).

Various systemic changes including increased blood pressure and heart rate occur during PLMS [50,51]. Most patients with PLMS are not aware of these changes and the associated arousals that disturb their sleep. There seems to be a close relationship between RLS and PLMD in children based on family history and long-term follow-up studies [44,51–53].

The exacerbating factors for RLS include sleep deprivation, irregular sleep schedules, low body iron stores, caffeine, nicotine, alcohol, and certain medications (eg, antihistamines, serotonergic antidepressants, and neuroleptics). The management of RLS and PLMD in children involves both nonpharmacologic and pharmacologic approaches; currently there are no FDA-approved medications for children. Although emerging literature supports medical therapy in children with RLS and PLMD, experiences with these medications are limited. Most children and adolescents with RLS and PLMD have low iron storage; therefore, iron therapy should be considered as the first line of treatment. A serum ferritin of greater than 50 ng/mL is considered an adequate therapeutic target in children [44]. Correcting iron deficiency in children with RLS/PLMD can be difficult because it not well-absorbed in the gastrointestinal tract. Systemic illness in children can further limit iron absorption. Compliance with oral iron therapy in children is difficult owing to its gastrointestinal side effects, such as constipation. Iron absorption can be enhanced by oral vitamin C and by not taking it within 2 hours of consuming calcium/dairy products. An alternative intravenous iron sucrose treatment has shown to be beneficial for children with RLS/PLMD who cannot tolerate oral iron preparations or when there is a need for a rapid replenishment of iron stores [44].

The literature supports the use of off-label medication in pediatric RLS. Clonidine is the most commonly used medication for children with sleep problems and it is particularly useful when there are severe sleep onset problems in children with RLS [54,55]. It is typically prescribed at a dose of 0.2 to 0.4 mg at bedtime. Gabapentin, an anticonvulsant, can improve sleep quality and decrease the sensory symptoms of RLS [44,55]. Ropinirole and pramipexole are dopamine agonists that are FDA approved for RLS in adults.

SUMMARY

In recent years, an increased understanding and awareness of sleep disorders in children have been achieved. Further understanding and research into the pathophysiology, epidemiology, clinical evaluation methods, sequelae, and supportive treatment options for children with sleep disorders are needed to effectively manage them in the clinical settings. Clarification of the important role that sleep disturbances play in children with medical, developmental, and mental health disorders is a goal for future research.

Acknowledgments

I would like to acknowledge Elizabeth Kociolek, MS, BA for her administrative support in composing this manuscript.

References

[1] Maski KP, Kothare SV. Sleep deprivation and neurobehavioral functioning in children. Int J Psychophysiol 2013;89:259–64.
[2] Ophoff D, Slaats MA, Boudewyns A, et al. Sleep disorders during childhood: a practical review. Eur J Pediatr 2018;177:641–8.
[3] Maski K, Owens JA. Insomnia, parasomnias and narcolepsy in children: clinical features, diagnosis and management. Lancet Neurol 2016;15(11):1170–81.
[4] International classification of sleep disorders. 3rd edition. Darien (IL): American Academy of Sleep Medicine; 2014.
[5] Ruoff C, Rye D. The ICSD-3 and DSM-5 guidelines for diagnosing narcolepsy: clinical relevance and practicality. Curr Med Res Opin 2016;32:1611–22.
[6] Thorpy MJ, Kriger AC. Delayed diagnosis of narcolepsy: characterization and impact. Sleep Med 2014;15(5):502–7.
[7] Scammell TE. Narcolepsy. N Engl J Med 2015;373:2654–62.
[8] Serra L, Montahna P, Mignot E, et al. cataplexy features in childhood narcolepsy. Mov Disord 2008;23:1012–20.
[9] Lecendreux M, Lavault S, Lopez R, et al. Attention-deficit/hyperactivity disorder (ADHD) symptoms in pediatric narcolepsy: a cross-sectional study. Sleep 2015;38:1285–95.
[10] Mignot EJ. History of narcolepsy at Stanford University. Immunol Res 2014;58:315–39.
[11] Iglowstein I, Jenni OG, Molinari L, et al. Sleep duration from infancy to adolescence: reference values and generational trends. Pediatrics 2003;111:302–7.
[12] Kotagal S, Krahn LE, Slocumb N. A putative link between childhood narcolepsy and obesity. Sleep Med 2004;5:147–50.
[13] Poli F, Pizza F, Mignot E, et al. High prevalence of precocious puberty and obesity in childhood narcolepsy with cataplexy. Sleep 2013;36:175–81.
[14] Thorpy MJ, Kriger AC. Delayed diagnosis of narcolepsy: characterization and impact. Sleep Med 2014;15(5):502–7.
[15] Andlauer O, Moore H, Jouhier L, et al. Nocturnal rapid eye movement sleep latency for identifying patients with narcolepsy/hypocretin deficiency. JAMA Neurol 2013;70:891–902.

[16] Littner MR, Kushida C, Wise M, et al. Practice parameters for clinical use of the multiple sleep latency test and the maintenance of wakefulness test. Sleep 2005;28:113–21.
[17] Mignot E, Lammers GJ, Ripley B, et al. The role of cerebrospinal fluid hypocretin measurement in the diagnosis of narcolepsy and other hypersomnias. Arch Neurol 2002;59: 1553–62.
[18] Ivanenko A, Tauman R, Gozal D. Modafinil in the treatment of excessive daytime sleepiness in children. Sleep Med 2003;4:579–82.
[19] Lecendreux M, Poli F, Oudiette D, et al. Tolerance and efficacy of sodium oxybate in childhood narcolepsy with cataplexy: a retrospective study. Sleep 2012;35:709–11.
[20] Bhattarai J, Sumerall S. Current and future treatment options for narcolepsy: a review. Sleep Sci 2017;10:19–27.
[21] Marcus CL, Brooks LJ, Draper KA, et al. Diagnosis and management of childhood obstructive sleep apnea syndrome. Pediatrics 2012;140(3):576–84.
[22] Da Silva Gusmao Cardoso T, Pompeia S, Miranda MC. Cognitive and behavioral effects of obstructive sleep apnea syndrome in children: a systematic literature review. Sleep Med 2018;46:46–55.
[23] Amini Z, Kotagal S, Lohse C, et al. Effect of obstructive sleep apnea treatment on lipids in obese children. Children 2017;44(4).
[24] Dehlink E, Tan HL. Update on paediatric obstructive sleep apnoea. J Thorac Dis 2016;8(2): 224–35.
[25] Bhattacharjee R, Kheirandish-Gozal L, Spruyt K, et al. Adenotonsillectomy outcomes in treatment of obstructive sleep apnea in children: a multicenter retrospective study. Am J Respir Crit Care Med 2010;182:676–83.
[26] Chan CCK, Au CT, Lam HS, et al. Intranasal corticosteroids for mild childhood obstructive sleep apnea-a randomized, placebo-controlled study. Sleep Med 2015;16:358–63.
[27] Noller MW, Guilleminault C, Gouveia CJ, et al. Mandibular advancement for pediatric obstructive sleep apnea: a systematic review and meta-analysis. J Craniomaxillofac Surg 2018;46:1296–302.
[28] Eckert D, Jordan A, Merchia P, et al. Central sleep apnea. Chest 2007;131(2):595–607.
[29] Zhao J, Gonzalez F, Mu D. Apnea of prematurity: from cause to treatment. Eur J Pediatr 2011;170(9):1097–105.
[30] Zee P, Attarian H, Videnovic A. Circadian rhythm abnormalities. American Academy of Neurology, 2013. Continuum (Minneap Minn) 2013;19(1):132–47.
[31] Meltzer L, Crabtree V. Pediatric sleep problems, a clinician's guide to behavioral interventions. Washington, DC: American Psychological Association; 2015.
[32] Sateia MJ, Buysse DJ, Krystal AD, et al. Clinical practice guideline for the pharmacologic treatment of chronic insomnia in adults: an American Academy of Sleep Medicine clinical practice guideline. J Clin Sleep Med 2017;13(2):307–49.
[33] Braam W, Smits MG, Didden R, et al. Exogenous melatonin for sleep problems in individuals with intellectual disability: a meta-analysis. Dev Med Child Neurol 2009;51(5):340–9.
[34] Weiss M, Wasdell M, Bomben M, et al. Sleep hygiene and melatonin treatment for children and adolescents with ADHD and initial insomnia. J Am Acad Child Adolesc Psychiatry 2006;45(5):512–9.
[35] Gagnon K, Godbout R. Melatonin and comorbidities in children with autism spectrum disorder. Curr Dev Disord Rep 2018;5:197–206.
[36] Irfan M, Schenck CH, Howell MJ. Non-rapid eye movement sleep and overlap parasomnias. Continuum (Minneap Minn) 2017;23:1035–50.
[37] Kotagal S. Sleep-wake disorders of childhood. Continuum (Minneap Minn) 2017;23(4): 1132–50.
[38] Berry R, Wagner M. Sleep medicine pearls. Fundamentals 35 – parasomnia. Philadelphia: Elsevier Inc; 2015.
[39] Reynolds K, Alfano C. Things that go bump in the night: frequency and predictors of nightmares in anxious and nonanxious children. Behav Sleep Med 2016;14:442–56.

[40] Morin C, Espie C. The Oxford handbook of sleep and sleep disorders. New York: Oxford University Press, Inc.; 2012.
[41] Picchietti D, Allen RP, Walters AS, et al. Restless legs syndrome: prevalence and impact in children and adolescents – the Peds REST study. Pediatrics 2007;120(2):253–66.
[42] Mohri I, Kato-Nishimura K, Tachibana N, et al. Restless legs syndrome (RLS): an unrecognized cause for bedtime problems and insomnia in children. Sleep Med 2008;9(6):701–2.
[43] Kushida CA. Clinical presentation, diagnosis, and quality of life issues in restless legs syndrome [review]. Am J Med 2007;120(1 Suppl 1):S4–12.
[44] Picchietti MA, Picchietti DL. Advances in pediatric restless legs syndrome: iron, genetics, diagnosis and treatment. Sleep Med 2010;11:643–51.
[45] Pullen SJ, Wall CA, Angstman ER, et al. Psychiatric comorbidity in children and adolescents with restless legs syndrome: a retrospective study. J Clin Sleep Med 2011;7:587–96.
[46] Picchietti DL, Bruni O, De Weerd A, et al. Pediatric restless legs syndrome diagnostic criteria: an update by the International Restless Legs Syndrome Study Group. Sleep Med 2013;14:1253–9.
[47] Allen RP. Restless legs syndrome: diagnostic criteria, special considerations, and epidemiology: a report from the restless legs syndrome diagnosis and epidemiology workshop at the National Institutes of Health. Sleep Med 2003;4(2):101–19.
[48] Iber C, Ancoli-Israel S, Chesson A, et al. Quan The AASM manual for the scoring of sleep and associated events: rules, terminology and technical specifications. 1st edition. Westchester (IL): American Academy of Sleep Medicine; 2007.
[49] Martinez S, Guilleminault C. Periodic leg movements in prepubertal children with sleep disturbance. Dev Med Child Neurol 2004;46(11):76570.
[50] Pennestri MH, Montplaisir J, Colombo R, et al. Nocturnal blood pressure changes in patients with restless legs syndrome. Neurology 2007;68(15):1213–8.
[51] Walters AS, Rye DB. Review of the relationship of restless legs syndrome and periodic limb movements in sleep to hypertension, heart disease stroke. Sleep 2009;32(5):589–97.
[52] Winkelman JW. Periodic limb movements in sleep—endophenotype for restless legs syndrome? N Engl J Med 2007;357:703–5.
[53] Picchietti DL, Rajendran RR, Wilson MP, et al. Pediatric restless legs syndrome and periodic limb movement disorder: parent–child pairs. Sleep Med 2009;10:925–31.
[54] Newcorn JH, Schulz K, Harrison M, et al. Alpha 2 adrenergic agonists. Neurochemistry, efficacy, clinical guidelines use children. Pediatr Clin North Am 1998;45(5):1022–99.
[55] Kotagal S, Silber MH. Childhood-onset restless legs syndrome. Ann Neurol 2004;56(6):803–7.

Advances in Pediatrics 66 (2019) 161–176

ADVANCES IN PEDIATRICS

Tall Stature in Children

Alexander K.C. Leung, MBBS, FRCPC, FRCP(UK & Irel), FRCPCH[a,*],
Alexander A.C. Leung, MD, MPH, FRCPC, MRCP (UK)[b,c],
Kam Lun Hon, MD[d]

[a]Department of Pediatrics, The University of Calgary, The Alberta Children's Hospital, #200, 233-16th Avenue North West, Calgary, Alberta T2M 0H5, Canada; [b]Department of Medicine, Community Health Sciences, and Oncology, The University of Calgary, 2500 University Drive, Northwest, Calgary, Alberta T2N 1N4, Canada; [c]Richmond Road Diagnostic and Treatment Centre, 1820 Richmond Road South West, Calgary, Alberta T2T 5C7, Canada; [d]Department of Pediatrics, The Chinese University of Hong Kong, 6/F, Clinical Sciences Building, Shatin, Hong Kong

Keywords

• Familial • Constitutional • Pathologic • Bone age • Growth hormone • Estrogen • Testosterone • Percutaneous epiphysiodesis

Key points

- Most tall children are healthy and simply have a familial tendency to tallness.
- Bone age determination is useful in the differential diagnosis of the various causes of tall stature and prediction of adult height of an individual.
- Children with constitutional and familial tall stature rarely require therapeutic intervention.
- Hormonal administration of estradiol or testosterone to children should be used with caution and only if the benefits outweigh the risks.

INTRODUCTION

Tall stature in children is arbitrarily defined as a height greater than 2 standard deviations (97.7%) more than the mean height for a population of the same sex, age, and race [1–5]. By definition, 2.3% of children have tall stature [3]. Stature is determined by the complex interaction of genetic, hormonal, nutritional, and

Portions of this article are reprinted from Leung AK. Tall stature. In Leung AK. Common Problems in Ambulatory Pediatrics: Symptoms and Signs. New York: Nova Science Publishers, Inc, 2011, pp 303-311; with permission from Nova Science Publishers, Inc.

*Corresponding author. *E-mail address:* aleung@ucalgary.ca

https://doi.org/10.1016/j.yapd.2019.04.004

environmental factors [3,5,6]. The growth hormone (GH)–insulinlike growth factor-1 (IGF-1) axis is only 1 of many regulatory systems that control chrondrogenesis in the growth plate and ultimate adult height [7]. Many other hormones such as thyroid hormone, glucocorticoids, estrogens, and androgens regulate linear growth [7]. In some cases, genetic mutations may lead to tall stature [7]. Familial tall stature is the most common cause of tall stature, followed by constitutional tall stature. Many pathologic conditions, although uncommon, also present with tall stature. Some of these conditions are associated with severe comorbidities. It is, therefore, important to distinguish tall children who are otherwise healthy from those who have underlying pathology [4]. Furthermore, excessively tall stature, especially of girls, can cause serious psychological problems. Tall individuals may also experience backache or other musculoskeletal complaints.

MEASUREMENTS OF GROWTH

The child should stand straight, with the back of the head, back, buttocks, and heels touching a firm vertical structure such as the vertical bar of a stadiometer, with shoes off and interfering hair accessories removed [8]. The horizontal measuring bar of the stadiometer should be lowered to level with the child's head to obtain the measurement [4]. Alternatively, a firm object can be placed at a right angle on the top of the head and against the wall above the head for the measurement to be made. A child younger than 3 years of age should be measured on a firm horizontal platform that contains an attached yardstick, a fixed head plate, and a movable foot plate [8]. The child's feet should be held steady while the measurement is made [4].

The growth charts that have been widely used are those published by the World Health Organization (WHO) as well as those published by the Centers for Disease Control and Prevention and National Center for Health Statistics (CDC/NCHS) [9]. The former are based on a pooled sample from 6 participating countries (Brazil, Ghana, Oman, India, Norway, the United States [California]) where children are raised under optimal environmental conditions (ie, economically advantaged, breastfed infants, and children of nonsmoking mothers), whereas the latter are based on large surveys of multiethnic populations for children living in the United States [9,10]. The WHO standards define a pediatric population that is leaner and taller than the CDC/NCHS standards [9]. The CDC and the American Academy of Pediatrics (AAP) recommend using the WHO growth charts for children younger than 2 years and the CDC/NCHS growth charts for children older than 2 years [11]. Because there are significant differences in growth rates, adult heights, and age of onset of puberty among different ethnic groups, it would be of great advantage to use standards based on ethnicity, whenever possible, for the child being assessed [6,12]. Unfortunately, such standard growth charts are not always available for every ethnic group.

In addition to the height and weight, careful and precise measurement of arm span (distance between tips of the middle fingers with the arms raised and stretched to a horizontal position) and upper/lower segment ratio is important in the physical examination [1]. The lower body segment can be determined by measuring the distance from the symphysis pubis to the floor with the child standing erect against a wall [1]. The upper body segment value can be obtained by subtracting the lower body segment value from the child's height. The upper/lower segment ratio is then derived by dividing the upper segment value by the lower segment value. For North American children, the upper/lower segment ratio is approximately 1.7 at birth [4]. With growth of the limbs, the ratio declines gradually to 1.25 at around 3 years of age and to 1 at around 14 years of age, with little change thereafter [13]. In adult black individuals, the upper/lower segment ratio is approximately 0.85 to 0.9, as blacks have relatively long limbs. On the other hand, Asian children have shorter limbs and therefore have a higher upper/lower segment ratio [14]. Children with proportional overgrowth such as familial tall stature, constitutional tall stature, exogenous obesity, precocious puberty, Soto syndrome, Weaver syndrome, and fragile X syndrome have a normal upper/lower segment ratio [4,11]. On the other hand, children with Klinefelter syndrome, Marfan syndrome, and homocystinuria have disproportionally long lower extremities and therefore have a decreased upper/lower segment ratio [11].

CAUSES AND CLINICAL MANIFESTATIONS

Familial tall stature

Familial or genetic tall stature is the most common cause of tall stature [1,2,15,16]. These children are usually tall from early infancy, grow along the same percentile and reach a correspondingly tall adult height [3]. These children have a high normal growth rate and otherwise normal findings on physical examination. The height age is greater than bone age, which is compatible with the chronologic age [1,17]. These children have tall parents. Comparing the growth of the patient and the parents on a growth chart reveals that the tall stature is appropriate for that family.

Constitutional tall stature

Constitutional tall stature, also known as constitutional advancement of growth, is the second most common cause of tall stature [4,15,18]. Children with constitutional tall stature have normal length at birth. The growth velocity accelerates in early childhood and the tall stature is usually evident by the age of 2 to 4 years [1,19]. The growth velocity slows down after the child reaches 4 or 5 years. The growth curve is parallel to and above the normal curve, and the child grows along this percentile until puberty [11,19]. The height age corresponds to the slightly advanced bone age and is greater than the chronologic age [11,17]. Pubertal development usually begins in the early range of normal, and final adult height is often in the upper range of normal [11,17]. There is usually a family history of "early bloomers." A recent study suggested that there may be a greater expression of the growth receptor gene in these children [18].

Exogenous obesity

Children with exogenous obesity are usually tall for their age and have an early onset of puberty, especially in girls [5,20]. In these children, bone age is advanced and proportional to height age, and the adolescent growth spurt begins and ends early [3]. These children often attain normal adult height or are only slightly taller than average as adults [5,21]. Presumably, the tall stature and increased growth velocity is mediated by ghrelin, which is a GH secretagog, as well as insulin and IGF-1 [21,22].

Precocious puberty

True precocious puberty (gonadotropin-dependent precocious puberty) results from a premature increase in pituitary secretion of gonadotropins with a consequent increase in gonadal sex hormones, as in normal puberty [23]. The condition is more common in girls than in boys [23]. Pseudoprecocious puberty (gonadotropin-independent precocious puberty) results from autonomous gonadal or adrenal sex hormone secretion, independent of pituitary gonadotrophic secretion, or from iatrogenic administration of sex hormones [23]. In children with precocious puberty, acceleration of linear growth invariably occurs simultaneously with signs of premature sexual development. Rapid growth is accompanied by a rate of osseous maturation that is greater than expected for the chronologic age. The advanced bone age results in early epiphyseal closure [19,23]. Consequently, the ultimate adult height is less than it would have been otherwise [19,20,23].

Pituitary growth hormone excess

GH hypersecretion in children is usually caused by a GH-producing pituitary adenoma [16,20]. Circulating basal GH levels are easily detectable and are often greater than 15 μg/L (normal range, 0–3 μg/L for males and 0 to 8 μg/L for females) [24]. The diagnosis of GH excess is confirmed by dynamic testing with failure to suppress the serum GH level to less than 1 μg/L (with specific cutoffs dependent on laboratory assay) 2 hours after an oral glucose load of 1.75 g/kg (maximum 75 g) [25]. Because of the large intraindividual variability in serum GH levels, serum IGF-1 is the recommended screening test [3]. Before the epiphyses close, an excess of GH produces accelerated linear growth and results in gigantism. Bone age is often advanced, but may be normal or delayed if the disease interferes with pituitary gonadotropin secretion [5]. An excess of GH after the epiphyses fuse results in acromegaly, a disorder characterized by large hands and feet, overgrowth of the mandible and supra-orbital ridges, and coarse facial features [1]. Pituitary tumors are associated with headache, decreased visual acuity, visual field defects (typically bitemporal hemianopsia), and symptoms or signs suggesting increased intracranial pressure. Tumors may also be associated with deficiency of other pituitary hormones, such as thyrotropin, corticotropin, and gonadotropin, as well as prolactin excess [1].

Sotos syndrome (cerebral gigantism)

Children with Sotos syndrome are often large at birth, and their growth is most rapid during the first few years of life [1]. Height continues to be more than 2 standard deviations until puberty [3]. Thereafter, the growth velocity slows down and the growth curve remains parallel to and above the normal curve. Other features include macrocephaly, frontal bossing, prominent forehead, hypertelorism, coarse facial features, prominent ears, pointed chin, high arched palate, malar flushing, down-slanting palpebral fissures, large hands and feet, increased arm span compared with height, clumsiness, intellectual and developmental disability, and tendency to aggressive behavior [3,21,26,27]. The bone age is often advanced and compatible with the height of the patient [3,27]. Puberty usually occurs early with premature epiphyseal fusion and most children achieve normal adult height [5]. Biochemical studies, including serum GH levels, are normal. In most patients, the lateral and third ventricles are mildly dilated. Electroencephalograms (EEGs) are often abnormal. Seizures, scoliosis, cardiac anomalies, and renal anomalies occur in 15% to 30% of patients [3,27]. Most cases are sporadic [5]. Familial cases are usually consistent with an autosomal dominant mode of inheritance [6]. Mutations and deletions of nuclear receptor set domain containing protein 1 (*NSD1*) gene at chromosome 5q35 occur in more than 90% of patients with Sotos syndrome [3,21,27,28]. Most mutations are de novo [3].

Hyperthyroidism

Excessive thyroid hormone in early childhood leads to an acceleration in linear growth and proportional osseous maturation [3]. Presumably, the thyroid hormone works synergistically with IGF-1 to stimulate growth [21]. Craniosynostosis sometimes develops when hyperthyroidism appears early in life. Proper and timely treatment of hyperthyroidism restores euthyroidism and normalizes the growth rate so that the ultimate adult height is unaffected [3].

Marfan syndrome

Marfan syndrome is characterized by tall stature, arachnodactyly, upward subluxation or dislocation of lens, and aortic or mitral regurgitation [21]. The arm span is greater than the height with an arm span to height ratio greater than 1.05 [24]. The upper/lower segment ratio is diminished. Bone age is usually normal. Other clinical features include joint hyperextension, striae distensae, hypotonia, narrow facies, high arched palate, inguinal/femoral hernia, pectus excavatum/carinatum, kyphoscoliosis, megalocornea, and myopia. Retinal detachment, mitral valve prolapse, and aortic aneurysm and rupture are important complications. Marfan syndrome is inherited as an autosomal dominant trait. The condition results from a mutation in the fibrillin-1 (*FBN1*) gene on chromosome 15q [3,29,30].

Homocystinuria

Homocystinuria is an autosomal recessive disorder caused by a deficiency of cystathionine β-synthetase (CBS) with resultant excretion of large amounts of homocysteine in the urine [21]. Patients with this disorder have a phenotypic appearance similar to those with Marfan syndrome [19]. Additional features of homocystinuria include intellectual and developmental disability, malar flush, downward subluxation or dislocation of lens, an increased incidence of seizures, arterial and venous thrombosis, osteoporosis, and vertebral collapse [3,19]. The condition results from mutation of the gene that encodes CBS.

Klinefelter syndrome

Klinefelter syndrome is due to the presence of more than 1 X chromosome in a male patient. The most common abnormal karyotype is 47 XXY. Affected children are tall and have eunuchoid proportions with a long arm span and legs, a decreased upper/lower segment ratio, possibly because of a third copy of the *SHOX* gene [31]. Tall stature is present before puberty [21,28]. Genital abnormalities, such as hypogonadism, cryptorchidism, a small phallus, and hypospadias are sometimes present [32,33]. Sertoli cell function and spermatogenesis are often defective, with resultant subfertility/infertility. Gynecomastia is common during adolescence [33]. Cognitive impairment, which may be evident in learning disabilities, especially in expressive language, and behavioral difficulties, such as excessive shyness, aggressiveness, and antisocial behavior, are often present [1]. Other features include hypertelorism, hypotonia, and clinodactyly. Bone age may be normal or delayed, depending on the level of testosterone secretion [5]. The condition is associated with hypergonadotropic hypogonadism. Serum follicle-stimulating hormone (FSH) and luteinizing hormone (LH) levels are usually normal in prepubertal children, but are high in adolescents and adults [5]. Serum testosterone levels are usually in the low normal range [5]. Patients with Klinefelter syndrome are at risk for breast cancer, cholelithiasis, type 2 diabetes mellitus, and metabolic syndrome [34,35].

XYY syndrome

The presence of an extra Y chromosome predisposes an individual to tall stature [1]. Patients with 1 (47, XYY) or more (48, XYYY) extra Y chromosomes achieve a greater than average adult height. Other features include severe nodulocystic acne, macrocephaly, large teeth, hypertelorism, clinodactyly, radioulnar synostosis, hypotonia, incoordination, tremor, macroorchidism, subfertility, learning difficulties, delayed speech, autism spectrum disorder, impulsivity, attention deficit hyperactivity disorder, physical aggressiveness, violence, and antisocial behavior [5,36,37].

Trisomy X (47, XXX females)

Patients with trisomy X tend to be tall, most probably because of the extra X chromosome and an extra copy of the *SHOX* gene [21]. The height is usually normal until 4 years of age. Affected children have long legs, which are obvious before puberty [21]. Most of these patients have a normal phenotype and have normal sexual development; fertility is not an issue, although ovarian failure and amenorrhea have been reported in some cases [3]. Some patients have minimal dysmorphic features such as epicanthal folds, up-slanting palpebral fissures, hypertelorism, hypotonia, joint hyperextensibility, pes planus, clinodactyly, and syndactyly [21].

Fragile X syndrome

Fragile X syndrome is characterized by intellectual and developmental disability, large and protruding auricles, and tall stature [3,21]. Other features include hypotonia, long and narrow face, flexible fingers, delayed speech, autism, strabismus, hyperactivity, and mitral valve prolapse [3,6]. Heterozygous females may also exhibit these features, although to a lesser extent [3]. Males with fragile X syndrome have macroorchidism [3,21]. An increase in growth rate often occurs during the preadolescent period. The growth rate slows down after puberty, resulting in a normal height in adulthood [3]. Fragile X syndrome is an X-linked dominant disorder with variable expressivity [6]. The gene that when disrupted results in fragile X syndrome has been mapped to Xq27.3 [21]. The DNA segment shows a peculiar stretch of trinucleotide (cytidine, guanosine, guanosine [CGG]) repeats in the fragile X mental retardation gene 1 (*FMR1*) [3,21]. The hypermethylated CGG-repeat stretch results in constriction of the X chromosome [6]. Fragile X syndrome may also arise in patients with deletions and point mutations of the *FMR1* gene without CGG amplification [21].

Hypogonadal syndromes

Hypogonadal syndromes such as aromatase deficiency, estrogen resistance, androgen insensitivity, and Kallmann syndrome can cause tall stature and eunuchoid body proportions (long legs, lower upper/lower segment ratio) [3,19]. The lack of sex hormones delays osseous maturation and epiphyseal fusion [19]. This allows continued, although slow, growth to a later age and tall stature in adolescence and beyond [19].

Familial glucocorticoid deficiency

Familial glucocorticoid deficiency is an autosomal recessive disorder of adrenal unresponsiveness to adrenocorticotropic hormone (ACTH). Type 1 is caused by mutations in the ACTH melanocortin 2 receptor (*MC2R*) gene, whereas type 2 is caused by mutations in the melanocortin 2 receptor accessory protein (*MCAP*) [38]. The condition is characterized by glucocorticoid deficiency, high ACTH levels, and normal mineralocorticoid levels [38]. Clinically, the condition presents with tall stature with advanced bone age, hypoglycemic episodes, fatigability, weakness, anorexia, vomiting, abdominal pain, weight loss, and generalized hyperpigmentation [38].

Beckwith-Wiedemann syndrome

Beckwith-Wiedemann syndrome is characterized by macrosomia, macroglossia, visceromegaly, abdominal wall defects (omphalocele, umbilical hernia, diastasis recti), and neonatal hypoglycemia [3,17]. Other features include facial nevus flammeus, earlobe malformation, prominent occiput, hemihyperplasia, renal medullary hyperplasia, cardiovascular abnormalities, hypothyroidism, thyroxine-binding globulin deficiency, and increased risk for embryonal tumors, notably Wilms tumor and adrenal cortical carcinoma [3,17,28,39]. Postnatal gigantism is common. Bone age is advanced but is appropriate for height age. Adult height is usually higher than the range predicted by the family [5].

Most cases are associated with maternal hypomethylation of 11p15, paternal uniparental disomy at chromosome 11p15, unbalanced translocations leading to trisomy of the 11p15 locus, and, less commonly, from a mutation in *CDKN1C* gene in the maternal allele [17,26,28]. IGF-2 plays an important role in the expression of this phenotype [5].

McCune-Albright syndrome

McCune-Albright syndrome is characterized by polyostotic fibrous dysplasia of bone, café au lait spots typically with irregular margins giving them a "coast of Maine" appearance, and sexual precocity. There is a high frequency of testicular abnormalities in boys and ovarian abnormalities in girls [6]. The syndrome is caused by an activating mutation in the *GNAS* gene, which encodes the alpha subunit of the stimulatory G-protein complexes involved in G-protein signaling [6,17,40]. The tall stature in McCune-Albright syndrome is due to excess GH, thyroid hormone, or sex hormone, or a combination of these [28]. The adult height can be less than normal owing to early fusion of the epiphyses if the condition remains untreated.

Weaver syndrome

Weaver syndrome is characterized by accelerated linear growth, advanced bone age, camptodactyly, mild intellectual and developmental disability, and characteristic facial features, including micrognathia, hypertelorism, down-slanting palpebral fissures, strabismus, large and dysplastic ears, megacephaly, broad forehead, flat occiput, long and wide philtrum, and depressed nasal bridge [17]. The excessive growth is present at birth or has its onset during infancy [21]. The syndrome is caused by missense and truncating mutations in enhancer of zeste homolog 2 (*EZH2*) or embryonic ectoderm development (*EED*) genes [41]. *EZH2* and *EED* are core components of the polycomb repressive complex 2 (*PRC2*), which possesses histone methyltransferase activity and catalyzes trimethylation of histone 3 at lysine 27 [41].

Proteus syndrome

Proteus syndrome is characterized by overgrowth of various body parts, macrocephaly, frontotemporal exostosis, multiple hyperpigmented warty nevi, and subcutaneous vascular tumors. In most individuals, the overgrowth starts in the first few years of life. The overgrowth can be generalized (whole body), unilateral (hemihyperplasia), or localized (macrodactyly). The syndrome is caused by activating mutations of *AKT1* and *PTEN* genes [6].

Congenital generalized lipodystrophy

Congenital generalized lipodystrophy is an autosomal recessive disorder [5]. Children with congenital generalized lipodystrophy have accelerated linear and muscular growth together with advanced bone age. Affected children have a generalized loss of subcutaneous and visceral fat. Acromegaloid changes, large hands and feet, prominent mandible, acanthosis nigricans, penile/clitoral enlargement, prominent superficial veins, hirsutism, alopecia, hepatomegaly, and hypertrophic cardiomyopathy can be present [1,5,21]. There is an increased risk for hyperlipidemia, insulin resistance, hyperinsulinism, and nonketotic diabetes mellitus [21].

Simpson-Golabi-Behmel syndrome

Simpson-Golabi-Behmel syndrome is characterized by prenatal and postnatal overgrowth (tall stature, macrocephaly, macroglossia, visceromegaly), distinctive craniofacial features ("coarse" or "bulldog" face, hypertelorism, broad nasal bridge, macrognathia, cleft lip/palate, macrostomia), and multiple congenital abnormalities (cardiovascular malformations, central nervous system malformations, multicystic dysplastic kidneys, congenital diaphragmatic hernia, omphalocele, polydactyly, broad hands and feet with hypoplastic/absent fingernails, vertebral segmentation defects, pectus excavatum) [6,17,21,42]. Other features include neonatal hypoglycemia and hypotonia. Affected individuals are at risk for embryonal tumors, notably Wilms tumor, neuroblastoma, and hepatoblastoma [21]. The bone age is advanced. Simpson-Golabi-Behmel syndrome is an X-linked recessive disorder. The classic form (type I) is caused by mutations in glypican-3 gene (*GPC3*) at Xq28. The extremely rare and lethal form (type II) is caused by mutations in the gene at Xp22 [21,42].

CLINICAL EVALUATION

In most cases, a diagnosis can be established from a careful history and physical examination. Familiarity with the many diseases and syndromes associated with tall stature is important; in some cases, the diagnosis can be established immediately.

The most important historical information in the evaluation of a child with tall stature is the family history of the pattern of growth and the age of onset of puberty in parents and siblings. In familial tall stature, the child's height is consistent with the midparental height [4]. On the other hand, in pathologic tall stature, the child's projected height usually far exceeds the midparental height [4]. The midparental height can be calculated by averaging the parents' heights after first adding 13 cm to the mother's height if the patient is a boy or subtracting 13 cm from the father's height if the patient is a girl [4]. Any familial conditions associated with tall stature should be noted. All previous heights, weights, and head circumferences (if applicable) should be obtained and plotted on a growth chart. The size at birth and the period of growth acceleration should be noted [43]. If the growth records of the parents are available, they should also be plotted for comparison.

A functional inquiry is important and in some cases reveals the underlying cause of tall stature. Any medical, social, or psychological problems associated with tall stature should be noted. Developmental, behavioral, and learning problems are associated with many syndromes.

A careful and precise measurement of the height, weight, head circumference, arm span, and upper/lower segment ratio is necessary. Children with familial tall stature and constitutional tall stature have a normal upper/lower segment ratio and arm span, whereas those with pathologic conditions such as Marfan syndrome and Klinefelter syndrome have an increased arm span and a decreased upper/lower segment ratio [4]. An obese child with no other abnormal physical findings suggests obesity as the cause of the tall stature. The body mass index, calculated by dividing the weight in kilograms by the height in meters squared (kg/m^2), is a widely accepted measure of adiposity. The stage of puberty should be assessed. A patient with absent or markedly delayed puberty may have hypogonadism, be it primary or secondary [21]. On the other hand, early pubertal changes suggest true precocious puberty or pseudoprecocious puberty.

A complete physical examination should be performed. Any dysmorphic features and abnormal physical findings (eg, heart murmur, organomegaly, pectus excavatum, scoliosis) should be noted. Coarse facial features, large hands and feet, and overgrowth of the mandible suggest GH excess or Sotos syndrome. Individuals with Sotos syndrome have, in addition, frontal bossing, macrocephaly, clumsiness, and intellectual and developmental disability. Superior subluxation of lens suggests Marfan syndrome, whereas inferior subluxation of lens suggests homocystinuria [4]. Macroorchidism is found in patients with fragile X syndrome, whereas signs of hypogonadism are found in patients with Klinefelter syndrome.

DIAGNOSTIC STUDIES

If the history and physical examination point to familial tall stature or constitutional tall stature, no investigation is usually necessary as long as the child is developing normally [16]. Bone age determination can help to confirm the diagnosis and is useful in estimating the probable adult height of the individual. The most commonly used tool to assess bone age is the atlas developed by Greulich and Pyle [44,45]. In this method, the appearance of different epiphyseal centers on the left hand and wrist radiograph is compared with the standards in the atlas [46,47]. If the bone age is delayed or advanced, then the projected height should be recalculated based on the bone age rather than the chronologic age [5]. The table developed by Bayley and Pinneau can be used to predict the adult height based on the child's bone age and chronologic age [5,48]. The Bayley and Pinneau method tends to overestimate the adult height in those with a bone age of 14 years or less, whereas the height predictions are accurate thereafter [49]. On the other hand, the Tanner-Whitehouse mark II method gives a good estimation of final height up to the bone age of 13 years in boys and 12 years in girls but tends to overestimate thereafter [44,45,49].

A significantly advanced bone age is sometimes seen in patients with true precocious puberty, adrenal or gonadal neoplasms, and congenital adrenal hyperplasia. Bone age is mildly or moderately advanced in patients with exogenous obesity, pituitary GH excess, hyperthyroidism, Sotos syndrome, Beckwith-Wiedemann syndrome, Weaver syndrome, and congenital generalized lipodystrophy [1,3,4]. Bone age is mildly advanced in children with constitutional tall stature and consistent with the height age, normal in children with familial tall stature, and delayed in patients with a hypogonadal syndrome.

Serum IGF-1 levels should be obtained to screen for GH excess [20,21]. The definitive test for the diagnosis of excessive GH secretion is the failure of serum GH to decrease to less than 1 μg/L (with specific cutoffs dependent on the laboratory assay) after an oral glucose load (1.75 g/kg; maximum 75 g) [21]. Magnetic resonance imaging (MRI) evaluation of the pituitary should be performed if there is evidence of GH excess.

If there is evidence of precocious puberty, determination of serum FSH, LH, estradiol, testosterone, dehydroepiandrosterone (DHEA), dehydroepiandrosterone sulfate (DHEAS), androstenedione, and 17α-hydroxyprogesterone may help to distinguish true (central) precocious puberty from pseudoprecocious puberty [23,43,50].

A karyotype is needed because trisomy X (XXX females) and XYY males may have tall stature as the sole manifestation [19,21]. Chromosome analysis should be performed in the presence of dysmorphic features especially with development delay and when the presentation is atypical and the diagnosis difficult. Fluorescence in situ hybridization can be used to detect small chromosomal abnormalities such as duplications and deletions. This approach is only useful when the clinicians is considering a specific deletion or duplication for a differential diagnosis. For example, *NSD1* and *FBN1* gene sequencing should be considered if Soto syndrome and Marfan syndrome are suspected, respectively [6]. Analysis of *FMR1* and CGG number should be considered if fragile X syndrome is considered [6].

Other laboratory tests and diagnostic imaging studies (Table 1) should be performed if suggested by the history or physical examination.

COMPLICATIONS

Some tall children, especially girls, are teased or ridiculed by their peers [17]. The psychologic stress can be severe enough to cause social withdrawal and depression in later life [51]. Anxiety and depression are more frequent among girls than boys and have an adverse effect on quality of life [24,52]. The incidence of spinal deformities, such as scoliosis or kyphosis, is increased in tall children [17]. Tall children can have difficulties purchasing appropriately sized clothes [43]. Tall girls sometimes have difficulties finding compatible male partners. Other complications can be related to the underlying disease. There is increasing evidence that some tall people are at increased risk for breast cancer, ovarian cancer, prostatic cancer, colon cancer, lung cancer, thyroid cancer, and melanoma; cancer incidence increases with increasing adult height for most cancer sites [53–58]. The exact cause of an increase in cancer risk is not known but might be related to the underlying disease and genes associated with tall stature.

MANAGEMENT

The underlying cause should be treated whenever possible. Children with familial and constitutional tall stature rarely require therapeutic intervention [5,51]. Reassurance is the cornerstone of management for those with normal variant tall stature. Psychologic counseling may be necessary if emotional stress

Table 1
Laboratory tests and diagnostic imaging studies helpful in the evaluation of a child with tall stature

Suspected diagnosis	Suggested tests
Precocious puberty	Serum FSH, LH, estradiol, testosterone, DHEA, DHEAS, androstenedione, 17α-hydroxyprogesterone, human chorionic gonadotropin; gonadotropin response to gonadotropin-releasing hormone; MRI of the sella
Ovarian or adrenal tumor	Serum estradiol, testosterone, DHEAS, androstenedione; abdominal ultrasonography or CT
Congenital adrenal hyperplasia	Serum electrolytes; serum testosterone, DHEAS, androstenedione, testosterone, 17α-hydroxyprogesterone, 11-deoxycortisol; ACTH
Pituitary growth hormone excess	Serum IGF-1-3; GH suppression test; MRI of the sella
Sotos syndrome	Skull radiography, cranial CT, or MRI; electroencephalography; renal ultrasonography; echocardiography
Hyperthyroidism	Serum free thyroxine, triiodothyronine, and thyroid-stimulating hormone
Homocystinuria	Plasma cystine, homocysteine, and methionine; urinary homocysteine
Beckwith-Wiedemann syndrome	Serum glucose, insulin; renal ultrasonography; echocardiography; tumor surveillance justified
Marfan syndrome	Spine radiography; echocardiography
Simpson-Golabi-Behmel syndrome	Spine radiography; renal ultrasound; echocardiography; tumor surveillance justified
Klinefelter syndrome	Serum FSH, LH, testosterone; karyotype; tumor surveillance justified
Hypogonadal syndromes	Serum FSH, LH, estradiol, or testosterone; tumor surveillance justified
Familial glucocorticoid deficiency	Serum cortisol, ACTH

Abbreviations: ACTH, adrenocorticotropic hormone; CT, computerized tomography; DHEA, dehydroepiandrosterone; DHEAS, dehydroepiandrosterone sulfate; FSH, follicle-stimulating hormone; IGF, insulinlike growth factor; LH, luteinizing hormone; MRI, magnetic resonance imaging.

Adapted from Leung AK. Tall stature. In: Leung AK, ed. Common Problems in Ambulatory Pediatrics: Symptoms and Signs. New York: Nova Science Publishers, Inc, 2011, p. 309, with permission.

is associated with the tall stature. Treatment may be considered for children, especially girls, who have severe psychologic problems because of their height and when the predicted adult height is excessively tall (greater than 4 standard deviations greater than the population mean) [52].

For girls, estrogen treatment can be considered to reduce the final height. Estrogen acts by accelerating epiphyseal fusion. It also has indirect effects on the GH-IGF-1 axis. Satisfactory results can often be obtained by starting treatment before the bone age reaches 12 years [3]. In this regard, high-dose ethinyl estradiol can be given, starting at doses of around 100 to 300 μg per day with titration, if needed, for a maximum dose of 500 μg per day [43,59]. Conjugated estrogens may also be used. Cyclic progesterone (eg, medroxyprogesterone acetate at a dose of 10 mg per day for 7 days), may be added [6,17]. Therapy is continued until the growth curve has leveled off and epiphyseal fusion is documented radiologically. The usual duration of treatment is approximately 2 years. A recent retrospective observational study of 60 Danish girls with constitutional tall stature treated with oral 17β-estradiol for a duration of 1.7 years showed an adult height reduction of 1.6 ± 2.1 cm [60]. Side effects of estradiol therapy are infrequent and include nausea, migraine headache, weight gain, leg cramps, transient hypertension, increased areolar pigmentation, benign breast disease, galactorrhea, ovarian cysts, hyperlipidemia, glucose intolerance, cholelithiasis, thromboembolism, post-therapeutic menstrual irregularities or amenorrhea, and increased risk of breast cancer [1,6].

Treating excessively tall boys with testosterone has been studied less extensively because boys do not usually complain of tall stature. Intramuscular injection of supraphysiologic amounts of testosterone enanthate at doses of 250 to 500 mg every 2 weeks for approximately 6 to 12 months has been shown to be effective [1,6,43,61]. Testosterone acts by accelerating bone maturation and epiphyseal fusion through aromatization to estrogen, thereby reducing the ultimate adult height. For most patients, therapy is initiated with the first signs of puberty, before the bone age reaches 14 years, until the epiphyses are completely closed [61]. Adverse effects include acne vulgaris, aggressive behavior, weight gain, edema, headache, hypertension, transient decrease in testicular volume, painful erections, myalgia, and increased risk of prostatic cancer [3,6,43,61].

Because of the greater social acceptance of tall stature and recognition of adverse effects associated with treatment, sex steroids should be used with caution and only after a thorough discussion of the potential side effects with the patient and parents.

A preliminary study showed that nocturnal infusion of octreotide, a somatostatin analogue, reduces GH secretion and leads to a significant reduction in height prediction in tall children [62]. A subsequent study, however, showed that long-term treatment with a somatostatin analogue does not reduce the final adult height in a manner sufficient to justify its use in the treatment of children with tall stature [63]. Pirenzepine and bromocriptine have been evaluated in the treatment of tall stature, but had little effect on adult height [64,65].

Percutaneous epiphysiodesis around the knees can be considered to reduce adult height in extremely tall boys and girls [43,66–68]. The procedure involves damaging the growth plates of the distal femur and proximal tibia and fibula with a drill and curettage, thereby preventing further longitudinal bone growth [19,43,67]. In general, the procedure should be performed before bone age 12.5 years in girls and 14 years in boys [19,43]. Complications include wound infection, peroneal nerve injury, joint effusion, and valgus deformity of the knee [67]. Overall, the complication rates are low with no significant decrease in knee function [66,67]. Although invasive, some have reported high patient satisfaction with the procedure [67].

References

[1] Leung AK. Tall stature. In: Leung AK, editor. Common problems in ambulatory pediatrics: symptoms and signs. New York: Nova Science Publishers, Inc; 2011. p. 303–11.
[2] Leung AK. Evaluating tall children. Can Fam Physician 1995;41:457–68.
[3] Albuquerque EV, Scalco RC, Jorge AA. Management of endocrine disease: diagnostic and therapeutic approach of tall stature. Eur J Endocrinol 2017;176(6):R339–53.
[4] Nwosu BU, Lee MM. Evaluation of short and tall stature in children. Am Fam Physician 2008;78:597–604.
[5] Richmond EJ, Rogol AD. The child with tall stature and/or abnormally rapid growth. UpToDate. Available at: https://www.uptodate.com/contents/the-child-with-tall-stature-and-or-abnormally-rapid-growth. Accessed May 8, 2019.
[6] Meazza C, Gertosio C, Giacchero R, et al. Tall stature: a difficult diagnosis? Ital J Pediatr 2017;43(1):66.
[7] Baron J, Sävendahl L, De Luca F, et al. Short and tall stature: a new paradigm emerges. Nat Rev Endocrinol 2015;11(12):735–46.
[8] Leung AK. Evaluation of the child with short stature. J Singapore Paediatr Soc 1987;29(3–4):120–7.
[9] Phillips SM, Shulman RJ, Measurement of growth in children. UpToDate. Available at: https://www.uptodate.com/contents/measurement-of-growth-in-children. Accessed May 8, 2019.
[10] Christesen HT, Pedersen BT, Pournara E, et al. Short stature: comparison of WHO and National Growth Standards/References for Height. PLoS One 2016;11(6):e0157277.
[11] Barstow C, Rerucha C. Evaluation of short and tall stature in children. Am Fam Physician 2015;92(1):43–50.
[12] Leung AK, Siu TO, Lai PC, et al. Physical growth parameters of Chinese children in Calgary. Can Fam Physician 1987;33:396–400.
[13] Pearson VV. In: Gunn VL, Nechyba C, editors. The Johns Hopkins Hospital Harriet Lane Handbook. 16th edition. Toronto: Mosby; 2002. p. 277.
[14] Leung AK, Leung AA. Evaluation and management of short stature in children. Consultant 2018;58:195–208, 210. Available at: https://www.consultant360.com/article/consultant360/pediatrics/evaluation-and-mamagement-short-stature-children.
[15] Stalman SE, Pons A, Wit JM, et al. Diagnostic work-up and follow-up in children with tall stature: a simplified algorithm for clinical practice. J Clin Res Pediatr Endocrinol 2015;7(4):260–7.
[16] Zargham S, Crotty JE. Tall stature. Pediatr Rev 2014;35(12):538–9.
[17] Iughetti L, Bergomi A, Bernasconi S. Diagnostic approach and therapy of overgrowth and tall stature in childhood. Minerva Pediatr 2003;55:563–82.
[18] Pagani S, Radetti G, Meazza C, et al. Analysis of growth hormone receptor gene expression in tall and short stature children. J Pediatr Endocrinol Metab 2017;30(4):427–30.
[19] Davies JH, Cheetham T. Investigation and management of tall stature. Arch Dis Child 2014;99(8):772–7.
[20] Narayanaswamy V, Rettig KR, Bhowmick SK. Excessive growth. Clin Pediatr 2008;47:705–10.
[21] Sotos JF, Argente J. Overgrowth disorders associated with tall stature. Adv Pediatr 2008;55:213–54.
[22] Fennoy I. Effect of obesity on linear growth. Curr Opin Endocrinol Diabetes Obes 2013;20(1):44–9.
[23] Leung AK, McArthur RG. Recent advances in the treatment of isosexual precocious puberty: identifying all the problems. Can Fam Physician 1991;37:2597–604.
[24] Coutant R, Donzeau A, Decrequy A, et al. How to investigate a child with excessive growth? Ann Endocrinol (Paris) 2017;78(2):98–103.
[25] Katznelson L, Laws ER Jr, Melmed S, et al. Acromegaly: an endocrine society clinical practice guideline. J Clin Endocrinol Metab 2014;99(11):3933–51.

[26] Eugster E. Gigantism. In: De Groot LJ, Chrousos G, Dungan K, et al, editors. Endotext. South Dartmouth (MA): MDText.com, Inc; 2000 [Internet].
[27] Tatton-Brown K, Rahman N. Sotos syndrome. Eur J Hum Genet 2007;15:264–71.
[28] Kant SG, Wit JM, Breuning MH. Genetic analysis of tall stature. Horm Res 2005;64: 149–56.
[29] Nam HK, Nam MH, Ha KS, et al. A novel fibrillin-1 gene mutation leading to Marfan syndrome in a Korean girl. Ann Clin Lab Sci 2017;47(2):221–5.
[30] Sakai LY, Keene DR, Renard M, et al. FBN1: The disease-causing gene for Marfan syndrome and other genetic disorders. Gene 2016;591(1):279–91.
[31] Wikström AM, Dunkel L. Klinefelter syndrome. Best Pract Res Clin Endocrinol Metab 2011;25(2):239–50.
[32] Leung AK, Robson WL. Current status of cryptorchidism. Adv Pediatr 2004;51:351–77.
[33] Leung AK, Robson WL. Hypospadias: an update. Asian J Androl 2007;9(1):16–22.
[34] Al-Garni A, Leung AK, Kao CP. Cholelithiasis in an infant with Klinefelter's syndrome. South Med J 2002;95(9):1063–4.
[35] Groth KA, Skakkebæk A, Høst C, et al. Clinical review: Klinefelter syndrome - a clinical update. J Clin Endocrinol Metab 2013;98(1):20–30.
[36] Bardsley MZ, Kowal K, Levy C, et al. 47,XYY syndrome: clinical phenotype and timing of ascertainment. J Pediatr 2013;163(4):1085–94.
[37] Jo WH, Jung MK, Kim KE, et al. XYY syndrome: a 13-year-old boy with tall stature. Ann Pediatr Endocrinol Metab 2015;20(3):170–3.
[38] Shivaprasad KS, Dutta D, Jain R, et al. Familial glucocorticoid deficiency presenting with generalized hyperpigmentation in adolescence. Report of three siblings. Indian J Endocrinol Metab 2012;16(Suppl 2):S382–4.
[39] Leung AK, McArthur RG, Ross SA, et al. Thyroxine-binding globulin deficiency in Beckwith syndrome. J Pediatr 1979;95(5 Pt 1):752–4.
[40] Muir A. Precocious puberty. Pediatr Rev 2006;27:373–80.
[41] Imagawa E, Higashimoto K, Sakai Y, et al. Mutations in genes encoding polycomb repressive complex 2 subunits cause Weaver syndrome. Hum Mutat 2017;38(6):637–48.
[42] Tenorio J, Arias P, Martínez-Glez V, et al. Simpson-Golabi-Behmel syndrome types I and II. Orphanet J Rare Dis 2014;9:138.
[43] Hannema SE, Sävendahl L. The evaluation and management of tall stature. Horm Res Paediatr 2016;85(5):347–52.
[44] Acheson RM, Vicinus JH, Fowler GB. Studies in the reliability of assessing skeletal maturity from x-rays. 3. Greulich-Pyle Atlas and Tanner-Whitehouse method contrasted. Hum Biol 1966;38(3):204–18.
[45] Oestreich AE. Tanner-Whitehouse versus Greulich-Pyle in bone age determinations. J Pediatr 1997;131(1 Pt 1):5–6.
[46] Greulich WW, Pyle SI. Radiographic atlas of skeletal development of the hand and wrist. 2nd edition. Stanford (CA): Stanford University Press; 1959. p. 190.
[47] Pyle SI, Waterhouse AM, Greulich WW. Attributes of the radiographic standard of reference for the National Health Examination Survey. Am J Phys Anthropol 1971;35(3):331–7.
[48] Bayley N, Pinneau Sr. Tables for predicting adult height from skeletal age: revised for use with the Greulich-Pyle hand standards. J Pediatr 1952;40(4):423–41.
[49] Joss EE, Temperli R, Mullis PE. Adult height in constitutionally tall stature: accuracy of five different height prediction methods. Arch Dis Child 1992;67(11):1357–62.
[50] Leung AK, Robson WL. Premature adrenarche. J Pediatr Health Care 2008;22(4):230–3.
[51] Bruinsma FJ, Venn AJ, Patton GC, et al. Concern about tall stature during adolescence and depression in later life. J Affect Disord 2006;91(2–3):145–52.
[52] Edouard T. What treatment for a child with tall stature? Ann Endocrinol (Paris) 2017;78(2): 104–5.

[53] Abar L, Vieira AR, Aune D, et al. Height and body fatness and colorectal cancer risk: an update of the WCRF-AICR systematic review of published prospective studies. Eur J Nutr 2017; https://doi.org/10.1007/s00394-017-1557-1.
[54] Green J, Cairns BJ, Casabonne D, et al. Height and cancer incidence in the Million Women Study: prospective cohort, and meta-analysis of prospective studies of height and total cancer risk. Lancet Oncol 2011;12(8):785–94.
[55] Laron Z. To be or not to be "TALL"? Pediatr Endocrinol Rev 2012;9(4):696–7.
[56] Tripaldi R, Stuppia L, Alberti S. Human height genes and cancer. Biochim Biophys Acta 2013;1836(1):27–41.
[57] Wang F, Xu X, Yang J, et al. Height and lung cancer risk: a meta-analysis of observational studies. PLoS One 2017;12(9):e0185316.
[58] Wirén S, Häggström C, Ulmer H, et al. Pooled cohort study on height and risk of cancer and cancer death. Cancer Causes Control 2014;25(2):151–9.
[59] Venn A, Hosmer T, Hosmer D, et al. Oestrogen treatment for tall stature in girls: estimating the effect on height and the error in height prediction. Clin Endocrinol (Oxf) 2008;68(6): 926–9.
[60] Upners EN, Juul A. Evaluation and phenotypic characteristics of 293 Danish girls with tall stature: effects of oral administration of natural 17β-estradiol. Pediatr Res 2016;80(5): 693–701.
[61] Reinehr T, Gueldensupp M, Wunsch R, et al. Treatment of tall stature in boys: comparison of two different treatment regimens. Horm Res Paediatr 2011;76(5):343–7.
[62] Hindmarsh PC, Pringle PJ, Stanhope R, et al. The effect of a continuous infusion of a somatostatin analogue (octreotide) for two years on growth hormone secretion and height prediction in tall children. Clin Endocrinol (Oxf) 1995;42(5):509–15.
[63] Noordam C, van Daalen S, Otten BJ. Treatment of tall stature in boys with somatostatin analogue 201-995: effect on final height. Eur J Endocrinol 2006;154(2):253–7.
[64] Hindmarsh PC, Pringle PJ, Brook CG. Cholinergic muscarinic blockade produces short-term suppression of growth hormone secretion in children with tall stature. Clin Endocrinol (Oxf) 1988;29(3):289–96.
[65] Schoenle EJ, Theintz G, Torresani T, et al. Lack of bromocriptine-induced reduction of predicted height in tall adolescents. J Clin Endocrinol Metab 1987;65(2):355–8.
[66] Benyi E, Berner M, Bjernekull I, et al. Efficacy and Safety of percutaneous epiphysiodesis operation around the knee to reduce adult height in extremely tall adolescent girls and boys. Int J Pediatr Endocrinol 2010;2010:740629.
[67] Goedegebuure WJ, Jonkers F, Boot AM, et al. Long-term follow-up after bilateral percutaneous epiphysiodesis around the knee to reduce excessive predicted final height. Arch Dis Child 2017; https://doi.org/10.1136/archdischild-2017-313295.
[68] Odink RJ, Gerver WJ, Heeg M, et al. Reduction of excessive height in boys by bilateral percutaneous epiphysiodesis around the knee. Eur J Pediatr 2006;165(1):50–4.

Advances in Pediatrics 66 (2019) 177–187

ADVANCES IN PEDIATRICS

Updates on Hypertension and New Guidelines

Pamela S. Singer, MD, MS

Cohen Children's Medical Center, Donald and Barbara Zucker School of Medicine at Hofstra/Northwell, 269-01 76th Avenue, New Hyde Park, NY 11040, USA

Keywords

• Blood pressure • Hypertension • Pediatrics • Cardiovascular • Nephrology • Epidemiology

Key points

- Pediatric high blood pressure tracks into adulthood and can be a significant cause of morbidity and mortality; therefore, early recognition is critical for prevention.
- Recently updated practice guidelines provide new normative data for blood pressure in children, using only normal-weight subjects to provide a more accurate assessment of normal pediatric blood pressure values.
- Ambulatory blood pressure monitoring is a crucial diagnostic tool for pediatric hypertension and is the only way to identify white coat and masked hypertension.
- Therapeutic lifestyle modifications, including diet and exercise, are recommended as first-line treatment in most cases of high blood pressure.

GENERAL CONTENT

Epidemiology

Elevated blood pressure (BP) represents a major cause of morbidity and mortality in the United States. An estimated 32% of adults in the United States have hypertension (HTN), with another one-third having pre-HTN [1]. Adult BP has its roots in pediatrics, because children with higher BPs have an increased prevalence of HTN in adulthood [2]. Studies of the prevalence and risk factors for pediatric HTN have relied mainly on large-scale studies, such as National

The author has nothing to disclose.

E-mail address: psinger@northwell.edu

https://doi.org/10.1016/j.yapd.2019.03.009

Health and Nutrition Examination Survey (NHANES) and the Bogalusa Heart Study [2–7]. Prevalence estimates in these studies generally range from 3% to 5% for HTN, and higher for pre-HTN. Studies using repeated BP measurements have resulted in lower estimates [8,9].

Numerous nonmodifiable risk factors have been associated with pediatric high BP. Boys have been shown to have higher rates of high BP as compared to girls [9], as do Hispanics and non-Hispanic African Americans as compared with whites [7].

Although there has been a general increase in the prevalence of pediatric HTN over time, which has mirrored the increase in pediatric obesity [9,10], a study of NHANES data from 1999 to 2012 actually found a leveling off in prevalence of high BP between the 1999 to 2002 and 2009 to 2012 time periods [3,4].

Obesity has been shown in numerous studies to be a risk factor for elevated BP [11–13]. A study of 2585 pediatric NHANES subjects found average BP was 8 mm Hg higher in obese patients as compared with those who were normal weight [14]. The association between elevated weight and BP could be seen even in young, preadolescent children [15].

In addition to obesity, other medical conditions have been shown to be associated with increased risk of high BP. Specifically, premature infants are at increased risk of high BP, as are those with obstructive sleep apnea. These conditions are in addition to the more classically recognized secondary causes of HTN. Studies have shown an incidence of about 0.2% to 3% for HTN in the neonatal intensive care unit [16,17]. Although previously, umbilical artery catheters have been attributed as a major source of neonatal HTN, much of the elevated BP in this population is now likely due to improved survival of premature babies [17]. Prematurity is associated with decreased nephron mass, upregulation of the renin-angiotensin system, increased catecholamine release, and endothelial dysfunction [18]. In up to 50% of patients, no other clearly identifiable cause of HTN is elucidated [17]. Although outcomes are variable, in most cases, BP due to prematurity can normalize within the first 6 months of life [19]; however, prematurity remains a long-term risk factor for future high BP as well.

Diagnosis

Although data linking pediatric HTN to cardiovascular morbidity and mortality are lacking, HTN is a well-known contributor to adult cardiovascular disease [20] and intermediate markers of damage are visible in children [21]. Children with elevated BP have also been found to perform less well on tests of cognitive function, suggesting potential central nervous system end-organ damage [22]. These findings underscore the importance of early diagnosis of high BP in children, in order to prevent future damage. Despite a 2013 US Preventative Services Task Force guideline stating insufficient evidence to recommend routine BP measurement in asymptomatic children and adolescents [23], the new 2017 high BP clinical practice guidelines continue to recommend screening at least annually for children ≥3 years of age. Furthermore, children with known risk factors, including obesity, should be screened at all health care encounters, and those under 3 years of age with known risk factors should be screened at well child visits as well [24]. High-risk conditions include prematurity, history of congenital heart disease, patients with known structural or functional renal disease, transplant recipients, those on medications known to raise BP, such as stimulants for attention-deficit/hyperactivity disorder, and those with syndromes known to affect BP, such as neurofibromatosis and tuberous sclerosis.

The definition and diagnosis of pediatric HTN are based on age-, gender-, and height-specific normative BP data. This method is in contrast to absolute values used in the diagnosis of adult HTN. Although the Fourth Report [25] included subjects who were overweight and obese, the 2017 guidelines use only normal-weight children. This change has resulted in a lowering of normal BP cutoffs, because obesity-related high BP skewed previous data toward higher values. When using the new criteria, studies have shown increases in the percentage of children diagnosed with HTN [26]. In a recent analysis of pediatric NHANES participants, comparison of BP classification using both the 2017 guidelines and the 2004 Fourth Report showed an increased prevalence of HTN, 14.2% versus 11.8%, when using the newer criteria [11]. This increase was especially notable among overweight and obese children. Khoury and colleagues [27] showed an increase in prevalence of HTN from 8% to 13% in obese diabetic youth when using the new criteria.

The 2017 guidelines also aimed to align themselves more closely with adult HTN criteria [28]. Children between the ages of 1 and 13 are classified using age-/gender-/height-specific percentile values, whereas children 13 and older, whose pressures are more similar to adults, are classified according to adult criteria. Table 1, adapted from the new guidelines, summarizes the new pediatric BP classification system.

Full tables of new normative data are available at pediatrics.aappublications.org/content/140/3/e20171904.figures-only. If patients have an isolated elevated systolic or diastolic pressure, they are classified according to whichever value is higher. Normative values are based on upper-extremity auscultatory data. Oscillometric measurements are commonly used as an initial screen for BP; however, these devices are known to overestimate BP as compared with auscultation [29].

Because BP is known to vary, the classification of BP status should be made after multiple measurements at different times rather than based on a single value [7]. For asymptomatic patients found to have elevated BP on screening examination, repeat measurements spaced 6 months apart are recommended, with workup only if elevations are persistent on 3 occasions. For those with stage I HTN, a period of 3 months of persistent BP elevation should occur before further workup is initiated, and for those with measurements in the stage II HTN range, more urgent evaluation is advised [24].

When further evaluation of BP is required, ambulatory BP monitoring (ABPM) is recommended for the most accurate detection of true high BP. ABPM represents one of the major advances in pediatric BP management

Table 1
2017 Pediatric blood pressure classification

	Ages 1 to <13 y[a]	Ages ≥13 y
Normal BP	Systolic blood pressure (SBP) and diastolic blood pressure (DBP) <90th% for gender/age/height	SBP <120 and DBP <80 mm Hg
Elevated BP (previously termed pre-HTN)	SBP or DBP ≥90th% to <95th% for gender/age/height	SBP 120–129 mm Hg with DBP <80 mm Hg
Stage I HTN	SBP or DBP ≥95th% to <95th% + 12 mm Hg for gender/age/height	SBP 130–139 or DBP 80–89 mm Hg
Stage II HTN	SBP or DBP ≥95th% + 12 mm Hg for gender/age/height	SBP ≥140 or DBP ≥90 mm Hg

[a]If values exceed the corresponding values for children ≥13 y, the lower value is used.

over the past 20 years. As compared with office measurements, ABPM in children has shown higher tracking stability with future adult BP [30] and is a more sensitive marker of HTN as compared with casual BP measurement [31]. ABPM in children correlates with markers of target organ damage, including increased pulse wave velocity and carotid intima-medial thickness (cIMT) [32] and left ventricular hypertrophy (LVH) [33–36]. The relationship between ABPM and markers of CV damage is stronger than that with in-office BP measurement [37]. Although there are limited pediatric data on the correlation between intermediate markers of damage and hard cardiovascular outcomes, adult data show this relationship [38]. In ABPM, a small portable oscillometric device is worn for a 24-hour period, including during sleep. BP values are obtained and recorded at 20- to 30-minute intervals. Patients provide a diary, which includes hours of sleep and wake during the monitoring period; using those data, a report is generated that provides information of average awake and asleep BP, BP loads (percentage of time spent with high BP), and dipping status (BP change between awake and asleep periods).

ABPM can identify white coat HTN, which is found in up to half of children referred for elevated BP [39]. The diagnosis of white coat HTN can prevent unnecessary testing and associated costs of further HTN workup. However, those with white coat HTN should continue to be monitored because they may be more likely to develop HTN in the future [40].

Normative values for ABPM based on sleep/wake status, gender, and height have been published [41,42]. Table 2 provides a classification scheme for ABPM results. ABPM classification relies on mean BPs during both sleep and wake periods as well as BP loads (percentage of time above the 95th% value). Other parameters, such as BP dipping (percentage difference between mean wake and mean sleep values), are also used in risk-stratification, however are not part of the classification scheme.

Table 2
Ambulatory blood pressure classification

White coat HTN	Clinic BP ≥95th% (SBP or DBP), ABPM mean awake and asleep SBP and DBP <95th%, loads all <25%
Pre-HTN	Mean awake and asleep SBP and DBP <95th%, at least 1 load ≥25%
Ambulatory HTN	Mean awake or asleep SBP or DBP ≥95th%, at least 1 load ≥25%
Severe ambulatory HTN	Mean awake or asleep SBP or DBP ≥95th%, at least 1 load >50%
Masked HTN	Normal clinic BP, ABPM mean awake or asleep SBP or DBP ≥95th%, at least 1 load ≥25%

It is important to note that ABPM classification does not line up fully with casual BP classification. For instance, severe ambulatory HTN is not equivalent to stage II HTN. Whereas casual BP classification is based on absolute BP values, ambulatory BP classification is the BP means as well as the percentage of time spent with high BP. Consultation with an HTN specialist is recommended for ABPM interpretation.

Workup

Whereas historically, pediatric HTN was thought to be largely due to secondary causes, newer studies have found that primary HTN is an equally important cause of high BP and is the predominant diagnosis in children over 6 years of age [43]. A positive family history for HTN was also an independent predictor of primary HTN [43], as is obesity [44].

Based on these data, the 2017 guidelines recommend against extensive secondary evaluation in children ≥6 years old, who have a positive family history for HTN and are overweight, and who do not have symptoms or findings concerning for specific secondary cause [24]. These recommendations are in contrast to the Fourth Report [25], which recommended at least complete blood count, comprehensive metabolic panel, renal ultrasound with Doppler, and echocardiogram in all children diagnosed with HTN. Of course, careful and accurate history and physical examination must be obtained to avoid a missed diagnosis of secondary cause. Furthermore, the 2017 guidelines do not explicitly define their recommendation regarding extent of evaluation.

Among those with secondary HTN, renal and renovascular disorders remain the most common causes. Evaluation of renovascular HTN is based on renin profiling (serum renin and aldosterone measurement) and renovascular imaging. The sensitivity of Doppler ultrasound varies based on age and weight, with best results noted in normal-weight children ≥8 years old [45,46]. Alternative imaging, such as computed tomography or magnetic resonance angiography, may be preferred in children not meeting these criteria. Other common causes include aortic coarctation, endocrine disorders, including hyperthyroidism and mineralocorticoid excess, monogenic HTN, and certain syndromes. Sleep apnea is another common risk factor for pediatric HTN and should be assessed in patients with signs of disordered sleep. Box 1 lists common causes of secondary HTN. Evaluation for secondary causes should be based on signs, symptoms, and index of suspicion. Management of secondary causes should focus on the underlying disorder and may differ from standard recommendations for primary HTN. Treatment of specific secondary causes is beyond the scope of this article.

Echocardiogram is recommended if there is a consideration of starting pharmacologic therapy for HTN in order to assess for the presence of LVH. Although there are many different echocardiographic methods and measurements used for determining left ventricular mass index and LVH [47,48], the current guidelines use left ventricular mass of greater than 51 g/m$^{2.7}$ in children older than 8 years, or greater than 115 g/body surface area in boys and greater than 95 g/BSA in girls less than that age. It is important to note that BSA-based measurements result in lower prevalence of left ventricular hypertrophy as compared with height-indexed 95th percentile [49,50]. However, less emphasis overall is placed on echocardiographic findings in the current guidelines, because evidence of LVH is not discussed as a clear indication for pharmacologic treatment as it is in the Fourth Report.

Additional markers of cardiovascular damage include increased cIMT as determined by carotid ultrasound, increased arterial stiffness as measured by increased pulse wave velocity, and impaired endothelial function as measured by flow-mediated dilatation. Although research on these methods in both the pediatric and the adult populations is ongoing [27], these tests are currently not commonly available in clinical practice, including among HTN specialists. However, they may continue to grow in importance given their ability to detect early cardiovascular damage in this population [51].

Treatment

Lifestyle modification is recommended for all patients with elevated BP as well as those with asymptomatic stage I HTN. Patients with stage II HTN, with symptomatic HTN, or with underlying chronic kidney disease (CKD) or diabetes mellitus (DM) may require pharmacologic treatment from the outset of diagnosis [24]. A combination of diet and exercise modifications is recommended, because this is more effective than either alone in lowering BP [52].

Dietary focus should be on fresh fruits and vegetables, lean proteins, and low-fat dairy products, key components of the DASH diet [53]. Although much of traditional literature focuses on sodium restriction in the management of HTN, recent adult studies have provided more conflicting evidence. The 2015 to 2020 Dietary Guidelines for Americans [54] recommend a sodium intake of less than 2300 mg/d, and in some cases less than 1500 mg/d. However, studies of the association between sodium intake and cardiovascular outcomes have shown varying effects, with many showing increased mortality at both the highest and the lowest intakes of sodium despite decreases in BP [55,56].

Box 1: Common causes of secondary hypertension

Renal

- Congenital anomalies of the kidney and urinary tract and obstructive uropathy
- Reflux nephropathy
- Cystic kidney disease
- Glomerulonephritis
- Renovascular disease (renal artery stenosis, fibromuscular dysplasia, arteritis)

Cardiovascular

- Aortic coarctation and midaortic syndrome

Endocrine

- Hyperthyroidism
- Hyperaldosteronism
- Congenital adrenal hyperplasia
- Apparent mineralocorticoid excess
- Hypercalcemia
- Pheochromocytoma

Monogenic

- Liddle syndrome
- Gordon syndrome

Oncologic

- Wilms tumor
- Neuroblastoma

Syndromic

- Neurofibromatosis I
- Tuberous sclerosis
- Turner syndrome
- Williams syndrome

Drugs

- Steroids
- Stimulants
- Caffeine
- Illicit drugs

Miscellaneous

- Prematurity
- Obstructive sleep apnea

In addition to dietary measures, increases in physical activity and decreased sedentary time are important measures to improve BP and overall cardiovascular health. Sedentary activities should be limited to fewer than 2 hours per day, and 30 to 60 minutes daily of cardiovascular activity is recommended. Although certain high-static and competitive sports participation may temporarily need to be restricted until BP is controlled, there are no restrictions on noncompetitive cardiovascular activity due to HTN [24,57]. Children and adolescents should not be prohibited from participating in these activities pending further evaluation.

Medication

For those who fail therapeutic lifestyle modifications, pharmacologic treatment may be needed. The 2017 guidelines go farther than previous reports in suggesting first-line agents for HTN. An angiotensin-converting enzyme inhibitor (ACEi) or angiotensin II receptor blocker is recommended as first line for anyone with CKD, DM, or proteinuria unless there is an absolute contraindication. In other cases of primary HTN, ACEi may also be used as a first-line agent, with consideration of a calcium-channel blocker or thiazide as first line in African American children because of decreased response to ACE inhibitors [58]. Beta-blockers are not recommended for first-line treatment because of their increased side-effect profile. Regardless of the medication initiated, dose maximization of a single agent should be used before adding additional medication. Although the Fourth Report recommended a BP goal of less than 95th% for gender/age/height except for those with underlying comorbid conditions, such as CKD and diabetes, the 2017 guidelines propose stricter goals of less than 90th% (or <130/80 mm Hg) for all patients with HTN. Even lower targets may be beneficial, as evidenced by the ESCAPE trial [59], which showed improved outcomes in those with lower BP goals.

SUMMARY

Early diagnosis of pediatric HTN is important to prevent both short- and long-term target organ damage and adverse outcomes. The recently published 2017 clinical practice guidelines serve as an update to the 2004 Fourth Report and provide recommendations on the diagnosis, workup, and management of pediatric high BP. The new guidelines provide updated normative BP data using normal-weight children, in order to more appropriately characterize ideal pediatric BP. Guidelines for evaluation of high BP have been modified to reduce unnecessary testing, and treatment focuses on lifestyle modifications before moving to pharmacologic therapy. The new guidelines propose stricter BP control goals because these may be associated with better long-term outcomes.

References

[1] Nwankwo T, Yoon SS, Burt V, et al. Hypertension among adults in the US: national health and nutrition examination survey, 2011-2012. NCHS data brief, no. 133. Hyattsville (MD): National Center for Health Statistics, Centers for Disease Control and Prevention, US Dept of Health and Human Services; 2013.

[2] Bao W, Threefoot SA, Srinivasan SR, et al. Essential hypertension predicted by tracking of elevated blood pressure from childhood to adulthood: the Bogalusa heart study. Am J Hypertens 1995;6(7):657–65.
[3] Xi B, Zhang M, Liu F, et al. Trends in elevated blood pressure among US children and adolescents: 1999-2012. Am J Hypertens 2016;29(2):217–25.
[4] Jackson SL, Zhang Z, Wiltz JL, et al. Hypertension among youths – United States, 2001-2016. MMWR Morb Mortal Wkly Rep 2018;67(27):758–62.
[5] May AL, Kuklina EV, Yoon PW. Prevalence of cardiovascular disease risk factors among US adolescents, 1999-2008. Pediatrics 2012;129(6):1035–41.
[6] McNiece KL, Poffenbarger TS, Turner JL, et al. Prevalence of hypertension and pre-hypertension among adolescents. J Pediatr 2007;150(6):640–4.
[7] Din-Dzietham R, Liu Y, Bielo MV, et al. High blood pressure trends in children and adolescents in national surveys, 1963 to 2002. Circulation 2007;116(13):1488–96.
[8] Becton LJ, Egan BM, Hailpern SM, et al. Blood pressure reclassification in adolescents based on repeat clinic blood pressure measurements. J Clin Hypertens 2013;15(10): 717–22.
[9] Rosner B, Cook NR, Daniels S, et al. Childhood blood pressure trends and risk factors for high blood pressure: the NHANES experience 1988-2008. Hypertension 2013;62(2): 247–54.
[10] Sorof J, Daniels S. Obesity hypertension in children: a problem of epic proportions. Hypertension 2002;40(4):441–7.
[11] Sharma AK, Metzger DL, Rodd CJ. Prevalence and severity of high blood pressure among children based on the 2017 American Academy of Pediatrics guidelines. JAMA Pediatr 2018;172(6):557–65.
[12] Li L, Perez A, Wu LT, et al. Cardiometabolic risk factors among severely obese children and adolescents in the United States, 1999-2012. Child Obes 2018;12(1):12–9.
[13] Skinner AC, Perrin EM, Moss LA, et al. Cardiometabolic risks and severity of obesity in children and young adults. N Engl J Med 2015;373(14):1307–17.
[14] Betz HH, Eisenmann JC, Laurson KR, et al. Physical activity, BMI, and blood pressure in US youth: NHANES 2003-2006. Pediatr Exerc Sci 2018;30(3):418–25.
[15] Messiah SE, Vidot DC, Gumurkar S, et al. Obesity is significantly associated with cardiovascular disease risk factors in 2- to 9-year olds. J Clin Hypertens 2014;16(12):889–94.
[16] Blowey DL, Duda PJ, Stokes P, et al. Incidence and treatment of hypertension in the neonatal intensive care unit. J Am Soc Hypertens 2011;5(6):478–83.
[17] Starr MC, Flynn JT. Neonatal hypertension: cases, causes, and clinical approach. Pediatr Nephrol 2018; https://doi.org/10.1007/s00467-018-3977-4.
[18] Lurbe E, Garcia-Vicent C, Torro I, et al. First-year blood pressure increase steepest in low birthweight newborns. J Hypertens 2007;25(1):61–6.
[19] Seliem WA, Falk MC, Shadbolt B, et al. Antenatal and postnatal risk factors for neonatal hypertension and infant follow-up. Pediatr Nephrol 2007;12:2081–7.
[20] Yoon PW, Gillespie CD, George MG, et al. Control of hypertension among adults – national health and nutrition examination survey, United States, 2005-2008. MMWR Suppl 2012;61(02):19–25.
[21] Rao G. Diagnosis, epidemiology, and management of hypertension in children. Pediatrics 2016;138(2) [pii:e20153616].
[22] Lande MB, Kaczorowski JM, Auinger P, et al. Elevated blood pressure and decreased cognitive function among school-age children and adolescents in the United States. J Pediatr 2003;143(6):720–4.
[23] Moyer VA. Screening for primary hypertension in children and adolescents: U.S. preventative services task force recommendation statement. Pediatrics 2013;132:907.
[24] Flynn JT, Kaelber DC, Baker-Smith CM, et al. Clinical practice guideline for screening and management of high blood pressure in children and adolescents. Pediatrics 2017;140(3): 3–72.

[25] The fourth report on the diagnosis, evaluation, and treatment of high blood pressure in children and adolescents. Pediatrics 2004;114(supplement 2):555–76.
[26] Bell CS, Samuel JP, Samuels JA. Prevalence of hypertension in children. Hypertension 2019;73(1):148–52.
[27] Khoury M, Khoury PR, Dolan LM, et al. Clinical implications of the revised AAP pediatric hypertension guidelines. Pediatrics 2018;142(2) [pii:e20180245].
[28] Whelton PK, Carey RM, Aronow WS, et al. 2017 ACC/AHA/AAPA/ABC/ACPM/AGS/APhA/ASH/ASPC/NMA/PCNA guideline for the prevention, detection, evaluation, and management of high blood pressure in adults: a report of the American college of cardiology/American heart association task force on clinical practice guidelines. J Am Coll Cardiol 2018;71:e127–248.
[29] Chio SS, Urbina EM, Lapointe J, et al. Korotkoff sound versus oscillometric cuff sphygmomanometers: comparison between auscultatory and DynaPulse blood pressure measurements. J Am Soc Hypertens 2011;5(1):12–20.
[30] Li Z, Snieder H, Harschfield GA, et al. A 15-year longitudinal study on ambulatory blood pressure tracking from childhood to early adulthood. Hypertens Res 2009;32(5):404–10.
[31] Maggio AB, Aggoun Y, Marchand LM. Associations among obesity, blood pressure, and left ventricular mass. J Pediatr 2008;152(4):489–93.
[32] Conkar S, Yilmaz E, Hacikara S, et al. Is daytime systolic load and important risk factor for target organ damage in pediatric hypertension? J Clin Hypertens 2015;17(10):760–6.
[33] Sorof JM, Cardwell G, Franco K, et al. Ambulatory blood pressure and left ventricular mass index in hypertensive children. Hypertension 2002;39(4):903–8.
[34] Andrade H, Pires A, Noronha N, et al. Importance of ambulatory blood pressure monitoring in the diagnosis and prognosis of pediatric hypertension. Rev Port Cardiol 2018;37(9):783–9.
[35] Stabouli S, Kotsis V, Rizos Z, et al. Left ventricular mass in normotensive, prehypertensive and hypertensive children and adolescents. Pediatr Nephrol 2009;24(8):1545–51.
[36] Ozcakar ZB, Yalcinkaya F, Tutar E, et al. Hypertension and left ventricular hypertrophy in pediatric peritoneal dialysis patients: ambulatory blood pressure monitoring and echocardiographic evaluation. Nephron Clin Pract 2006;104(2):c101–6.
[37] Dolan E, Stanton A, Thijs L. Superiority of ambulatory over clinic blood pressure measurement in predicting mortality: the Dublin outcome study. Hypertension 2005;46(1):156–61.
[38] Levy D, Garrison RJ, Savage DD, et al. Prognostic implications of echocardiographically determined left ventricular mass in the Framingham heart study. N Engl J Med 1990;322(22):1561–6.
[39] Swartz SJ, Srivaths PR, Croix B, et al. Cost-effectiveness of ambulatory blood pressure monitoring in the initial evaluation of hypertension in children. Pediatrics 2008;122(6):1177–81.
[40] Westerstahl M, Forss M, Persson L, et al. Hypertension outcomes and cardiovascular status in young adults with childhood-diagnosed white coat hypertension. Arch Dis Child 2018;103(1):113–4.
[41] Soergel M, Kirschstein M, Busch C, et al. Oscillometric twenty-four-hour ambulatory blood pressure values in healthy children and adolescents: a multicenter trial including 1141 subjects. J Pediatr 1997;130(2):178–84.
[42] Wuhl E, Witte K, Soergel M, et al, German Working Group on Pediatric Hypertension. Distribution of 24-h ambulatory blood pressure in children: normalized reference values and role of body dimensions. J Hypertens 2002;20(10):1995–2007.
[43] Gupta-Malhotra M, Banker A, Shete S, et al. Essential hypertension vs. secondary hypertension among children. Am J Hypertens 2015;28(1):73–80.
[44] Gomes RS, Quirino IG, Pereira RM, et al. Primary versus secondary hypertension in children followed up at an outpatient tertiary unit. Pediatr Nephrol 2011;26(3):441–7.
[45] Dillman JR, Smith EA, Coley BD. Ultrasound imaging of renin-mediated hypertension. Pediatr Radiol 2017;47(9):1116–24.

[46] Castelli PK, Dillman JR, Kershaw DB, et al. Renal sonography with Doppler for detecting suspected pediatric renin-mediated hypertension – is it adequate? Pediatr Radiol 2014;44(1): 42–9.
[47] Cho H, Choi HJ, Kang HG, et al. Influence of the method of definition on the prevalence of left-ventricular hypertrophy in children with chronic kidney disease: data from the Know-Ped CKD study. Kidney Blood Press Res 2017;42(3):406–15.
[48] Mirchandani D, Bhatia J, Leisman D, et al. Concordance of measures of left-ventricular hypertrophy in pediatric hypertension. Pediatr Cardiol 2014;35(4):622–6.
[49] Mahgerefteh J, Linder J, Silver EJ, et al. The prevalence of left ventricular hypertrophy in obese children varies depending on the method utilized to determine left ventricular mass. Pediatr Cardiol 2016;37(6):993–1002.
[50] Khoury PR, Mitsnefes M, Daniels SR, et al. Age-specific reference intervals for indexed left ventricular mass in children. J Am Soc Echocardiogr 2009;22(6):709–14.
[51] Stelcar A, Homsak E, Marcun Varda N. Assessment of early cardiovascular risk in children and adolescents with essential hypertension. Klin Padiatr 2017;229(5):286–92.
[52] Cai L, Wu Y, Wilson RF, et al. Effect of childhood obesity prevention programs on blood pressure: a systematic review and meta-analysis. Circulation 2014;129(18):1832–9.
[53] Asghari G, Yuzbashian E, Miriran P, et al. Dietary approaches to stop hypertension (DASH) dietary pattern is associated with reduced incidence of metabolic syndrome in children and adolescents. J Pediatr 2016;174:178–84.
[54] US Department of Health and Human Services and US Department of Agriculture. 2015–2020 Dietary Guidelines for Americans. 8th Edition. December 2015. Available at: http://health.gov/dietaryguidelines/2015/guidelines/. Accessed April 17, 2019.
[55] O'Donnell MJ, Yusuf S, Mente A, et al. Urinary sodium and potassium excretion and risk of cardiovascular events. JAMA 2011;306:2229–38.
[56] Singer PS, Cohen HW, Alderman MH. Assessing the associations of sodium intake with long-term all-cause and cardiovascular mortality in a hypertensive cohort. Am J Hypertens 2015;28(3):335–42.
[57] Demorest RA, Washington RL, Council on Sports Medicine and Fitness. Athletic participation by children and adolescents who have systemic hypertension. Pediatrics 2010;125(6):1287–94.
[58] Li JS, Baker-Smith CM, Smith PB, et al. Racial differences in blood pressure response to angiotensin-converting enzyme inhibitors in children: a meta-analysis. Clin Pharmacol Ther 2008;84(3):315–9.
[59] ESCAPE Trial group. Strict blood pressure control and progression of renal failure in children. N Engl J Med 2009;361(17):1639–50.

Advances in Pediatrics 66 (2019) 189–208

ADVANCES IN PEDIATRICS

Cerebral Palsy

Diagnosis, Epidemiology, Genetics, and Clinical Update

Abimbola Michael-Asalu, MBBS, MPH[a], Genevieve Taylor, MD[b], Heather Campbell, MD[b], Latashia-Lika Lelea, MD, MPH, MSc[c], Russell S. Kirby, PhD, MS[d,*]

[a]Department of Community and Family Health, College of Public Health, University of South Florida, 13201 Bruce B. Downs Boulevard, MDC56, Tampa, FL 33612, USA; [b]The University of North Carolina at Chapel Hill, 260 MacNider Building, CB# 7220, Chapel Hill, NC 27599-7220, USA; [c]University of Central Florida College of Medicine, UCF/HCA Consortium - Gainesville, North Florida Regional Medical Center, 6440 West Newberry Road, Suite 508, Gainesville, FL 32605, USA; [d]Strategic Area Faculty Lead for Population Health Science, College of Public Health, University of South Florida, 13201 Bruce B. Downs Boulevard, MDC56, Tampa, FL 33612, USA

Keywords

• Cerebral palsy • Diagnosis • Epidemiology • Genetics • Clinical management

Key points

- Cerebral palsy is one of the most common physical and developmental disabilities in childhood, with a prevalence of approximately 3 per 1000 births.
- Although preterm birth accounts for approximately 35% of cases of cerebral palsy, more cases occur among term births. Antepartum risk factors figure more prominently in cerebral palsy than peripartum complications.
- Although the cause and pathophysiology of cerebral palsy remain poorly understood, advances in molecular genetics and genomic research continually add to the knowledge base.
- Clinical management of children with cerebral palsy requires a multidisciplinary, family-centered approach, focusing not only on physical health and development but also on maintaining or improving the child's quality of life.

Disclosure: The authors have nothing to disclose.

*Corresponding author. *E-mail address:* rkirby@health.usf.edu

https://doi.org/10.1016/j.yapd.2019.04.002

INTRODUCTION

Cerebral palsy (CP) is a common physical and developmental disability varying in severity but with common developmental features [1]. CP was originally characterized by Little in 1861, and thoughts concerning its origins and clinical features have evolved in the 150 years since then. An international panel provided a consensus definition in 2006: "Cerebral palsy (CP) describes a group of permanent disorders of the development of movement and posture, causing activity limitation, that are attributed to non-progressive disturbances that occurred in the developing fetal or infant brain" [2]. As one of the most common developmental disorders, many pediatric health providers encounter patients and their families with this condition. This update reviews methods for diagnosis, data regarding prevalence and risk factors, recent research on the genetics of CP, and current approaches to clinical management.

DIAGNOSIS OF CEREBRAL PALSY

The diagnosis of CP relies on a combination of neurologic assessment, neuroimaging findings, and recognition of clinical risk factors. Diagnosis is thus often complicated and delayed, and typically occurs at the age of 1 to 2 years or beyond [3]. In recent years, earlier and accurate diagnosis of CP has become possible and highly desirable, because it allows earlier initiation of therapies that may improve long-term outcomes during the period of rapid brain growth and neuroplasticity. Moreover, contrary to concerns that attempts at earlier diagnosis may lead to false-positive screens and create unnecessary parental stress, population studies have shown that parents generally prefer to know if their child has CP or is at high risk for CP sooner rather than later, so that they can start therapies that may optimize their child's development [4,5].

The pathways to diagnosis of CP differ depending on whether a child has identifiable risk factors for CP in the neonatal period, which result in earlier screening and closer developmental surveillance. A wide array of developmental screening tools and neurologic assessments have been used to aid in the diagnosis of CP among high-risk newborns. A recent review by a multidisciplinary, international group of CP experts focused on the following tools with the best predictive validity for detection of CP before 5 months of age: neonatal magnetic resonance imaging (MRI) (86%–89% sensitivity), the Prechtl Qualitative Assessment of General Movements (GMA) (98% sensitivity), and the Hammersmith Infant Neurologic Examination (HINE) (90% sensitivity) [6]. These investigators recommend that infants with newborn-detectable risk factors for CP undergo a standardized neurologic examination, motor assessment, and neuroimaging to help make the diagnosis, ideally before 5 months of age. The diagnosis of CP is made when an infant has evidence of motor dysfunction as well as either abnormal neuroimaging or a clinical history suggestive of risk. If a clinician suspects CP but is unsure of the diagnosis, Novak and colleagues (2017) recommend the use of the label "high risk for CP" in place of more general terms like "high risk for developmental delay" so that children can be appropriately referred for CP-specific early intervention therapies.

The diagnosis of CP in children who lack risk factors often occurs later in life, when parents or general pediatricians realize that they are not achieving their expected motor milestones. Signs that warrant specific evaluation for CP include the inability to sit independently by 9 months of age, the presence of asymmetric movements or limb preference, or the inability of an infant to bear weight on the plantar surface of the feet [6]. This evaluation should consist of a standard neurologic examination (eg, the HINE); a neuromotor assessment; and, if possible, neuroimaging by MRI to identify brain lesions that may corroborate the diagnosis. Useful standardized neuromotor assessment tools in this population include the Developmental Assessment of Young Children, the Alberta Infant Motor Scale, the Motor Assessment of Infants, the Neuro Sensory Motor Development Assessment, and the Test of Infant Motor Performance [6].

Neuroimaging

Numerous studies have reported on the predictive validity of MRI and cranial ultrasonography for the diagnosis of CP, with MRI generally accepted as the more sensitive imaging modality [7–9]. Neonatal MRI findings that are particularly suggestive of high risk for CP include white matter injury (eg, cystic periventricular leukomalacia [CPVL], periventricular hemorrhagic infarction, progressive ventriculomegaly, neonatal stroke), injury to deep gray matter structures such as the basal ganglia, cerebellar hemorrhage, and developmental brain malformations (eg, lissencephaly, microgyria, cortical dysplasia) [5,6,10]. Some children with CP have normal MRI or cranial ultrasonography in the neonatal period. Clinicians may consider repeating the MRI closer to 2 years of age to detect more subtle signs of white matter injury that may have been missed on earlier neuroimaging. Consideration should also be given to underlying genetic or metabolic causes of CP for children with normal neuroimaging but persistent neurologic abnormality [8].

Imaging for patients with CP can be important not only in differentiating between various forms of brain injury leading to CP but also as a prognostic assessment to determine the risk of neurodevelopmental disability [11]. Using MRI at the time of diagnosis of CP can determine the type and extent of brain damage [11]. Vossough's [11] 2017 analysis of several studies reported that 50% to 94% of infants who had changes in the basal ganglia seen on MRI developed CP, intellectual disability, and seizures at 1 to 2 years of age. The morphology of the brain damage is strongly associated with the stage of brain development at which the injury or insult occurred (Jacobsson and Hagberg [12], 2004). Cerebral malformations occur during the first 20 weeks of pregnancy, periventricular leukomalacia (PVL) occurs between 24 and 34 weeks, and the damage to gray matter occurs after 34 weeks [12].

Neuromotor assessment

Although many neuromotor assessment tools exist and have been shown to have varying abilities to accurately identify children with CP, this article focuses on the 2 assessments that have been identified as having the highest predictive value for CP detection in early infancy [6]: the GMA and the HINE examinations. The accuracy of these motor assessment tools improves with serial examinations, which allow clinicians to establish an overall developmental trajectory for a given child, as opposed to relying on an assessment performed at a single point in time.

General movements assessment

The patterns of spontaneous movements in infants have long been studied as a way of identifying children with motor dysfunction [13]. Heinz Prechtl, an Austrian neurologist, developed the GMA, a tool that uses specific descriptions of the spontaneous movements of infants which change in a predictable way during normal development. A recent systematic review of the GMA identified 2 specific movement patterns that are highly sensitive and specific for the diagnosis of CP: cramped synchronous general movements (70% sensitivity, 90% specificity), characterized by rigid contraction and relaxation of the infant's trunk and extremities; and absent fidgety movements (97% sensitivity, 89% specificity), characterized by a lack of the normal small-amplitude fidgety movements that should be present in newborns from 10 to 20 weeks corrected age [14]. Other systematic reviews have also reported a high sensitivity and specificity of abnormalities on the GMA for the prediction of CP among high-risk newborns [7]. The GMA should be performed by providers who have completed standardized training to ensure accuracy and high interrater reliability [15].

Hammersmith infant neurologic examination

This examination has also been evaluated for its ability to aid in the diagnosis of CP. This tool, originally developed as a standardized neurologic examination to help detect movement disorders in infants aged 2 to 24 months, consists of 26 scored items that assess an infant's cranial nerve function, posture, movements, tone, and reflexes. A recent literature review found that a global HINE score less than 56 at 3 months and less than 65 at 12 months was highly sensitive and specific for the development of CP. Moreover, scores less than 40 were invariably associated with later severe nonambulatory CP [16]. Hay and colleagues [17] found that adding an asymmetry score, a tally of items on the neurologic examination that are different between right and left sides, to the overall HINE score allowed a reliable diagnosis of hemiplegia with a sensitivity and specificity of 91.8% and 100% respectively.

Differential diagnosis

A range of neurologic abnormalities from a variety of causes may contribute to the clinical diagnosis of CP. A small subset of children diagnosed with CP may have motor dysfunction related to an underlying neurogenetic or metabolic disorder. Some clinicians recommend genetic testing for children who have normal neuroimaging, a concerning family history, progressive symptoms, a lack of identified clinical risk factors for CP, or who otherwise do not fit the typical pattern of CP [8,18]. Testing may include chromosomal microarray, targeted gene sequencing, whole-exome, and/or whole-genome sequencing depending on the clinical scenario [18,19]. A recently published study by Takezawa and colleagues [20] found that 9 out of 17 cases (52.9%) of full-term children with a diagnosis of CP and nonspecific MRI findings had a pathogenic or likely pathogenic candidate gene variant found on whole-exome sequencing. Decisions concerning genetic testing should be made in conjunction with a pediatric geneticist.

Pediatricians should also be aware of another diagnosis that is being recognized with increasing frequency, particularly among preterm and very-low-birthweight survivors: developmental coordination disorder (DCD). This disorder is characterized by problems with coordination, balance, gross and fine motor skills, and visual-motor integration [21–23] without the neurologic abnormalities seen in children with CP. Although children with DCD generally have more mild motor impairment compared with children with CP, this disorder can have a significant impact on a child's functional abilities and quality of life. Children with DCD should be referred to physical and occupational therapy to address motor skill development.

CLASSIFICATION OF CEREBRAL PALSY

CP is a heterogeneous disorder encompassing a range of clinical phenotypes and types of motor impairments. Traditionally, CP has been classified by motor type, topography of motor impairment, or by degree of functional impairment. Four main motor types of CP have been described in the literature: spastic (by far the most common form, characterized by hypertonicity and muscular resistance to movement), dyskinetic (presents with athetosis or dystonia), ataxic (primarily presents with difficulties with coordination), and hypotonic (decreased muscle tone) CP [24]. Because of low interrater reliability and the tendency for the type of motor impairment to evolve over time or involve features of multiple subtypes, some CP registers simplify designation to spastic versus nonspastic CP [21]. In terms of topography, the term hemiplegia generally refers to involvement of 1 side of the body. Diplegia refers to involvement of the lower extremities to a greater extent than the upper extremities, and quadriplegia refers to involvement of all 4 extremities (although there may be differences in severity of involvement). It is important to distinguish between unilateral and bilateral neuromotor involvement because treatment strategies may differ.

The gold standard for describing motor function is the Gross Motor Function Classification System (GMFCS) [25], with motor classification descriptions that change slightly based on the age of the patient. The GMFCS uses an ordinal scale to provide clinicians with an assessment of the child's level of motor function at present, as well as what mobility aids or equipment the child may need in the future. It is generally thought that the GMFCS is not reliable until after age 2 to 5 years, so clinicians should be cautious about using children's GMFCS levels in early childhood to prognosticate their long-term functional outcome [6,26].

EPIDEMIOLOGY OF CEREBRAL PALSY

Because CP is often diagnosed in infancy or early childhood, it is difficult to obtain reliable prevalence estimates. Data from birth certificates or newborn hospital discharges underenumerate cases of CP. Birth certificates must be filed within 3 to 5 days after birth, before most diagnoses, and many diagnoses occur in specialty clinics or outpatient settings and are not captured in hospital discharge databases. Population surveillance using registries, active case-finding, or representative sample surveys is required to obtain population-based estimates. In the United States, the Autism and Developmental Disabilities Monitoring (ADDM) Network estimates the prevalence of CP among children 8 years of age in several catchment areas. Overall prevalence declined from 3.5 per 1000 8-year-old children in 2006 to 2.9 per 1000 in 2010 [27]. This incidence compares with estimates of 2.6 to 2.9 per 1000 children 2 to 17 years old from the 2011 to 2012 National Survey of Children's Health and the 2011 to 2013 National Health Interview Survey, respectively [28].

Risk factors

Although numerous risk factors for CP have been identified, many children with these risk factors (for example, premature birth) do not go on to develop CP, and nearly 50% of children who are ultimately diagnosed with CP are term-born children who have no identified risk factors in the neonatal period [24].

A 2013 systematic review described the following risk factors as significantly associated with CP in term infants: neonatal respiratory distress syndrome, meconium aspiration, instrumental or emergency cesarean section, birth asphyxia, neonatal seizures, hypoglycemia, and neonatal infections [29]. For many risk factors identified through epidemiologic investigation, direct causal relationships are not clear. For example, respiratory distress syndrome is caused by surfactant deficiency or dysfunction, which is overwhelmingly caused by prematurity. Term infants with respiratory distress syndrome may have inaccurately estimated gestational age and their underlying relative prematurity may be the true risk factor for CP, therefore this article does not discuss respiratory distress syndrome separately from prematurity. Similarly, instrumental or emergency cesarean section are likely associated with birth asphyxia and may not represent independent risk factors for development of CP. Hypoglycemia has not been definitively linked to CP and is not discussed further.

Maternal risk factors

Maternal sociodemographic characteristics and reproductive history are associated with CP. Maternal age less than 20 years or greater than 34 years, low maternal educational attainment, numerous pregnancies, nulliparity, short or long interpregnancy interval, and previous history of intrauterine fetal demise are risk factors for CP [12,30]. Although the crude odds for CP are higher among black non-Hispanic births compared with white non-Hispanic births, after controlling for gestational age as well as other maternal characteristics and socioeconomic factors black non-Hispanic infants were at slightly reduced risk for CP (adjusted odds ratio, 0.87; 95% confidence interval, 0.77–0.99) [30]. Mothers who have a child with CP have a higher risk of having another child with CP [12].

Antenatal risk factors

Assisted reproductive technology. Neonates conceived by in vitro fertilization (IVF) have an increased risk of CP because of the high frequency of twins, low birth weight, and prematurity [12]. Although the increased risk of CP in children born after IVF is most likely secondary to the increased risk of preterm birth and low birth weight, this is not entirely the case. The incidence of CP is higher in monozygous twins than it is in heterozygous twins, and this is thought to be caused by the anastomosis of the vasculature in the placenta in monozygotic twins [31]. If 1 twin dies in utero, the surviving twin may develop brain injury because of the release of thromboplastic substances or shifts in hemodynamics [31]. The death of that twin can also affect the neurologic development of the surviving twin, and the surviving twin has a 20% overall risk of cerebral impairment [12].

Intrauterine growth restriction. Intrauterine growth restriction (IUGR) is thought to be associated with CP because it affects brain development, causes restriction in gray matter development, and increases neonatal morbidity and mortality [12]. IUGR has various causes, some known and some unknown. IUGR is most commonly caused by poor implantation of the placenta to the uterine wall leading to placental insufficiency, causing poor fetal growth and potentially leading to abnormal brain development [32]. In term neonates, IUGR is associated with up to a 10-fold to 30-fold increase in the risk of developing CP [32]. Studies in growth-restricted animal models have shown a reduction in oxygen delivery to the brain and delayed growth of the forebrain and cerebellum [12].

Intrauterine infection. Maternal fever and infection are associated with a significantly increased risk of CP [32]. Maternal infection during pregnancy can affect the fetal brain, causing white matter damage and thus increasing the risk of CP [32]. It is possible that some children with CP who do not have any recognized risk factors for CP development may have experienced an intrauterine infection. Many viral and bacterial infections have mild or nonspecific maternal signs and symptoms and go undiagnosed, therefore not giving any indication for the need to send the placenta to pathology after delivery for further inspection that may indicate an inflammatory disorder [32]. Similarly, infections in neonates may show no clinically detectable signs at birth but may present as CP, developmental delay, or sensorineural hearing loss later in life [12]. TORCH (toxoplasmosis, rubella, cytomegalovirus, and herpes simplex virus) infections are well-known infections that can occur in utero and are associated with long-term neurodevelopmental disabilities, including CP [12]. These infections account for about 5% or less of CP cases in industrialized countries [12].

Chorioamnionitis is an independent risk factor for CP and is associated with a 4-fold increased risk of CP in term infants [33]. It is thought that placental infection may cause or exacerbate brain injury because of hypoxia-ischemia, which leads to an increase in inflammatory cytokine levels in the fetus [33]. High levels of inflammatory cytokines have been implicated in the pathogenesis of preterm birth, as well as in the development of intraventricular hemorrhage and PVL in preterm children [12]. In children born with CP, an increased prevalence of abnormalities in the placenta and cord has been observed, highlighting the importance of obtaining placental histology as well as arterial cord gases in those infants that are delivered in poor condition [32].

Peripartum risk factors

Premature birth. Preterm birth (<37 weeks' gestation) is one of the most important risk factors for CP [12]. Children born prematurely account for about 35% of cases of CP, with higher prevalence of CP at earlier gestational ages [32]. With advancements in neonatal care, babies born very premature are more likely to survive; however, extreme prematurity puts them at an increased risk for CP because of underdevelopment of the brain as well as lack of lung maturity increasing their risk of postnatal hypoxia [9]. PVL and intraventricular hemorrhage (IVH) are the two major disorders affecting very preterm infants that are associated with CP [31].

Meconium aspiration. Meconium aspiration may occur when the fetus has its first bowel movement, referred to as meconium, while in utero; when the neonate is born and starts breathing there is increased risk of aspiration caused by fluid and secretions present in the mouth at birth. If the neonate aspirates the meconium-stained amniotic fluid, this can lead to respiratory distress and aspiration pneumonia, which can lead to hypoxia, pulmonary hypertension, and cardiorespiratory failure in severe cases [31]. Among term infants experiencing severe meconium aspiration, 41% may develop mild deficits such as speech delay or mild hypotonicity without motor or cognitive deficits, 7% may develop CP, and 14% may develop other severe long-term developmental disabilities [34].

Hypoxic-ischemic encephalopathy. Birth asphyxia is a much less frequent cause of CP than was previously thought. Birth asphyxia may account for less than 3% to greater than 50% of cases of CP depending on how birth asphyxia is defined [35]. The definition of asphyxia was previously less rigorous and often referred only to the need for oxygen after birth [36]. The term hypoxic-ischemic encephalopathy (HIE) refers more specifically to neonatal encephalopathy resulting from an acute intrapartum hypoxic event. The diagnosis of HIE is made through a combination of neurologic examination findings and biochemical evidence of metabolic acidosis on cord blood gas or arterial blood gas obtained within an hour of birth. Other supporting evidence for HIE may include low Apgar scores, seizures, and brain MRI findings suggestive of an ischemic insult to the watershed areas of the brain or to the deep structures, such as germinal matrix hemorrhage, which is caused by reperfusion of ischemic brain tissue leading to increased venous pressure and rupture of weak capillaries, PVL, passive ventriculomegaly, and thinning of the corpus callosum [37]. Other findings include electroencephalogram findings, or evidence of multisystem organ failure [38]. An Australian study of a cohort of 235 neonates with CP found that in only 1% could CP be associated with birth asphyxia when criteria from the American College of Obstetricians and Gynecologists (ACOG) and the international CP task force were used in a cohort of 213 infants of the 235 cases [39]. Although other studies report slightly higher risk, this risk may be mitigated by the use of therapeutic hypothermia [40]. Davidson and colleagues [41] found that recent hypothermia treatment protocols showed a significant improvement in outcomes; however, it is only partially effective, and more research is needed to further reduce the burden of injury. The hypothermia protocols advise systemically cooling patients with HIE within the first 6 hours of life to 34.5° ± 0.5°C for cooling the head, or 33.5° ± 0.5°C for whole-body cooling with continued treatment for 48 to 72 hours [41].

Neonatal seizures. Neonatal seizures may occur in infants with HIE but also may be a presenting sign of perinatal stroke or central nervous system (CNS) infection, both of which are associated with increased risk of CP. About 30% of infants with perinatal arterial ischemic strokes develop CP, with unilateral spastic CP as the most common subtype. A 2018 analysis of 188 infants with perinatal arterial ischemic stroke suggests the middle cerebral artery is most commonly involved, and findings on initial MRI correlate with later neurodevelopment [42].

Risk factors for postneonatally acquired cerebral palsy

Postneonatal CP is often described as injury outside of the neonatal period and before 5 years of age, accounting for fewer than 10% of CP cases [39,43]. Almost all cases of postneonatal CP are caused by head trauma, near-drowning events, or meningitis [39,44]. In the United States, CP cases with documented postneonatal causes accounted for 6% to 10% of all cases in the ADDM Network data [27]. Many postneonatally acquired cases of CP could be prevented through public health programs designed to reduce likelihood of child injury.

PREVENTION

Although many neonatal measures to prevent CP have been studied, very few have been shown to be effective [43]. Of 96 randomized controlled trials reviewed in a 2018 Cochrane Review, therapeutic hypothermia and caffeine were the only effective interventions. This article briefly reviews several of the more commonly used interventions.

Therapeutic hypothermia

Therapeutic hypothermia initiated within 6 hours of birth and lasting 72 hours decreases the risks of CP in term and late preterm infants with moderate to severe HIE by approximately one-third. Hypoxic-ischemic brain injury is characterized by several cellular-based events, which include failure of the Na+/K+ ATP-dependent pump from deranged metabolism; accretion of excitatory amino acids (EAAs); production of cytotoxic oxygen free radicals; and generation of the reactive oxygen species nitric oxide, which leads to cell membrane and cytosol organelle damage. The cumulative effects of these events is neuronal depolarization and cerebral edema. Further complicating brain swelling is the disruption of the blood-brain barrier with associated leaks. Hypothermia has been shown to reduce cerebral metabolism, accumulation of EAAs, suppression of nitric oxide, and the leakiness of the blood-brain barrier [45]. This neuroprotective effect is likely caused by the inhibition of a variety of inflammatory and apoptotic cellular processes that occur following an ischemic insult. It has been estimated that for every 8 infants treated with therapeutic hypothermia, 1 case of CP is prevented. Whole-body cooling and selective head cooling with mild systemic hypothermia seem to be equally effective [40].

Recent studies have sought to refine therapeutic hypothermia practices. An attempt to optimize therapeutic hypothermia suggested cooling for longer than 72 hours, and cooling to lower than 33.5°C did not reduce death or moderate to severe disability at age 18 months [46]. Another study supported late initiation of therapeutic hypothermia from 6 to 24 hours after birth, reporting 76% probability of any reduction in death or disability [47]. The investigation of potential adjuvant therapies is a subject of active research with ongoing studies evaluating the used of xenon, erythropoietin, antiepileptic drugs (such as topiramate), melatonin, magnesium sulfate, and umbilical cord stem cells [43]. Another current clinical trial is investigating therapeutic hypothermia in preterm infants from gestational age 33 to 35 weeks with moderate to severe HIE [48].

Caffeine

Preterm infants are often treated with caffeine for apnea of prematurity or to facilitate extubation. Caffeine, like other methylxanthines, increases respiratory drive and decreases the number of apneic events. The Caffeine for Apnea of Prematurity Trial compared caffeine versus placebo in very-low-birth-weight infants initiated during the first 10 days of life [49]. Post hoc analysis of the study suggests caffeine reduces the incidence of CP in very-low-birth-weight infants treated with caffeine specifically to facilitate extubation (relative risk, 0.54) [50]. However, post hoc analysis of the same study suggested no clear differences in CP following overall treatment or prophylaxis with caffeine for apnea of prematurity [43].

Avoidance of early postnatal corticosteroids

Postnatal corticosteroids are used to decrease inflammation in order to decrease rates of bronchopulmonary dysplasia and facilitate extubation. Despite the pulmonary benefits, early (<8 days) use of dexamethasone after birth has been associated with increased rates of CP [43,51]. The 2010 American Academy of Pediatrics policy statement on postnatal corticosteroid use for bronchopulmonary dysplasia recommends the avoidance of early high-dose dexamethasone because of the association with CP [52].

The risks and benefits of postnatal corticosteroids must be balanced for individual patients. A 2005 meta-analysis notes that among infants with less than 35% risk of bronchopulmonary dysplasia, corticosteroid treatment significantly increased the chance of death or CP, but among infants with more than 65% risk of bronchopulmonary dysplasia, treatment decreased the chance of death or CP [53]. In a recent randomized controlled trial, early low-dose hydrocortisone decreased survival without bronchopulmonary dysplasia and no association with CP was noted [54]. The risks and benefits of hydrocortisone remain unclear in meta-analyses and is an area of ongoing research [43,55].

Antenatal steroids

In a population-based case-control study by Jacobsson and colleagues [56], antenatal corticosteroids were associated with a decrease in the risk of CP. Betamethasone has been shown to reduce PVL in preterm infants; however, dexamethasone has not shown the same outcome [56]. Betamethasone helps to reduce the severity of respiratory distress syndrome as well as decrease the risk of IVH [57].

Magnesium

Administration of magnesium sulfate during the antenatal period is important for neuroprotection in preterm infants [58]. Magnesium given before preterm delivery is associated with a significant reduction in the risk of CP at 2 years of age [58]. Magnesium sulfate reduces inflammatory effects by reducing oxidative stress as well as proinflammatory cytokines [58]. Based on Chollat and Marret's [58] (2018) findings, the use of magnesium sulfate antenatally did not result in adverse neonatal outcomes, including respiratory distress, the need for mechanical ventilation, and necrotizing enterocolitis. However, reduction in CP with antenatal use of magnesium sulfate occurred only in infants of nonobese women, which suggests that adjustment of magnesium dosage based on maternal weight may be required for adequate neuroprotection.

PATHOGENESIS

The cause of CP is multifactorial and remains incompletely understood. CP can be a result of a brain insult or injury that occurs during the prenatal, perinatal, or postnatal periods. The old views of CP being caused by asphyxial injury during delivery are not supported by evidence [31]. Platt and colleagues [31] (2017) found that a prenatal cause was most likely to be responsible for about 50% to 55% of quadriplegic CP, a perinatal cause in 30%, and a postnatal cause in 15% to 20%. Different brain structures show varying levels of susceptibility to insult or injury at different gestational ages, which further supports the idea that CP can develop at any point through pregnancy caused by multiple injuries throughout development. Despite advances in diagnostic techniques, a specific cause is found for no more than 50% to 75% of CP cases.

Many pathways can lead to development of CP. Intrauterine hypoxia affecting the fetal brain is one of the most common prenatal risk factors associated with CP [31]. Hypoxia in utero typically occurs because of placental insufficiency toward the end of pregnancy or because of anomalies in the placenta and cord, or placental abruption leading to decrease in oxygen delivery to the fetus [31]. During the second and third trimesters of pregnancy, the main causes of CP are placental problems or other problems that can cause chronic endometrial hypoxia [31]. Chronic hypoxia of the fetus over a long period of time can lead to an abnormal head circumference in the fetus, indicating abnormal brain development [31]. Fetal hypoxia can occur during labor as well; however, it requires severe hypoxia or prolonged anoxia to cause deterioration in the CNS because of the protective mechanisms the fetus has that protect it from repeated episodes of mild hypoxia during contractions and the process of labor [31].

Another hypothesis regarding the pathogenesis of CP is the inflammatory/cytokine hypothesis. It suggests that when maternal infection or fever occurs it causes an increase in cytokine levels in the fetal blood and brain and these cytokines can cause periventricular white matter damage as well as preterm birth [12]. Interleukin (IL)-6 and IL-8, as well as other proinflammatory cytokines, have been found to have an association with CP in preterm children [12]. IL-6 in the amniotic fluid has been shown to be related to intraventricular hemorrhage and increased levels of IL-6, IL-1 alpha, and TNF-alpha are related to PVL [12].

THE GENETICS OF CEREBRAL PALSY

CP is considered a complex disease because of the convoluted interactions between environmental and genetic factors. Although the diagnosis and classification of CP are mainly clinical, and its cause varies greatly, there is considerable evidence that many cases of CP have genetic underpinnings [59]. The prevalence of congenital anomalies in children with CP is about 11% to 32%, significantly higher than the general population prevalence of 2% to 3% [60]. Higher rates of CP have been observed in monozygotic than in dizygotic twins, and there is a 2 to 5 times higher risk of CP in consanguineous compared with outbred families [60].

Genomic insights are a gateway to understanding the neurogenetic routes that cause CP and have the potential to influence patient care. Suspicion of CP's genetic basis stems from its syndromic presentations and its association with twinning (especially the monozygotic variant), consanguinity, and congenital anomalies [61–63]. Human genome sequencing, including whole-exome sequencing, X-chromosome exome sequencing, and chromosomal analysis in population studies, has led to the identification of various gene mutations that are linked to the development of CP, indicating that no single CP gene exists but that multiple genes are involved [64,65]. This genetic heterogeneity underscores the complexity of the contribution of genes to the development of CP.

Numerous Mendelian disorders inherited as autosomal dominant, recessive, as well as X-linked can present with characteristics that are distinct to CP. Some of these conditions are rare as individual disorders, but others are not all that uncommon as a group and should be taken into account when assessing children with CP [60]. Several known single-gene causes of CP were discovered through studying families with 2 or more individuals with CP; these include mutations in the KANK1, AP4M1, and GAD1 genes [32].

Plausible genetic variants associated with CP can be grouped into several categories, which are discussed later.

Single-gene mutations

The many genes that have been identified as being related to CP encode proteins with a variety of functions [66]. KANK1 controls actin polymerization and its heterozygous deletion often leads to a spastic CP phenotype [62]. Also linked to spastic CP are mutations in subunits of the Adaptor protein 4 complex (subunits B1, E1, M1, and S1), which are responsible for vesicle formation and selection of inclusion molecules to be transported across cells [67]. ADD3 mutation has also been linked to spastic CP and its function is related to that of KANK1 [64]. The GAD1 gene is responsible for cytogenetic production of the gamma-aminobutyric acid neurotransmitter and its homozygous mutation causes CP [61,62]. ITPR1, KCNC3, and SPTBN2 all code specific ion channels in body cells and their mutations are linked to ataxic CP [64,68].

Candidate cerebral palsy genes

According to McMichael and colleagues [69], gene mutations thought to be associated with CP together with numerous newly identified associated genes were found in 14% of unselected CP cohorts using whole-exome sequencing. De novo candidate CP genes identified were AGAP1, JHDM1D, MAST1, NAA35, RFX2, and WIPI2, whereas known hemizygous X-linked variants were L1CAM and PAK3 and, in novel genes, CD99L2 and TENM1, inherited from an unaffected mother. This diverseness implies that newer and less familiar mutations can potentially contribute to the development of CP, further emphasizing the complexity of the genetics in CP etiopathogenesis.

Copy number variants

Copy number variants (CNVs) are variations in the structure of DNA sequences, which can be duplications or deletions greater than 1000 base pairs. CNVs can either occur de novo (observed in an affected individual and not in the parents of the individual) or inherited from either parent, who can be affected or not affected. This variability in expressivity makes it difficult to determine the link between a single gene and CP. Various CNVs have been associated with specific subclasses of CP, of which several percentages in different studies have either occurred de novo or been inherited. CNVs that have been associated with the development of CP include: GRIK2, LAMA1, DMD, PTPRM, and DIP2C, associated with hemiplegic CP [70]; SPAST, MEF2C, WDR45, KANK1, NKX2-1, and tripXq28 [62,64]; PARK2, PACRG and HSPA4, WNT4, RAPGEF1 [59,64]; MC2R, CTNND2, SPG6/NIPA1, associated with spastic paraplegia; and DAAM1, MCPH1, NIPA2 [71].

Single nucleotide polymorphisms

Single nucleotide polymorphisms refer to a substitution of nucleotide base pairs on specific positions in a gene and has been implicated in heterogeneity seen in different populations. It is also responsible for occurrence of some diseases (cystic fibrosis, sickle cell disease) and differences observed in susceptibility to diseases processes and responses to illnesses and medications. Although several studies have tried to find associations between CP and several single nucleotide polymorphs, no strong associations were found, and conflicting results abound across studies [64]. The link between mutations in genes causing hereditary thrombophilia (eg, antithrombin, proteins C and S) and CP as a result of its tendency to cause hypercoagulative states and therefore perinatal stroke and CP was small [72]. A case-control study of more than 1400 Chinese participants found that IL-6 gene polymorphisms on IL-6 synthesis and the risk of CP was related to sex and gestational age [73].

As study into the neurobiology of CP continues, the use of lower eukaryotes, as opposed to current large-animal models, seems to be the way forward. These lower eukaryotes have a high percentage of gene/protein analogues to humans, are less costly, and are more genetically pliable in nature, providing potent insights into how CP-associated variations in human gene/proteins affect normal physiology and cause disorders [64]. Overall, a thorough understanding of the interplay between genes and environmental risk factors on the clinical manifestations of CP will require more studies of larger populations. This research should be accompanied by comprehensive evaluations of their applicability in prenatal diagnosis and prevention, as well as for clinical diagnosis and management.

MANAGEMENT OF CEREBRAL PALSY

Historically, many interventions, ranging from activity-based rehabilitation interventions to use of antispasticity medications, have been used to ameliorate symptoms and improve motor outcomes in children with CP. However, high-quality evidence about the efficacy of these interventions is largely lacking, because few interventions have been rigorously studied [74,75]. Novak and colleagues [74] conducted a systematic review in which they deemed the following interventions effective: botulinum toxin, diazepam, or selective dorsal rhizotomy for muscle spasticity; casting to improve ankle function; hip surveillance to maintain hip joint integrity; goal-directed therapies based in the home; bisphosphonates to improve bone density; pressure care to reduce risk of pressure ulcers; and anticonvulsants if needed for seizure disorders. Goals Activity Motor Enrichment (GAME) is a specific early intervention program that involves goal-directed activities and parental coaching and has been shown in a randomized trial to improve motor and cognitive skills of children with CP at 1 year of age compared with usual care [76]. There is robust evidence that infants with hemiplegia who receive early constraint-induced movement therapy, which encourages use of the affected extremity by restraining the unaffected one, improves hand functioning, at least in the short term [77]. Evidence for other intervention strategies continues to evolve, but experts advocate early initiation of therapies as soon as signs of CP are recognized in order to optimize motor development during the period of neuroplasticity in early childhood.

The management of CP requires a multidisciplinary approach and clinicians must also address other comorbidities that may coexist with motor impairment. Children with CP may be followed by a range of specialists, including orthopedic surgeons, urologists, neurologists, physiatrists, gastroenterologists, sleep medicine specialists, and developmental pediatricians, in addition to physical therapists, occupational therapists, developmental therapists, speech therapists, and feeding specialists.

Addressing quality of life in patients with cerebral palsy

Much of CP management has focused on improving motor function, but an understanding of what affects quality of life most is important when devising care plans. Quality of life is often evaluated using the framework of the World Health Organization's International Classification of Functioning, Disability and Health, which includes the following domains: body structure and function, activity limitation, participation, environmental factors, and personal factors [36]. Many of these topics were addressed by a recent systematic review describing comorbidities in children with CP. Common comorbidities, in declining level of frequency, included pain, inability to walk, hip displacement, bladder control problems, sleep disorders, dribbling, and dependence on tube feeding [78]. The high percentage of children with pain is especially striking, because pain is often associated with poor quality of life across domains [79]. Associated developmental and behavior impairments included intellectual disability (1 in 2), inability to talk (1 in 4), epilepsy (1 in 4), behavior disorder (1 in 4), blindness (1 in 10), and deafness (1 in 25) [78].

Some clinicians assume children with CP have worse quality of life than their typically developing peers. Quality-of-life assessments done in 500 children with CP aged 8 to 12 years across Europe evaluated self-reported quality-of-life measures in domains of physical well-being, psychological well-being, moods and emotions, self-perception, autonomy, relationships with parents, social support, school environment, financial resources, and social acceptance. Self-reported quality-of-life scores were broadly similar to those of typically developing children except for equivocal differences in schooling and physical well-being in children with severe motor impairments [80].

Quality of life is most difficult to assess in severely affected individuals with impaired communication. For these individuals, assessments must rely on information from caregivers. When comparing parent-reported quality of life for children with CP in Europe, poor gross motor function and low intelligence quotient were associated with low quality of life in most domains. However, parents of less severely impaired children rated the following domains lower than parents of children with very severe impairments: moods and emotions, self-perception, social acceptance, and school environment [81]. Caregiver assessments may be influenced by confounding factors. For example, high levels of parental stress correspond with poor parent-reported quality of life in all domains [81].

Ability to complete activities of daily living and function within society are important domains affecting an individual's quality of life. Although CP is caused by a fixed nonprogressive neurologic injury, an individual's motor performance and daily activity performance often improves over time, although at a slower pace than typically developing individuals. A 2018 study tracked motor performance in 421 individuals aged 1 to 20 years and reported the age at which individuals reached 90% of the average maximal performance level [82]. Individuals with CP who were able to walk (GMFCS levels I to III) continued to improve in motor performance until age 6 to 8 years. For those without intellectual disability who were able to walk, limits of daily activity performance were similar to typically developing peers, but it took longer for individuals with CP to achieve these limits. These individuals continued to improve through age 11 to 14 years (self-care activities), 26 to 32 years (domestic activities), and 22 to 26 years (community activities). In comparison, typically developing individuals reach 90% of the average maximal performance level for self-care, domestic activity, and community activity at about 7, 18, and 15 years of age, respectively. Individuals who are severely affected functionally (GMFCS IV and V) had poorer motor performance and attained significantly lower limits of daily activity performance. Individuals with CP and intellectual disability also reached lower maximal daily activity performance levels and at an earlier age than typically developing peers [82].

SUMMARY

CP is a heterogeneous disorder with many well-recognized risk factors in the prenatal, perinatal, and early postnatal periods. CP is the most common physical disability of childhood, and all pediatricians should be aware of the general strategies for diagnosis and treatment. The diagnosis may be made in infants as early as 6 months of age through a combination of neurologic assessment, neuroimaging findings, and recognition of clinical risk factors. Management of CP and its associated comorbidities is complex and requires a multidisciplinary approach. Further research is needed to identify strategies for prevention of CP and to inform clinicians about which interventions are most effective in improving the functional outcomes of children with CP.

References

[1] Graham HK, Rosenbaum P, Paneth N, et al. Cerebral palsy. Nat Rev Dis Primers 2016;2: 15082.

[2] Rosenbaum P, Paneth N, Leviton A, et al. A report: the definition and classification of cerebral palsy April 2006. Dev Med Child Neurol Suppl 2007;109:8–14.
[3] Herskind A, Greisen G, Nielsen JB. Early identification and intervention in cerebral palsy. Dev Med Child Neurol 2015;57(1):29–36.
[4] Baird G, McConachie H, Scrutton D. Parents' perceptions of disclosure of the diagnosis of cerebral palsy. Arch Dis Child 2000;83(6):475–80.
[5] Spittle AJ, Morgan C, Olsen JE, et al. Early diagnosis and treatment of cerebral palsy in children with a history of preterm birth. Clin Perinatol 2018;45(3):409–20.
[6] Novak I, Morgan C, Adde L, et al. Early, accurate diagnosis and early intervention in cerebral palsy: advances in diagnosis and treatment. JAMA Pediatr 2017;171(9):897–907.
[7] Bosanquet M, Copeland L, Ware R, et al. A systematic review of tests to predict cerebral palsy in young children. Dev Med Child Neurol 2013;55(5):418–26.
[8] Ashwal S, Russman BS, Blasco PA, et al. Practice parameter: diagnostic assessment of the child with cerebral palsy: report of the Quality Standards Subcommittee of the American Academy of Neurology and the Practice Committee of the Child Neurology Society. Neurology 2004;62(6):851–63.
[9] Korzeniewski SJ, Birbeck G, DeLano MC, et al. A systematic review of neuroimaging for cerebral palsy. J Child Neurol 2008;23(2):216–27.
[10] Palmer FB. Strategies for the early diagnosis of cerebral palsy. J Pediatr 2004;145(2 Suppl): S8–11.
[11] Vossough A. Brain imaging: magnetic resonance imaging. In: Pateliadis CP, editor. Cerebral palsy: a multidisciplinary approach, 3rd Ed. Cham, Switzerland: Springer International Publishing; 2018. p. 113–31.
[12] Jacobsson B, Hagberg G. Antenatal risk factors for cerebral palsy. Best Pract Res Clin Obstet Gynaecol 2004;18(3):425–36.
[13] Prechtl HF. Qualitative changes of spontaneous movements in fetus and preterm infant are a marker of neurological dysfunction. Early Hum Dev 1990;23(3):151–8.
[14] Kwong AKL, Fitzgerald TL, Doyle LW, et al. Predictive validity of spontaneous early infant movement for later cerebral palsy: a systematic review. Dev Med Child Neurol 2018;60(5):480–9.
[15] Einspieler C, Prechtl HF. Prechtl's assessment of general movements: a diagnostic tool for the functional assessment of the young nervous system. Ment Retard Dev Disabil Res Rev 2005;11(1):61–7.
[16] Romeo DM, Ricci D, Brogna C, et al. Use of the Hammersmith Infant Neurological Examination in infants with cerebral palsy: a critical review of the literature. Dev Med Child Neurol 2016;58(3):240–5.
[17] Hay K, Nelin M, Carey H, et al. Hammersmith infant neurological examination asymmetry score distinguishes hemiplegic cerebral palsy from typical development. Pediatr Neurol 2018;87:70–4.
[18] Lee RW, Poretti A, Cohen JS, et al. A diagnostic approach for cerebral palsy in the genomic era. Neuromolecular Med 2014;16(4):821–44.
[19] MacLennan A, Gecz J, Perez-Jurado L. A genomic cause of cerebral palsy should not change the clinical classification. Ann Clin Transl Neurol 2018;5(8):1011.
[20] Takezawa Y, Kikuchi A, Haginoya K, et al. Genomic analysis identifies masqueraders of full-term cerebral palsy. Ann Clin Transl Neurol 2018;5(5):538–51.
[21] Spittle AJ, Orton J. Cerebral palsy and developmental coordination disorder in children born preterm. Semin Fetal Neonatal Med 2014;19(2):84–9.
[22] Williams J, Lee KJ, Anderson PJ. Prevalence of motor-skill impairment in preterm children who do not develop cerebral palsy: a systematic review. Dev Med Child Neurol 2010;52(3):232–7.
[23] Edwards J, Berube M, Erlandson K, et al. Developmental coordination disorder in school-aged children born very preterm and/or at very low birth weight: a systematic review. J Dev Behav Pediatr 2011;32(9):678–87.

[24] McIntyre S, Morgan C, Walker K, et al. Cerebral palsy–don't delay. Dev Disabil Res Rev 2011;17(2):114–29.
[25] Palisano R, Rosenbaum P, Walter S, et al. Development and reliability of a system to classify gross motor function in children with cerebral palsy. Dev Med Child Neurol 1997;39(4): 214–23.
[26] Palisano RJ, Avery L, Gorter JW, et al. Stability of the gross motor function classification system, manual ability classification system, and communication function classification system. Dev Med Child Neurol 2018;60(10):1026–32.
[27] Durkin MS, Benedict RE, Christensen D, et al. Prevalence of cerebral palsy among 8-year-old children in 2010 and preliminary evidence of trends in its relationship to low birthweight. Paediatr Perinat Epidemiol 2016;30(5):496–510.
[28] Maenner MJ, Blumberg SJ, Kogan MD, et al. Prevalence of cerebral palsy and intellectual disability among children identified in two U.S. National Surveys, 2011-2013. Ann Epidemiol 2016;26(3):222–6.
[29] McIntyre S, Taitz D, Keogh J, et al. A systematic review of risk factors for cerebral palsy in children born at term in developed countries. Dev Med Child Neurol 2013;55(6): 499–508.
[30] Durkin MS, Maenner MJ, Benedict RE, et al. The role of socio-economic status and perinatal factors in racial disparities in the risk of cerebral palsy. Dev Med Child Neurol 2015;57(9): 835–43.
[31] Platt MJ, Pateliadis CP, Häusler M. Aetiological factors. In: Pateliadis CP, editor. Cerebral palsy: a multidisciplinary approach, 3rd Ed. Cham, Switzerland: Springer International Publishing; 2018. p. 49–58.
[32] MacLennan AH, Thompson SC, Gecz J. Cerebral palsy: causes, pathways, and the role of genetic variants. Am J Obstet Gynecol 2015;213(6):779–88.
[33] Millichap J. Chorioamnionitis: a risk factor for cerebral palsy. Pediatr Neurol Briefs 2003;17(12):91.
[34] Beligere N, Rao R. Neurodevelopmental outcome of infants with meconium aspiration syndrome: report of a study and literature review. J Perinatol 2008;28(Suppl 3):S93–101.
[35] Ellenberg JH, Nelson KB. The association of cerebral palsy with birth asphyxia: a definitional quagmire. Dev Med Child Neurol 2013;55(3):210–6.
[36] Colver A, Fairhurst C, Pharoah PO. Cerebral palsy. Lancet 2014;383(9924):1240–9.
[37] Bano S, Chaudhary V, Garga UC. Neonatal hypoxic-ischemic encephalopathy: a radiological review. J Pediatr Neurosci 2017;12(1):1–6.
[38] American College of Obstetricians and Gynecology. Executive summary: Neonatal encephalopathy and neurologic outcome, second edition. Report of the American College of Obstetricians and Gynecologists' Task Force on Neonatal Encephalopathy. Obstet Gynecol 2014;123(4):896–901.
[39] Strijbis EM, Oudman I, van Essen P, et al. Cerebral palsy and the application of the international criteria for acute intrapartum hypoxia. Obstet Gynecol 2006;107(6):1357–65.
[40] Jacobs SE, Berg M, Hunt R, et al. Cooling for newborns with hypoxic ischaemic encephalopathy. Cochrane Database Syst Rev 2013;(1):CD003311.
[41] Davidson JO, Wassink G, van den Heuij LG, et al. Therapeutic hypothermia for neonatal hypoxic–ischemic encephalopathy–where to from here? Front Neurol 2015;6:198.
[42] Wagenaar N, Martinez-Biarge M, van der Aa NE, et al. Neurodevelopment after perinatal arterial ischemic stroke. Pediatrics 2018;142(3) [pii:e20174164].
[43] Shepherd E, Salam RA, Middleton P, et al. Neonatal interventions for preventing cerebral palsy: an overview of Cochrane Systematic Reviews. Cochrane Database Syst Rev 2018;(6):CD012409.
[44] Maudsley G, Hutton JL, Pharoah PO. Cause of death in cerebral palsy: a descriptive study. Arch Dis Child 1999;81(5):390–4.
[45] Wassink G, Davidson JO, Dhillon SK, et al. Therapeutic hypothermia in neonatal hypoxic-ischemic encephalopathy. Curr Neurol Neurosci Rep 2019;19(2):2.

[46] Shankaran S, Laptook AR, Pappas A, et al. Effect of depth and duration of cooling on death or disability at age 18 months among neonates with hypoxic-ischemic encephalopathy: a randomized clinical trial. JAMA 2017;318(1):57–67.
[47] Laptook AR, Shankaran S, Tyson JE, et al. Effect of therapeutic hypothermia initiated after 6 hours of age on death or disability among newborns with hypoxic-ischemic encephalopathy: a randomized clinical trial. JAMA 2017;318(16):1550–60.
[48] ClinicalTrials.gov: Preemie hypothermia for neonatal encephalopathy. Available at: https://clinicaltrials.gov/ct2/show/NCT01793129?cond=preterm+therapeutic+hypothermia&rank=1. Accessed December 2, 2018.
[49] Schmidt B, Roberts RS, Davis P, et al. Long-term effects of caffeine therapy for apnea of prematurity. N Engl J Med 2007;357(19):1893–902.
[50] Henderson-Smart DJ, De Paoli AG. Prophylactic methylxanthine for prevention of apnoea in preterm infants. Cochrane Database Syst Rev 2010;(12):CD000432.
[51] O'Shea TM, Kothadia JM, Klinepeter KL, et al. Randomized placebo-controlled trial of a 42-day tapering course of dexamethasone to reduce the duration of ventilator dependency in very low birth weight infants: outcome of study participants at 1-year adjusted age. Pediatrics 1999;104(1 Pt 1):15–21.
[52] Watterberg KL. Policy statement–postnatal corticosteroids to prevent or treat bronchopulmonary dysplasia. Pediatrics 2010;126(4):800–8.
[53] Doyle LW, Halliday HL, Ehrenkranz RA, et al. Impact of postnatal systemic corticosteroids on mortality and cerebral palsy in preterm infants: effect modification by risk for chronic lung disease. Pediatrics 2005;115(3):655–61.
[54] Baud O, Trousson C, Biran V, et al. Association between early low-dose hydrocortisone therapy in extremely preterm neonates and neurodevelopmental outcomes at 2 years of age. JAMA 2017;317(13):1329–37.
[55] ClinicalTrials.gov: Hydrocortisone for BPD. Available at: https://clinicaltrials.gov/ct2/show/NCT01353313. Accessed December 3, 2018.
[56] Jacobsson B, Hagberg G, Hagberg B, et al. Cerebral palsy in preterm infants: a population-based case-control study of antenatal and intrapartal risk factors. Acta Paediatr 2002;91(8):946–51.
[57] Malaeb SN, Stonestreet BS. Steroids and injury to the developing brain: net harm or net benefit? Clin Perinatol 2014;41(1):191–208.
[58] Chollat C, Marret S. Magnesium sulfate and fetal neuroprotection: overview of clinical evidence. Neural Regen Res 2018;13(12):2044–9.
[59] Oskoui M, Gazzellone MJ, Thiruvahindrapuram B, et al. Clinically relevant copy number variations detected in cerebral palsy. Nat Commun 2015;6:7949.
[60] Moreno-De-Luca A, Ledbetter DH, Martin CL. Genetic [corrected] insights into the causes and classification of [corrected] cerebral palsies. Lancet Neurol 2012;11(3):283–92.
[61] Levenson D. Genetic factors may underlie many cerebral palsy cases. Hoboken (NJ): Wiley-Blackwell; 2015.
[62] van Eyk CL, Corbett MA, Maclennan AH. The emerging genetic landscape of cerebral palsy. Handb Clin Neurol 2018;147:331–42.
[63] Tollanes MC, Wilcox AJ, Lie RT, et al. Familial risk of cerebral palsy: population based cohort study. BMJ 2014;349:g4294.
[64] Fahey MC, Maclennan AH, Kretzschmar D, et al. The genetic basis of cerebral palsy. Dev Med Child Neurol 2017;59(5):462–9.
[65] Schaefer GB. Genetics considerations in cerebral palsy. Semin Pediatr Neurol 2008;15(1):21–6.
[66] Ebrahimi-Fakhari D, Cheng C, Dies K, et al. Clinical and genetic characterization of AP4B1-associated SPG47. Am J Med Genet A 2018;176(2):311–8.
[67] Abou Jamra R, Philippe O, Raas-Rothschild A, et al. Adaptor protein complex 4 deficiency causes severe autosomal-recessive intellectual disability, progressive spastic paraplegia, shy character, and short stature. Am J Hum Genet 2011;88(6):788–95.

[68] Parolin Schnekenberg R, Perkins EM, Miller JW, et al. De novo point mutations in patients diagnosed with ataxic cerebral palsy. Brain 2015;138(Pt 7):1817–32.
[69] McMichael G, Bainbridge MN, Haan E, et al. Whole-exome sequencing points to considerable genetic heterogeneity of cerebral palsy. Mol Psychiatry 2015;20(2):176–82.
[70] Zarrei M, Fehlings DL, Mawjee K, et al. De novo and rare inherited copy-number variations in the hemiplegic form of cerebral palsy. Genet Med 2018;20(2):172–80.
[71] McMichael G, Girirajan S, Moreno-De-Luca A, et al. Rare copy number variation in cerebral palsy. Eur J Hum Genet 2014;22(1):40–5.
[72] Torres VM, Saddi VA. Systematic review: hereditary thrombophilia associated to pediatric strokes and cerebral palsy. J Pediatr (Rio J) 2015;91(1):22–9.
[73] Bi D, Chen M, Zhang X, et al. The association between sex-related interleukin-6 gene polymorphisms and the risk for cerebral palsy. J Neuroinflammation 2014;11:100.
[74] Novak I, McIntyre S, Morgan C, et al. A systematic review of interventions for children with cerebral palsy: state of the evidence. Dev Med Child Neurol 2013;55(10):885–910.
[75] Ward R, Reynolds JE, Bear N, et al. What is the evidence for managing tone in young children with, or at risk of developing, cerebral palsy: a systematic review. Disabil Rehabil 2017;39(7):619–30.
[76] Morgan C, Novak I, Dale RC, et al. Single blind randomised controlled trial of GAME (Goals - Activity - Motor Enrichment) in infants at high risk of cerebral palsy. Res Dev Disabil 2016;55:256–67.
[77] Sakzewski L, Ziviani J, Boyd RN. Efficacy of upper limb therapies for unilateral cerebral palsy: a meta-analysis. Pediatrics 2014;133(1):e175–204.
[78] Novak I, Hines M, Goldsmith S, et al. Clinical prognostic messages from a systematic review on cerebral palsy. Pediatrics 2012;130(5):e1285–312.
[79] Colver A, Rapp M, Eisemann N, et al. Self-reported quality of life of adolescents with cerebral palsy: a cross-sectional and longitudinal analysis. Lancet 2015;385(9969):705–16.
[80] Dickinson HO, Parkinson KN, Ravens-Sieberer U, et al. Self-reported quality of life of 8-12-year-old children with cerebral palsy: a cross-sectional European study. Lancet 2007;369(9580):2171–8.
[81] Arnaud C, White-Koning M, Michelsen SI, et al. Parent-reported quality of life of children with cerebral palsy in Europe. Pediatrics 2008;121(1):54–64.
[82] van Gorp M, Roebroeck ME, Swan Tan S, et al. Activity performance curves of individuals with cerebral palsy. Pediatrics 2018;142(5) [pii:e20173723].

Advances in Pediatrics 66 (2019) 209–229

ADVANCES IN PEDIATRICS

ELSEVIER
MOSBY

Pediatric Multiple Sclerosis

A Review

Megan M. Langille, MD[a,*], Alice Rutatangwa, DO, MS[b], Carla Francisco, MD[b]

[a]Pediatrics, University of California Los Angeles, Harbor UCLA, 1000 West Carson Street, Box 468, Torrance, CA 90509, USA; [b]Pediatric Neurology and Multiple Sclerosis Clinic, University of California, San Francisco, Pediatric Brain Center, 550 16th Street, 4th Floor Box 0137, San Francisco, CA 94158, USA

Keywords

• Pediatric multiple sclerosis • McDonald criteria • Disease-modifying treatment

Key points

- Risk factors, including diet, genetics, body mass index, microbiome, and infections, are actively being explored.
- Cognitive issues can be a prominent part of multiple sclerosis (MS) in children and deserve special attention.
- Diagnostic criteria for adults with MS have changed in 2017; some evidence shows these changes are valid for pediatric-onset multiple sclerosis.
- Treatment options and paradigms are expanding for patients with MS, and this has implications on pediatric MS treatment.

Multiple sclerosis (MS) is a chronic, inflammatory condition that affects the central nervous system (CNS). Study of pediatric-onset multiple sclerosis (POMS) is relevant to adult-onset multiple sclerosis (AOMS) because children are temporally closer to the exposure of environmental influences and risk factors.

DEMOGRAPHICS

Between 3% and 10% of MS cases are diagnosed before the age of 18 years [1–6]. MS in prepubertal children is rare and makes up less than 1% of cases [3,7]. Age at first attack is 11 to 13 years in most POMS studies [8]. Sex ratios are

The authors have nothing to disclose.

*Corresponding author. *E-mail address:* MLangille@dhs.lacounty.gov

https://doi.org/10.1016/j.yapd.2019.03.003
0065-3101/19/Published by Elsevier Inc.

equal in prepubertal children. As children age, the distribution shows clear female predominance, similar to AOMS. The skew toward female sex distribution with age suggests a possible connection between sex hormones and disease expression [7].

As seen in adults, there is a correlation with higher latitude and increased risk for MS in pediatric cohorts [9–11]. Studies show that when people emigrate from an area of low MS risk to an area of high MS risk during childhood (up to age 15 years), they assume the risk of their new home [12–14]. Several studies report higher rates of non-Caucasian patients in POMS cohorts in the United States compared with adult cohorts, which are primarily Caucasian with Northern European ancestry. The cause for this is unknown; it could reflect changing population trends in the United States, or the increased migration of people from lower-incident MS areas to the relatively higher incident area of North America [4,5,15].

OTHER DEMYELINATING CONDITIONS OF CHILDHOOD

Acute disseminated encephalomyelitis

Acute disseminated encephalomyelitis (ADEM) is typically a monophasic demyelinating condition characterized by multifocal neurologic deficits and some degree of encephalopathy. Although ADEM can occur at any age, it is more common in young children, and the mean age of presentation is 5 to 8 years [16]. Rarely, ADEM can be multiphasic with recurrence; however, this should prompt further workup to rule out other diagnoses. Historically, the definition of ADEM varied widely both in research and in clinical use. In 2007, the International Pediatric Multiple Sclerosis Study Group proposed a consensus definition for ADEM, and criteria were updated in 2013 (Box 1). Examples of MRI in ADEM are shown in Fig. 1 and Table 1.

Multiphasic ADEM is defined as 2 episodes consistent with ADEM separated by 3 months but not followed by any further events. Relapses beyond a second event are not consistent with ADEM and indicate a chronic, relapsing disorder. The initial ADEM event can be considered the first attack of a chronic disease if it is followed by attacks without encephalopathy [17].

Radiologically isolated syndrome

Radiologically isolated syndrome (RIS) has only been reported in the last 10 years and describes people who are asymptomatic and have a brain MRI (due to car crash, headache, and such) with CNS demyelination as seen in

Box 1: Acute disseminated encephalomyelitis criteria based on International Pediatric Multiple Sclerosis Study Group 2013 revision

- A first demyelinating, multifocal clinical attack of the CNS with inflammatory cause
- Encephalopathy not explained by fever
- Brain MRI with demyelinating findings during acute illness
- Absence of new clinical and MRI findings on follow-up

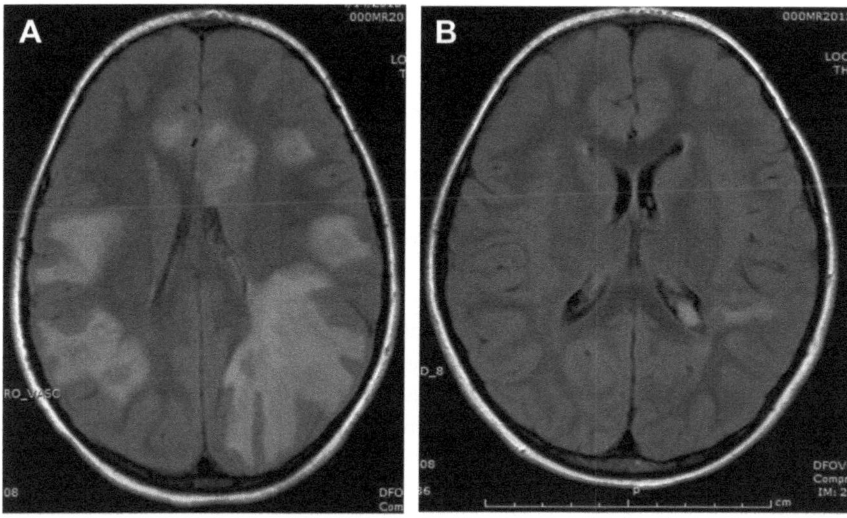

Fig. 1. ADEM MRI T2 fluid-attenuated inversion recovery (MS Flare). A 5-year-old girl with ADEM. (*A*) MRI from presentation shows large, confluent areas of T2-FLAIR signal abnormality predominantly in the subcortical and periventricular white matter in the bilateral parietal, frontal, temporal, and left occipital lobes. (*B*) Follow-up scan 3 months later with resolution of most of the abnormal signal.

MS, including ovoid and well-circumscribed lesions [18,19]. RIS is described in adults, but recently Makhani and colleagues [20] reported on a pediatric cohort with RIS followed with serial scans [18,19,21]. Forty-two percent developed a clinical attack consistent with CNS demyelination within a median of 2 years after the first MRI scan. Evolution of the MRI findings was seen in 61%, in line with findings in adults. Increased risk of developing a clinical event was seen in those with spinal cord lesions on MRI and positive oligoclonal bands in the cerebrospinal fluid (CSF) [21].

Neuromyelitis optica spectrum disorder

Neuromyelitis optica spectrum disorder (NMOSD) is a chronic, relapsing, autoimmune demyelinating disease that affects the CNS and, in particular,

Table 1
MRI findings in multiple sclerosis versus acute disseminated encephalomyelitis

POMS	AOMS	ADEM
• Can have larger and more diffuse lesions than in adults, especially younger children • More likely to have infratentorial lesions	• Periventricular lesions • Black holes • Well-circumscribed lesions • Asymmetric lesions	• Diffuse, fluffy, or ill-defined lesions • Can be symmetric • Can involve the basal ganglia or thalamus • Tend to spare PV areas

Abbreviation: PV, periventricular.

the optic nerves and spinal cord. In 2004, a highly specific autoimmune antibody for neuromyelitis optica (NMO) targeted against the aquaporin-IV water channel was described. Pediatric onset makes up just 3% to 5% of all NMOSD cases [22]. Pediatric patients can present with bilateral or unilateral optic neuritis, longitudinally extensive transverse myelitis, or brainstem symptoms (Fig. 2). Rarely, children can exhibit multifocal deficits and encephalopathy, which can be confused with ADEM [23]. Prompt identification of NMOSD is important because treatment differs from MS, and attacks are often severe with poor recovery.

Myelin oligodendrocyte glycoprotein antibody

Anti-myelin oligodendrocyte glycoprotein (MOG) antibodies are present in some patients with acquired demyelinating syndrome (ADS) (this has not been defined anywhere), including young children with monophasic ADEM and older children with recurrent optic neuritis, transverse myelitis, and antibody-negative NMOSD. MOG is a glycoprotein with a role in myelination of the nerves of the CNS [24,25]. Children are more likely to be positive than adults with the same diagnosis [26–28]. There has been debate about whether the presence of anti-MOG antibodies constitutes a separate demyelinating condition or is seen as part of other conditions. Recent investigations helped clarify clinical characteristics of relapsing anti-MOG$^+$ patients. In children who are positive, a substantial amount, one-third, experienced a relapse within 2 years of initial presentation [29].

However, many children with monophasic ADEM are anti-MOG$^+$. Following MOG titer may be helpful in guiding management. Risk of recurrent

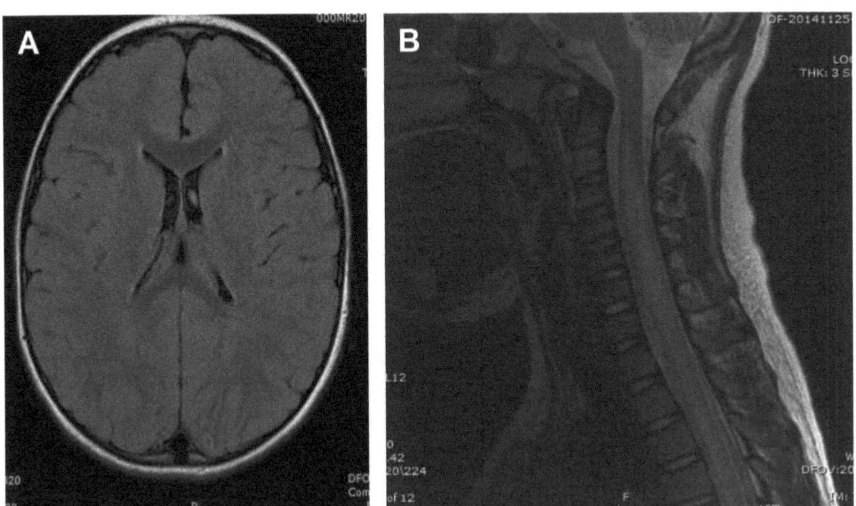

Fig. 2. Pediatric NMO case. (*A*) Note normal brain MRI. (*B*) Longitudinally extensive cord lesion.

demyelinating disease is very low if the anti-MOG antibody titer decreases over time [30,31]. Thus, a persistently high titer could serve as a marker for relapsing disease. Persistence of high titer has been described in children with recurrent optic neuritis and NMOSD. It is rare to find anti-MOG antibodies in children with MS [30,31]. In 1 study, 3 patients with MS had anti-MOG$^+$ antibodies at disease onset but had undetectable levels over time [31].

Children with monophasic disease and anti-MOG$^+$ antibodies generally respond acutely to high-dose pulse steroids. Ideal treatment strategies for children with relapsing anti-MOG are still under investigation; some studies report success with immunosuppressant medications.

DIAGNOSIS

The diagnosis of MS rests on at least one clinical episode and objective findings on examination or imaging reflecting a CNS inflammatory demyelinating event lasting at least 24 hours in the absence of fever or infection. The McDonald criteria allow diagnosis based on clinical grounds alone, but also propose that MRI, and now CSF, can serve as markers for dissemination in space (DIS) and/or time (DIT). McDonald criteria have been revised over time (2001, 2005, 2010, and 2017); the changes generally allow earlier diagnosis so patients can start on treatment more quickly than in the past.

The 2010 McDonald criteria have been evaluated in POMS patients and found to have high sensitivity, specificity, and positive predictive value (PPV, 76%) for children older than 11 [32]. In young children with a non-ADEM-like presentation, the PPV was only 55%. The low PPV in younger children suggest caution must be used when employing the criteria in this group. Also, the criteria are not suitable for application in patients with ADEM-like presentations because although no child with ADEM met clinical criteria for MS, 10 did meet the 2010 MRI criteria.

In 2017, the International Panel on Diagnosis of Multiple Sclerosis made revisions to the 2010 McDonald criteria [33,34]. Changes include accepting both symptomatic and asymptomatic lesions for DIS/DIT. The caveat to this, MRI lesions in the optic nerve of a patient with optic neuritis, is excluded. Cortical lesions on MRI can be used to establish DIS. CSF-specific oligoclonal bands can fulfill DIT, which previously required enhancing and nonenhancing MRI lesions, or an additional clinical attack of a different CNS site. The criteria require testing with MRI or CSF-specific oligoclonal bands, depending on the number of clinical attacks with objective clinical evidence [32]. For example, if someone has 1 clinical event, criteria for DIS and DIT must be met. DIS could be met by either an additional clinical attack implicating a different CNS site or by MRI showing 1 lesion in 2 or more of the areas typically affected in MS; DIT could be met by CSF-specific oligoclonal bands or another attack. Tables 2 and 3 provide the McDonald criteria for DIS/DIT and highlight 2017 revisions.

A study was conducted on 324 pediatric patients with ADS to evaluate the 2017 McDonald criteria and compare it with the 2010 McDonald criteria

Table 2
McDonald criteria

DIS	DIT
One T2 lesion in at least 2 of the areas commonly affected by MS: Periventricular Infratentorial Spinal cord Juxtacortical **Cortical**	• Asymptomatic *or* **symptomatic**[a] lesions, contrast-enhancing lesions, and nonenhancing lesions *OR* • A new T2- or contrast-enhancing lesion on follow-up scan done at any time *OR* • **CSF-specific oligoclonal bands OR** • Wait for additional attack

DIS and DIT 2017 revisions are set in bold type.
[a]Excludes lesions in optic nerve in symptomatic optic neuritis patients.

Table 3
McDonald criteria for diagnosis[a]

Clinical presentation	Additional evidence for MS diagnosis
• ≥2 clinical attacks and objective clinical evidence >2 lesions • ≥2 attacks, objective clinical evidence of 1 lesion with historical evidence of a prior attack in a different location	None. *DIS and DIT are met*
≥2 attacks and objective clinical evidence of 1 lesion	Fulfills DIT DIS needed • ≥1 **symptomatic** or asymptomatic lesion in PV, juxtacortical, infratentorial, spinal cord, or **cortical location** *OR* • Await second attack
One attack and objective clinical evidence of >2 lesions	Fulfills DIS DIT needed • Enhancing and nonenhancing **symptomatic** or asymptomatic typical MS lesions *OR* • New T2 or enhancing lesion on follow scan *OR* • **CSF-specific oligoclonal bands *OR*** • Await further clinical attack
One attack and objective clinical evidence of 1 lesion	DIT needed • Enhancing and nonenhancing **symptomatic** or asymptomatic typical MS lesions *OR* • New T2 or enhancing lesion on follow scan OR • **CSF-specific oligoclonal bands** *OR* • Await further clinical attack DIS needed • ≥1 **symptomatic** or asymptomatic lesion in PV, juxtacortical, infratentorial, spinal cord, or **cortical location** *OR* • Await second attack in different location

2017 revisions are set in bold type.
[a]Assumes patient has typical MS symptoms at onset.

[35]. At the time of the first attack, the 2017 criteria performed well in identifying children with MS. The presence of oligoclonal bands to establish DIT increased the number of diagnoses. As in 2010, the 2017 McDonald criteria had a lower PPV for children under 11 years of age, suggesting caution when applying the criteria in young children. Also, 2017 McDonald criteria should not be applied to ADEM-like presentation; the diagnosis of MS in these children requires at least 1 non-ADEM relapse and the accrual of clinically silent new lesions [35].

RISK FACTORS FOR THE DEVELOPMENT OF PEDIATRIC

Genetics

Epidemiologic studies have shown about 2% to 5% risk of MS in first-degree relatives and 25% to 30% in monozygotic twins [36]. Most of these genetic risk factors are associated with immune regulation genes [37]. Genome-wide association studies have identified more than 200 susceptibility genes associated with adult MS, including at least 13 major histocompatibility complex (MHC) loci [38,39]. About one-third of the adult MS genetic variants are associated with POMS, suggesting a shared genetic inheritance. The first genetic risk factor identified in Caucasians with MS is *HLA-DRB1*15:01*, in the MHC class II. Presence of the variant increases MS risk about 3-fold. A similar association is seen in POMS [37,40].

Environmental factors

Infection

Prior infection with Epstein-Barr virus has consistently been associated with an increased risk for pediatric MS [41]. For individuals with prior herpes simplex (HSV)-1 infection, the contribution to POMS risk depends on *HLA-DRB1*1501* status [41,42].

Diet and dietary micronutrients

Several studies have assessed dietary factors associated with risk of developing MS, including average caloric intake and consumption of fats, proteins, carbohydrates, sugars, fruits, vegetables, dairy, fiber, vitamins, iron, salt, and beverages. Notably, only low levels of vitamin D and low-iron intake have shown significant associations with pediatric MS [43,44].

Gut microbiome

The composition of gut microbiota in pediatric MS displays some differences compared with healthy controls. A study showed differences in gut microbial taxa enrichments and depletions between cases and controls demonstrating alteration of the gut microbiota in POMS patients toward a more inflammatory environment [45].

Obesity

Many studies show a high percentage of POMS patients are overweight. At least 49% of 1 cohort of children with MS were overweight or obese [46]. Higher body mass indexes (BMIs) are associated with an increased risk of developing POMS in postpubertal girls [47]. Overweight or obese girls had an earlier age of disease onset compared with those with a lower BMI [48].

Smoking exposure

One study showed parental smoking at home doubles the risk for first episode of MS [49]. Second-hand cigarette smoke exposure is more common in POMS (37% exposed) compared with monophasic ADS (29.5% exposed). Cigarette smoke exposure combined with *HLA-DRB1*1501*-positive status increased the odds of pediatric MS by 3.7 times compared with monophasic ADS [50].

MRI FINDINGS IN PEDIATRIC-ONSET MULTIPLE SCLEROSIS

There are notable differences in MRI findings in POMS versus AOMS patients. Waubant and colleagues [51] examined both initial MRI scans and follow-up scans comparing pediatric and adult cohorts. They found the POMS group had an initial scan with higher total number of T2-hyperintense foci and more large (≥1 cm) foci compared with the adults. A greater portion of children had gadolinium-enhancing foci (68.4% vs 21.2%) and T2-hyperintense foci in the posterior fossa (68.3% vs 31.4%). When follow-up scans were compared, the children still had a greater number of new T2-hyperintense foci and gadolinium-enhancing foci than the adults; however, several children showed greater than 50% reduction of previously seen T2-hyperintensities compared with their adult counterparts (22.5% children vs 0% adults). Fig. 3 and Table 4 provide POMS MRI characteristics.

These findings suggest POMS patients have higher MRI disease burden at presentation and higher disease activity on follow-up scans. Pediatric patients have more frequent radiologic involvement of the infratentorial region than adults. MRI findings match the clinical findings, that is, that POMS patients have symptoms of cerebellum or brainstem involvement more often than AOMS [52]. Pediatric patients demonstrated more ill-defined and larger T2-hyperintense foci on initial scans, suggesting that the inflammatory process in children is from more edematous reactions; however, these differences could be due to the immature blood-brain barrier and microglia in children. There was resolution (>50%) of previously seen T2-hyperintense signal in a greater percentage of pediatric patients compared with adults, suggesting less destructive or more reversible lesions in children [51]. This finding could be explained by less axonal loss and demyelination or by better remyelination in children than adults. Despite the resolution of lesions, however, the fact that pediatric patients have a higher MRI disease burden, greater occurrence of new lesions early in MS onset, and higher frequency of infratentorial lesions is concerning. These same features have been associated with more rapid disability in AOMS patients.

Traditionally, MS is considered a disease of the white matter, but MRI has shown gray matter involvement in both pediatric and adult patients. Relative to healthy controls, pediatric patients have lower gray matter volume, total brain

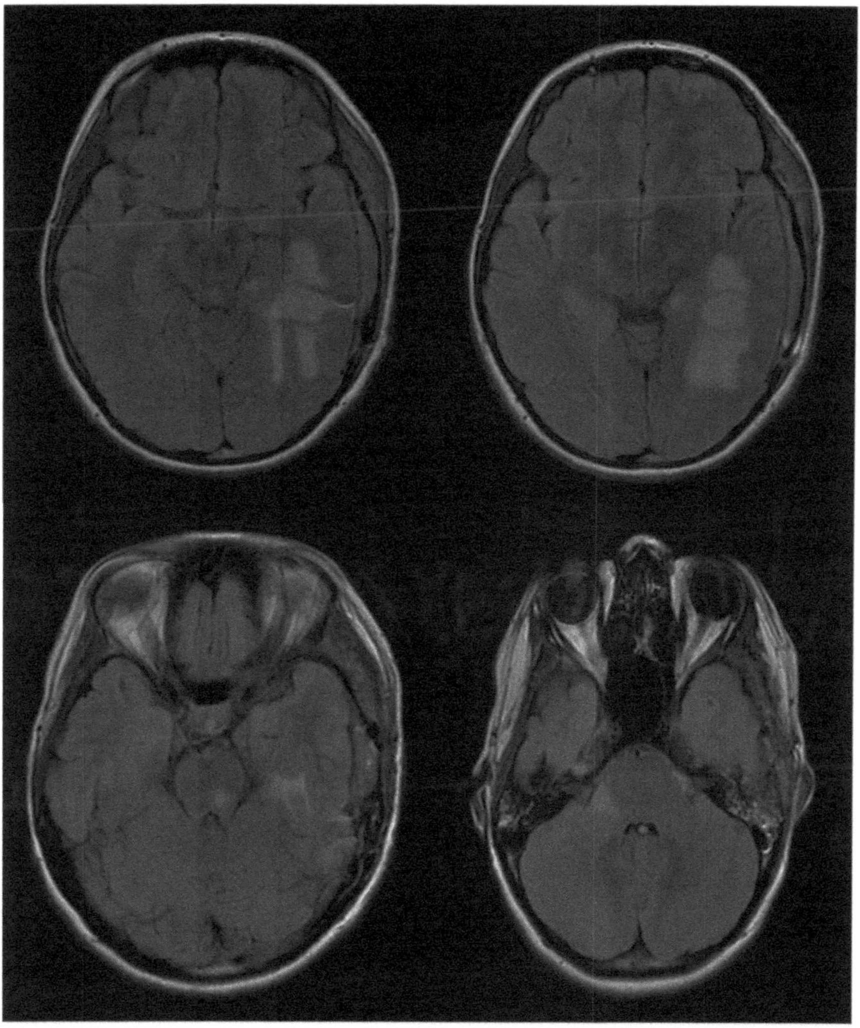

Fig. 3. Teen girl with MS. Note the large confluent lesions and infratentorial lesions.

volume, and thalamic volume [53,54]. One study showed that thalamic volume changes correlated with clinically identified cognitive impairment [54].

CLINICAL COURSE AND PROGNOSIS

MS is often broken up into different subtypes; relapsing remitting MS (RRMS) is characterized by discrete neurologic attacks followed by some amount of recovery between attacks (Table 5). The overwhelming majority of POMS cases are RRMS, more than 98%. Primary progressive MS (PPMS) has gradual and progressive accumulation of disability in absence of neurologic attacks or relapses. In adults, about 15% of cases are PPMS. If a child experiences a

Table 4
Clinical course of pediatric-onset multiple sclerosis versus adult-onset multiple sclerosis

	POMS		
Sex	Prepubertal M:F	Postpubertal F > M	AOMS F > M
Clinical symptoms	Multifocal symptoms are more common, seizures, brainstem symptoms more common	Monofocal more common, brainstem symptoms more common	Examples of typical MS presentations include unilateral optic neuritis, focal supratentorial, brainstem, or cerebellar syndromes, or partial myelopathy
Relapses	More severe relapses Increased number of relapses earlier in disease course		Poorer recovery potential from relapse
Disability	Time to disability is longer, but age at disability is younger than adults		After EDSS 4 progression is similar in POMS and AOMS
MS subtype	98% RRMS		85% RRMS, 15% PPMS

Abbreviations: F, female; M, male.

progressive course without remission, this should raise concern for alternative diagnosis and prompt further workup [7].

Studies show POMS patients suffer more frequent relapses early in their disease course compared with AOMS [55]. One study showed this increase in

Table 5
Multiple sclerosis subtype

RRMS	• Most common disease course • Clinical attacks or relapses occur and are followed by some amount of recovery and remission • Over time, disability can become permanent, but no progression of disability is seen during remission periods • Considered active or not active depending on whether relapses are occurring and worsening/not worsening if disability has increased
Secondary progressive MS (SPMS)	• People initially have RRMS, and over time most transition to SPMS • Characterized by progressive worsening of disability measures • Active or not active depending on whether relapses occur and MRI progresses
PPMS	• Very rare in children; should prompt further workup if children have progressive course • Worsening disability and neurologic dysfunction from onset without early relapses • Considered active if occasional relapses occur or MRI activity or not active • Considered with progression or without progression depending on disability assessments

relapse rate persisted for more than 5 years after disease onset. Also, they found that POMS patients had a shorter interval between first and second attack [56]. Another study found pediatric patients have more severe relapses compared with adults. Despite more frequent and severe relapses, pediatric patients show greater potential for complete recovery from relapses, especially early in their disease course [56–60].

POMS patients take longer to reach disability levels, but because they are younger at disease onset, they reach disability 7 to 12 years younger than adults. The European Database for MS enrolled patients from 1967 to 1997 and followed them through 2003. A total of 394 patients with disease onset before age 16 were studied, and time to reach expanded disability status scale (EDSS) score of 4 (limited ability to walk 500 meters unassisted) was 20 years, whereas the time to same EDSS score for adult-onset patients was 8 years [7]. After this point, progression rates are similar between adults and POMS. Long-term follow-up data of POMS and disability status occurred before the current treatment strategies. It is hoped that modern treatment options, which include more powerful immunosuppressant medication, could help improve prognosis in the future. Risk factors for poor outcome in pediatric patients include shorter time between relapses (<1 year), incomplete recovery after first attack, and brainstem involvement in initial attack.

Cognitive effects in pediatric MS patients are significant and fairly common, seen in as many as one-third of patients [60]. Correlation of cognitive deficits and imaging findings, like brain atrophy, has been reported. Lower IQ scores have correlated with younger age at disease onset. In a longitudinal study of POMS, 25% of patients had cognitive decline from baseline at 1 year and 75% had decline after 2 years [61]. Care should be taken to monitor for these issues. School concessions and strategies can be addressed through a child's individual education plan.

TREATMENT

Today, there are more medications for MS than ever before, which can allow more individualized management, but also increases the complexity of treatment and concern for serious side effects. The concept of NEDA, or no evidence of disease activity, measured by lack of clinical and radiologic progression is an ultimate goal of MS treatment. In studies evaluating NEDA, roughly 50% of adult patients followed for 2 years in any clinical trial were able to achieve NEDA, and only 7% remain NEDA at 7-year follow-up [62]. NEDA has not been longitudinally evaluated in POMS so it is not possible to say if it is a realistic goal for every patient [63].

Treatment of POMS patients with disease-modifying therapies (DMT) has largely been based on extrapolation of adult data and expert experience, because there has been a lack of clinical trials in pediatric patients until recently. Still, published case series support reduction in relapses with first-line injectable agents like Glatiramer acetate and interferons. These medications reduce relapses in adults by as much as 30%, and case series report similar efficacy in pediatric patients with similar safety profiles [64–66]. Dose and common side effects are listed in Table 6.

Table 6
Disease-modifying treatments

Medication	Trade name	Mechanism of action	Dose and route	Side effects	Screening laboratory tests	Monitoring laboratory tests
Injectable immunomodulator						
IFN-β-1a	Rebif	• Inhibits lymphocyte trafficking in CNS • Enhances suppressor T-cell activity • Reduces proinflammatory cytokine production	22 or 44 μg SC TIW	Flulike reactions, elevated transaminases, depression, injection site reactions Serious AE are rare	• CBC • LFT • TSH	• CBC • LFT • TSH
IFN-β-1a	Avonex		30 μg IM every week			
IFN-β-1b	Betaseron		250 μg SC every other day			
Pegylated IFN-β-1a	Plegridy		125 μg SC every 14 d			
Glatiramer acetate	Copaxone	• Promotes Th2 cell activity • Shifts toward anti-inflammatory state	20 mg SC qd 40 mg SC TIW	Injection site reactions Serious AE are rare	None	None
Oral immunomodulator						
Fingolimod	Gilenya	• Sphingosine 1-phosphate receptor modulator • Leads to down-regulation in LN and prevents activated lymphocytes from leaving LN	0.5 mg po qd	Bradycardia, macular edema, infection, lymphopenia, increased LFT	• CBC • LFT • VZV antibodies • ECG • OCT/ophthalmology examination • ECG • Vaccinate if needed	• First-dose monitoring • Follow-up OCT/ophthalmology examination • CBC • LFT • Periodic skin examination

Teriflunomide	AUBAGIO	• Lymphocytopenia in T and B cells • Disrupts pyridine synthesis	• 14 mg po qd • 7 mg po qd	GI symptoms, alopecia, increased LFT, increase BP, peripheral neuropathy	• CBC • LFT • QuantiFERON gold • Pregnancy test	• ALT monthly for 6 mo • Then LFT periodically • CBC
DMF	Tecfidera	• Nrf2 pathway • Shift to Th2 or anti-inflammatory • Cytokine profile • Promotes antioxidant	240 mg po bid	Flushing, nausea, stomach upset, UTI, lymphopenia PML has been reported	• CBC • LFT	• CBC • LFT
Infusion immunosuppressant						
Natalizumab	Tysabri	• mAb against alpha 4 integrin • Prevents lymphocytes from crossing BBB	300 mg IV every 4 wk (adult dose) 3–5 mg/kg IV every 4 wk (children)	PML, infusion reaction, hepatotoxicity	• JC virus antibody/ index • CBC • LFT	• JC virus antibody/ index • CBC • LFT
Ocrelizumab	Ocrevus	• mAb against CD 20 on B cells	600 mg IV every 6 mo	Infusion reaction, UTI, URT infection Malignancy	• QuantiFERON gold • Hepatitis panel • VZV antibodies • Vaccinations if needed	• CD 19/20 counts every 3 mo • Standard cancer screening
Rituximab	Rituxan	• mAb against CD 20 on B cells	750 mg/m2/ dose IV (maximum 1 g) × 2 doses spaced 2 wk apart every 6 mo	Infusion reactions, PML (not in MS but has been seen in other conditions)	• QuantiFERON gold • Hepatitis panel • VZV • Vaccinations if needed • CBC, cell subsets, CMP	• CD19/20 counts every 3 mo

(*continued on next page*)

Table 6
(continued)

Medication	Trade name	Mechanism of action	Dose and route	Side effects	Screening laboratory tests	Monitoring laboratory tests
Alemtuzumab	LEMTRADA	• mAb against CD 52, causes long-term depletion of CD52+ lymphocytes	12 mg IV 5 consecutive daily infusions. 1 y later 3 consecutive daily infusions	Lymphopenia, infusion reactions, risk of secondary autoimmune conditions, malignancy (thyroid cancers, melanoma)	• Skin examination baseline • VZV antibodies • Hepatitis panel (high-risk groups) • QuantiFERON gold • Vaccinations if needed	• PCP and HSV prophylaxis • Thyroid studies every 3 mo • CBC, creatinine, UA monthly • Skin examination yearly

Abbreviations: AE, adverse events; ALT, alanine aminotransferase; BBB, blood-brain barrier; CBC, complete blood count; CMP, complete metabolic panel; ECG, electrocardiogram; GI, gastrointestinal; IM, intramuscularly; LFT, liver function test; LN, lymph nodes; mAb, monoclonal antibody; OTC, optical coherence tomography; PCP, pneumocystis carinii pneumonia; SC, subcutaneous; T1W, T1 weighted; Th2, T-helper 2; TSH, thyroid stimulating hormone; UA, urinalysis; URT, upper respiratory tract; UTI, urinary tract infection; VZV, varicella-zoster virus.

TREATMENT MODELS

Two treatment models for MS therapy are escalation and induction therapy. Induction therapy generally refers to the use of powerful cell-depleting treatments. Experimental models of MS as well as other immune-mediated diseases suggest these treatments could help "reset" the immune system and control inflammation from the outset [67]. A limiting factor is the potential toxicity and serious adverse events. Escalation therapy refers to sequentially advancing treatment as needed based on efficacy. There is insufficient evidence in both the adult and pediatric MS population to favor one model over the other. For an individual patient, there are many factors to consider, including personal risk tolerance and prior disease activity [63].

INADEQUATE TREATMENT RESPONSE

Despite initiation of first-line therapies, continued relapses and/or accrued disability necessitate switching from a first-line to a second-line agent in a significant number of POMS patients [68]. In a study of more than 250 POMS patients, 28% were switched to second therapy after a mean of 1.3 years due to disease progression. However, the concept of traditional first- and second-line therapies is blurring because there is more attention paid to the individualized needs of patients [63]. A recent paper examining treatment practices in POMS has reported increased use of oral medications like DMF, Fingolimod, and infusion treatments in pediatric patients. Seventeen percent of treatment-naïve pediatric patients were started on a newer agent as first therapy [69].

In 2012, the International Pediatric MS Study Group proposed criteria for inadequate treatment of patients taking a DMT for at least 6 months: (1) no reduction in relapse rate, or new T2 lesions or contrast enhancing lesions; and/or (2) 2 or more relapses within 12 months [70].

MEDICATIONS

Oral

Fingolimod is given as a once-daily oral medication. It sequesters lymphocytes in the lymph nodes by binding to sphingosine-1-phosphate receptors and therefore indirectly prevents activated lymphocytes from crossing into the CNS. It is the first Food and Drug Administration (FDA) -approved DMT for pediatric patients with MS aged 10 years and older. It performed well in clinical trials; when compared with interferon-β-1a, there was an 82% reduction in annualized relapse rates in the Fingolimod group as well as reduction in new lesions and brain atrophy. Serious adverse events were similar to adult studies, namely leukopenia, seizures, and allergic reactions [71,72]. Additional safety concerns include bradycardia, disseminated herpes zoster infection in absence of immunity, and progressive multifocal leukoencephalopathy (PML) risk.

Dimethyl fumarate (DMF) was approved by the FDA in 2013. It is administered as an oral medication given twice a day. Mechanism of action is still unclear; it has cytokine modulatory effects and is known to lower lymphocyte counts. Side effects include stomach upset and flushing, which often will abate with time. There have been rare cases of PML in persons taking DMF.

Teriflunomide is an oral once-daily pill. The active metabolite leflunomide has been used in rheumatoid arthritis since 1998. It reduces activation and proliferation of lymphocytes by inhibition of pyrimidine synthesis [73]. In clinical trials in adults, it was superior to placebo and comparable to interferon-β-1ba. Side effects include nausea, diarrhea, hair thinning, and elevation of transaminases. Teratogenicity potential is also of great concern [74].

Infusion

Natalizumab is a humanized monoclonal antibody that targets a protein located on leukocytes causing the blood-brain barrier to block T and B lymphocytes from crossing over into the CNS. It is given as an IV infusion once a month, and the typical adult dose is 300 mg. Young children may be given a dose of 3 to 5 mg/kg per dose. Impressive reduction in both clinical relapses and MRI progression was seen in adult studies (68% reduction in annualized relapse rate and 82% reduction in new T2 lesions) [75]. Natalizumab use in POMS has been reported in retrospective series and prospective studies and generally has been well tolerated and demonstrated reduction in clinical relapses for patients with aggressive disease [76].

PML caused by reactivation of the JC virus (John Cunningham virus, a type of human polyomavirus) is a serious, potentially life-threatening complication. The TOUCH program restricts prescribing, infusing, or dispensing privileges to providers, pharmacies, and infusion centers enrolled in the program in an effort to mitigate PML risk. Overall incidence of PML in Natalizumab patients is 4.22 in 1000 patients. Risk factors for PML include positive JC virus antibody titer, prior immunosuppressant use, and duration of Natalizumab therapy [63,77].

Rituximab is an anti-CD20 chimeric monoclonal antibody that targets B cells and has been widely used in pediatric autoimmune diseases. There has been increasing recognition of the role of B cells in MS pathologic condition because of varied effector functions, including interactions with T cells [78]. Rituximab has been used off label for MS patients for many years. In one review of pediatric patients with various inflammatory/autoimmune conditions including MS and NMOSD, treatment with Rituximab showed benefit in 87% of patients [79]. A report of 14 MS patients with mean age of 16.5 years treated with Rituximab showed a favorable safety profile with no serious infections and no new relapses after median treatment of 2 years [80].

Ocrelizumab is a related B-cell suppressor therapy that has gained attention as the first FDA-approved therapy for PPMS and is also approved for

Table 7
Clinical trials in pediatric multiple sclerosis

Drug	Trial name	Phase	Outcome/notes	Expected date of completion
DMF (Tecfidera)	CONNECT	3		2025
DMF (Tecfidera)	FOCUS	2	• Safety date • Reduction in T2 lesions during treatment period • Small sample size • Short treatment period	2018
Teriflunomide (AUBAGIO)	TERIKids	3		2021
Alemtuzumab (LEMTRADA)	LEMKids	3	• Will only enroll children who had breakthrough disease on another agent	2025
Fingolimod (Gilenya)	PARADIGMS	3	• Reduction in relapses over comparator • FDA approved for pediatric MS 10 y and older	2017

RRMS. It is a fully humanized monoclonal antibody against CD20. Side effects include risk of infection and infusion reactions, and in trials, an increased risk of breast cancer was seen. It is dosed at 600 mg IV every 6 months.

Alemtuzumab is a humanized monoclonal antibody to $CD52^{+}$ cells that depletes certain lymphocytes. Effects are sustained for up to 1 year after treatment. By depleting T and B lymphocytes, it may help "erase" the memory cells responsible for attacking the CNS. One-third of patients experienced new-onset autoimmune diseases. These diseases may not present until several years after treatment so surveillance and monitoring must be continued for years beyond treatment [73].

CLINICAL TRIALS

Several pediatric trials are ongoing or recently completed (Table 7).

FINAL THOUGHTS

- As research into environmental and genetic risk factors progresses, it may broaden the understanding of MS pathophysiology.
- Evidence shows that 2017 McDonald criteria apply well to older children presenting with typical MS symptoms and could facilitate swift diagnosis and initiation of DMT
- Pediatric MS-specific clinical trials will give new information about treatment of POMS, and follow-up studies may be helpful to better understand long-term prognosis.

References

[1] Ahlgren C, Oden A, Lycke J. High nationwide prevalence of multiple sclerosis in Sweden. Mult Scler 2011;17(8):901–8.
[2] Banwell B, Ghezzi A, Bar-Or A, et al. Multiple sclerosis in children: clinical diagnosis, therapeutic strategies, and future directions. Lancet Neurol 2007;6(10):887–902.
[3] Boiko A, Vorobeychik G, Paty D, et al. Early onset multiple sclerosis - A longitudinal study. Neurology 2002;59(7):1006–10.
[4] Chitnis T, Glanz B, Jaffin S, et al. Demographics of pediatric-onset multiple sclerosis in an MS center population from the Northeastern United States. Mult Scler 2009;15(5):627–31.
[5] Langer-Gould A, Zhang JL, Chung J, et al. Incidence of acquired CNS demyelinating syndromes in a multiethnic cohort of children. Neurology 2011;77(12):1143–8.
[6] Ness JM, Chabas D, Sadovnick AD, et al. Clinical features of children and adolescents with multiple sclerosis. Neurology 2007;68(16 Suppl 2):S37–45.
[7] Renoux C, Vukusic S, Mikaeloff Y, et al. Natural history of multiple sclerosis with childhood onset. N Engl J Med 2007;356:2603–13.
[8] Otallah S, Banwell B. Pediatric multiple sclerosis: an update. Curr Neurol Neurosci Rep 2018;18(76):2–10.
[9] Taylor BV, Lucas RM, Dear K, et al. Latitudinal variation in incidence and type of first CNS demyelinating events. Mult Scler 2010;16(4):398–405.
[10] Lossius A, Riise T, Pugliattie M, et al. Season of infectious mononucleosis and risk of MS at different latitudes; the EnyIMS Study. Mult Scler 2014;20(6):669–74.
[11] Spelman T, Gray O, Trojano M, et al. Seasonal variation in relapse rate in MS is latitude dependent. Ann Neurol 2014;76(6):880–90.
[12] Dean G, Kurtzke JF. On the risk of multiple sclerosis according to age at immigration to South Africa. Br Med J 1971;3:725–9.
[13] McLeod JG, Hammond SR, Kurtzke JF. Migration and multiple sclerosis in immigrants to Australia from United Kingdom and Ireland: a reassessment. I. Risk of MS by age at immigration. J Neurol 2011;258:1140–9.
[14] Berg-Hansen P, Moen S, Sandvik L, et al. Prevalence of multiple sclerosis among immigrants in Norway. Mult Scler 2015;21(6):695–702.
[15] Belman AL, Krupp LB, Olsen CS, et al. Characteristics of children and adolescents with MS. Pediatrics 2016;138(1):e20160120.
[16] Pohl D, Hennemuth I, von Kries R, et al. Paediatric multiple sclerosis and acute disseminated encephalomyelitis in Germany: results of a nationwide survey. Eur J Pediatr 2007;166: 405–12.
[17] Krupp LB, Banwell B, Tenembaum S. Consensus definitions proposed for pediatric multiple sclerosis and related disorders. Neurology 2007;68(suppl 2):S7–12.
[18] Okuda DT, Mowry EM, Beheshtian A, et al. Incidental MRI anomalies suggestive of multiple sclerosis: the radiologically isolated syndrome. Neurology 2009;72:800–5.
[19] Lebrun C, Bensa C, Debouverie M, et al. Unexpected MS: follow-up of 30 patients with magnetic resonance imaging and clinical conversion profile. J Neurol Neurosurg Psychiatry 2008;79:195–8.
[20] Makhani N, Lebrun C, Siva A, et al. RIS in children: clinical and radiologic outcomes. Neurol Neuroimmunol Neuroinflamm 2017;4(6):e395.
[21] Siva A, Saip S, Altintas A, et al. MS risk in radiologically uncovered asymptomatic possible inflammatory-demyelinating disease. Mult Scler 2009;15:918–27.
[22] Tenembaum S, Chitnis T, Nakashima I, et al. NMOSD in children and adolescents. Neurology 2016;87:S59–66.
[23] Wingerchuk DM, Banwell B, Bennett JL, et al. International consensus diagnostic criteria for NMOSD. Neurology 2015;85(2):177–89.
[24] Pham-Dinh D, Mattei MG, Nussbaum JL, et al. Myelin/oligodendrocyte glycoprotein is a member of a subset of the immunoglobulin superfamily encoded within the major histocompatibility complex. Proc Natl Acad Sci U S A 1993;90(17):7990–4.

[25] Pham-Dinh D, Allinquant B, RubergM, et al. Characterization and expression of the cDNA coding for the human myelin/oligodendrocyte glycoprotein. J Neurochem 1994;63(06): 2353–6.
[26] Mader S, Gredler V, Schanda, et al. Complement activating antibodies to myelin oligodendrocyte glycoprotein in neuromyelitis optica and related disorders. J Neuroinflammation 2011;8:184.
[27] Höftberger R, Sepulveda M, Armanque T, et al. Antibodies to MOG and AQP4 in adults with neuromyelitis optica and suspected limited forms of the disease. Mult Scler 2015;21: 866–74.
[28] Baumann M, Hennes E, Schanda K, et al. Children with multiphasic disseminated encephalomyelitis and antibodies to the myelin oligodendrocyte glycoprotein (MOG): extending the spectrum of MOG antibody positive diseases. Mult Scler 2016;22:1821–9.
[29] Hennes EM, Baumann M, Schanda K, et al. Prognostic relevance of MOG antibodies in children with an acquired demyelinating syndrome. Neurology 2017;89(9):900–8.
[30] Baumann M, Sahin K, Lechner C, et al. Clinical and neuroradiological differences of paediatric acute disseminating encephalomyelitis with and without antibodies to the myelin oligodendrocyte glycoprotein. J Neurol Neurosurg Psychiatry 2015;86:265–72.
[31] Pröbstel AK, Dornmair K, Bittner R, et al. Antibodies to MOG are transient in childhood acute disseminated encephalomyelitis. Neurology 2011;77:580–8.
[32] Sadaka Y, Verhey LH, Shroff MM, et al. 2010 McDonald criteria for diagnosing pediatric multiple sclerosis. Ann Neurol 2012;72:211–23.
[33] Thompson AJ, Banwell BL, Barkhof F, et al. Diagnosis of multiple sclerosis: 2017 revisions of the McDonald criteria. Lancet Neurology 2017;17:162–73.
[34] Polman CH, Reingold SC, Banwell B, et al. Diagnostic criteria for multiple sclerosis: 2010 revisions to the McDonald criteria. Ann Neurol 2011;69:292–302.
[35] Fadda G, Brown RA, Longoni G, et al. MRI and laboratory features and the performance of international criteria in the diagnosis of multiple sclerosis in children and adolescents: a prospective cohort study. Lancet Child Adolesc Health 2018;2(3):191–204.
[36] Nielsen NM, Westergaard T, Rostgaard K, et al. Familial risk of multiple sclerosis: a nationwide cohort study. Am J Epidemiol 2005;162(8):774–8.
[37] Gianfrancesco MA, Stridh P, Shao X, et al. Genetic risk factors for pediatric-onset multiple sclerosis. Mult Scler 2017; https://doi.org/10.1177/1352458517733551.
[38] Patsopoulos N, on behalf of IMSGC. (2016 Oct 18). Abstract: 200 loci complete the genetic puzzle of multiple sclerosis. Presented at the American Society of Human Genetics Annual Meeting. Vancouver, B.C., Canada, October 18–22, 2016.
[39] Beecham AH, Patsopoulos NA, Xifara DK, et al. Analysis of immune-related loci identifies 48 new susceptibility variants for multiple sclerosis. Nat Genet 2013;45(11):1353–60.
[40] Disanto G, Magalhaes S, Handel AE, et al. HLA-DRB1 confers increased risk of pediatric-onset MS in children with acquired demyelination. Neurology 2011;76(9):781–6.
[41] Nourbakhsh B, Rutatangwa A, Waltz M, et al. Heterogeneity in association of remote herpesvirus infections and pediatric MS. Ann Clin Transl Neurol 2018;5(10):1222–8.
[42] Waubant E, Mowry EM, Krupp L, et al. Common viruses associated with lower pediatric multiple sclerosis risk. Neurology 2011;76(23):1989–95.
[43] Banwell B, Bar-Or A, Arnold DL, et al. Clinical, environmental, and genetic determinants of multiple sclerosis in children with acute demyelination: a prospective national cohort study. Lancet Neurol 2011;10(5):436–45.
[44] Hunsberger M, O'Malley J, Block T, et al. Relative validation of Block Kids Food Screener for dietary assessment in children and adolescents. Matern Child Nutr 2015;11(2):260–70.
[45] Tremlett H, Fadrosh DW, Faruqi AA, et al. Gut microbiota in early pediatric multiple sclerosis: a case–control study. Eur J Neurol 2016;23(8):1308–21.
[46] Yamamoto E, Ginsberg M, Rensel M, et al. Pediatric-onset multiple sclerosis: a single center study. J Child Neurol 2018;33(1):98–105.

[47] Langer-Gould A, Brara SM, Beaber BE, et al. Childhood obesity and risk of pediatric multiple sclerosis and clinically isolated syndrome. Neurology 2013;80(6):548–52.
[48] Chitnis T, Graves J, Weinstock-Guttman B, et al. Distinct effects of obesity and puberty on risk and age at onset of pediatric MS. Ann Clin Transl Neurol 2016;3(12):897–907.
[49] Mikaeloff Y, Caridade G, Tardieu M, et al. Parental smoking at home and the risk of childhood-onset multiple sclerosis in children. Brain 2007;130(10):2589–95.
[50] Lavery AM, Collins BN, Waldman AT, et al. The contribution of secondhand tobacco smoke exposure to pediatric multiple sclerosis risk. Mult Scler 2019;25(4):515–22.
[51] Waubant E, Chabas DC, Okuda DT, et al. Difference in disease burden and activity in pediatric patients on brain magnetic resonance imaging at time of MS onset vs adults. Arch Neurol 2009;66(8):967–71.
[52] Chabas D, McCulloch C, Strober J, et al. Age modifies MS phenotype at onset. Mult Scler 2008;14(suppl 1):S61.
[53] Mesaros S, Rocca MA, Absinta M, et al. Evidence of thalamic gray matter loss in pediatric multiple sclerosis. Neurology 2008;70:1107–12.
[54] Till C, Ghassemi R, Aubert-Broche B, et al. MRI correlates of cognitive impairment in childhood-onset multiple sclerosis. Neuropsychology 2011;25:319–32.
[55] Gorman MP, Healy BC, Polgar-Turcsanyi M, et al. Increased relapse rate in pediatric-onset compared with adult-onset multiple sclerosis. Arch Neurol 2009;66:54–9.
[56] Benson LA, Healy BC, Gorman MP, et al. Elevated relapse rates in pediatric compared to adult MS persist for at least 6 years. Mult Scler Relat Disord 2014;3(2):186–93.
[57] Fay AJ, Mowry EM, Strober J, et al. Relapse severity and recovery in early pediatric multiple sclerosis. Mult Scler 2012;18:1008–12.
[58] Mowry EM, Pesic M, Grimes B, et al. Demyelinating events in early multiple sclerosis have inherent severity and recovery. Neurology 2009;72:602–8.
[59] O'Mahony J, Marrie RA, Laporte A, et al. Recovery from central nervous system acute demyelination in children. Pediatrics 2015;136:e115–23.
[60] Amato MP, Krupp LB, Charvet LE, et al. Pediatric multiple sclerosis: cognition and mood. Neurology 2016;87(9 Suppl 2):S82–7.
[61] Ghezzi A, Goretti B, Portaccio E, et al. Cognitive impairment in pediatric multiple sclerosis. Neurol Sci 2010;31(S2):215–8.
[62] Rotstein DL, Healy BC, Malik MT, et al. Evaluation of no evidence of disease activity in a 7 year longitudinal multiple sclerosis cohort. JAMA Neurol 2015;72:152–8.
[63] Chitnis T, Ghezzi A, Bajer-Kornek B, et al. Pediatric MS: escalation and emerging treatment. Neurology 2016;87(9):S103–9.
[64] Banwell B, Reder AT, Krupp L, et al. Safety and tolerability of interferon beta-1b in pediatric multiple sclerosis. Neurology 2006;66(4):472–6, 79.
[65] Waubant E, Hietpas J, Stewart T, et al. Interferon beta-1a in children with multiple sclerosis is well tolerated. Neuropediatrics 2001;32(4):211–3.
[66] Kornek B, Bernert G, Balassy C, et al. Glatiramer acetate treatment in patients with childhood and juvenile onset multiple sclerosis. Neuropediatrics 2003;34(3):120–6.
[67] Freedman M, Selchen D, Prat A, et al. Managing MS: treatment initiation, modification and sequencing. Can J Neurol Sci 2018;45:489–503.
[68] Yeh EA, Waubant E, Krupp LB, et al. Multiple sclerosis therapies in pediatric patients with refractory MS. Arch Neurol 2011;68:437–44.
[69] Krysko K, Graves J, Rensel M, et al. Use of newer disease modifying therapies in pediatric MS in US. Neurology 2018;00:e1–10.
[70] Chitnis T, Tenenbaum S, Banwell B, et al. Consensus statement: evaluation of new and existing therapeutics for pediatric MS. Mult Scler 2012;18:116–27.
[71] Chitnis T, et al. PARADIGMS: a randomised double-blind study of fingolimod versus interferon β-1a in paediatric multiple sclerosis. Poster presented at ECTRIMS, Paris, France, October 25–28, 2017. Preliminary data from the PARADIGMS trial.

[72] FDA expands approval of Gilenya to treat multiple sclerosis in pediatric patients. Available at: https://www.fda.gov/NewsEvents/Newsroom/PressAnnouncements/ucm607501.htm?utm_campaign=05112018_FDA%20approve. Accessed December 10, 2018.
[73] Ingwersen J, Aktas O, Hartung P. Advances in and algorithms for the treatment of RRMS. Neurotherapeutics 2016;13:47–57.
[74] Kieseier B, Benamor M. Pregnancy outcomes following maternal and paternal exposure to teriflunomide during treatment for RRMS. Neurol Ther 2014;3:133–8.
[75] Polman CH, O'Connor PW, Havrdova E, et al. A randomized, placebo controlled trial of natalizumab for relapsing MS. N Engl J Med 2006;354:99–910.
[76] Alroughani R, Ahmed SF, Behbehani R, et al. The use of natalizumab in pediatric patients with active relapsing MS: a prospective study. Pediatr Neurol 2017;70:56–60.
[77] Schwab N, Schneider-Hohendorf T, Melzer N, et al. Natalizumab-associated PML: challenges with incidence, resulting risk and risk stratification. Neurology 2017;88:1197–205.
[78] Sabatino J, Zamvil S, Hauser S. B cell therapies in MS. Cold Spring Harb Perspect Med 2019; https://doi.org/10.1101/cshperspect.a032037.
[79] Dale RC, Brilot F, Duffy LV, et al. Utility and safety of rituximab in pediatric autoimmune and inflammatory CNS disease. Neurology 2014;83:142–50.
[80] Salzer J, Lycke J, Wickstrom R, et al. Rituximab in paediatric onset multiple sclerosis: a case series. J Neurol 2015;263:322–6.

Advances in Pediatrics 66 (2019) 231–244
ADVANCES IN PEDIATRICS

Resurgence of Syphilis

Joseph A. Puccio, MD*, Aileen Cannon, MD,
Kalyani Derasari, MD, Rodney Friend, MD
USF Morsani College of Medicine, 4202 East Fowler Avenue, SHS 100, Tampa, FL 33620, USA

Keywords

• Syphilis • HIV+ • PrEP • MSM • Women • Penicillin

Key points

- Since 2013, syphilis rates have been increasing for all age groups and races.
- Currently, men who have sex with men (MSM), and in particular MSM who are HIV+, have the highest rates of syphilis infection.
- As rates of syphilis increase in women, the number of infants being born with congenital syphilis has increased.

INTRODUCTION

Syphilis is a sexually transmitted infection (STI) caused by the spirochete bacterium *Treponema pallidum*. Syphilis has 4 stages: primary, secondary, latent (hidden), and tertiary (late). Primary syphilis is characterized by a painless sore called a chancre. The chancre is the site where the bacteria entered the body and usually appears within 3 weeks of contact but can take as long as 90 days. The chancre can take up to 6 weeks to heal and usually requires no treatment. The person is highly contagious during primary syphilis and continues to be contagious after the sore heals [1].

Two to six weeks after the appearance of the chancre a reddish brown, small, flat, or raised rash develops over the body including the palms of the hands and soles of the feet. This rash characterizes secondary syphilis and can last up to 2 months. As the bacteria spreads through the body, the person is still contagious and can experience fever; sore throat; fatigue; weight loss; lymphadenopathy; patchy hair loss of the eyebrows, eyelashes, or scalp hair; and neurologic symptoms including headache, neck stiffness, irregular pupils,

Disclosure Statement: The authors have nothing to disclose.

*Corresponding author. *E-mail address:* jpuccio@health.usf.edu

https://doi.org/10.1016/j.yapd.2019.03.006
0065-3101/19/

and unequal reflexes. Small open sores can also develop on mucous membranes. These sores may contain pus or can have a moist wartlike appearance (condyloma lata) [1].

If a person with these symptoms is untreated, all symptoms will resolve and the infection will become hidden. This is the latent phase and the infection can remain hidden for up to 20 years. During latency, the person may continue to be contagious. It is also common to experience a relapse of secondary syphilis several times during latency. During the latent stage a woman can pass syphilis to her fetus causing a miscarriage, stillbirth, or birth to an infant infected with congenital syphilis [1].

Tertiary syphilis can develop anytime 1 year after initial infection. Tertiary syphilis is associated with the most morbidity of any stage of syphilis and can consist of any of the following: large internal or superficial sores known as gummata, cardiovascular symptoms, and neurologic symptoms. Neurosyphilis, often seen in tertiary syphilis, can occur during any stage of the infection, especially in immunocompromised patients [1].

HISTORY AND EPIDEMIOLOGY

Numerous theories have attempted to explain the origins of syphilis. The pre-Columbian hypothesis and the Unitarian hypothesis propose that syphilis has been infecting humans since 3000 BC after the spirochete experienced numerous mutations from those that cause pinta (*Treponema carateum*), Yaws (*Treponema pertenue*), and endemic syphilis (*Treponema Pallidum endemicum*). The mutations were in response to geographic and climate changes and interactions with different populations. However, the Columbian theory proposes that syphilis was brought to Europe by Columbus when he returned from the New World in 1493 [2–5].

The first descriptions of syphilis were transcribed in a poem, Syphilis sive morbus gallicus, by Girolamo Fracastoro in 1530. It euphemizes the shepherd Syphilis who is cursed with illness by the all-powerful Greek god, Apollo [4].

For centuries to follow, all sexually transmitted infections (STIs) were considered one malady. It was not until the nineteenth century that syphilis was determined to be a unique infectious agent after Ricord in 1831 determined that patients with syphilis only got syphilis after being in contact with other patients with syphilis and patients only got gonorrhea when in contact with others with gonorrhea [2,6].

In 1905 the etiologic agent for syphilis was discovered by Schaudinn, and Hoffman named the bacterium *T pallidum.* In 1906, dark-field microscopy was introduced by Landsteiner to detect spirochetes. In 1910, the first serologic test for syphilis was introduced by Wasserman [6]. In 1949, the first test to specifically diagnosis *T pallidum* infection was developed by Nelson and Mayer. This test was able to diagnosis syphilis and monitor treatment response in asymptomatic patients [6].

The treatment for syphilis has been very diverse and has involved inflicting significant pain on patients and serious adverse reactions. The earliest treatment was derived from a plant brought back to Europe from the New World called *Guaiacum Officinale*, commonly known as the guaiac tree. It was a very effective purgative agent and was thought to be a "blood Cleanser." By the mid-1500s oral or injected mercury was used to treat syphilis. Mercury is a potent diuretic and it was thought that syphilis could be removed from the body through excessive sweating and diuresis. By the late 1880s, bismuth became the preferred heavy metal used to treat syphilis, because it was less toxic than mercury and had a stronger bactericidal effect. By the early 1900s, arsenic compounds such salvarsan and neosalvarsan were the mainstay of syphilis treatment, and they were replaced in the early 1940s with penicillin [2,7]. Penicillin continues to be an effective first-line treatment for syphilis, and it was once thought that it would eradicate the bacterium [8].

A large autopsy study published by Yale University in 1947 concluded that approximately 10% of the US population was afflicted with syphilis [9]. Although penicillin was discovered in 1929, the first use of penicillin to treat syphilis was described by John Mahoney of the United Stated Public Health Service (USPHS) in 1943 [5,10,11]. The USPHS conducted the infamous "Tuskegee Study of the Untreated Syphilis in Negro Male" [5,11], an observational study of the natural history of syphilis. The subjects included 412 African-American men with syphilis and 192 without syphilis in rural Alabama. Both study groups were followed until 1973 or until autopsy results were available, and all received free meals, medical examinations, and burial insurance. However, infected subjects with positive serologies were not informed that they had syphilis and were not treated [11]. It was not until 1997 that the US government apologized for its role in the study.

Syphilis is an infection that does not discriminate. Over the years, all levels of society have been affected by syphilis, varying by social circumstances of the time [2]. In the United States, after World War I (WWI) rates of syphilis dropped dramatically after diagnostic tests and acceptable treatments with arsenic compounds became available. The number of syphilis cases increased following the return of soldiers from WWII, but with the discovery of penicillin in the 1940s, the increase quickly plateaued and throughout the 1950s new diagnoses decreased [8,12,13]. With the advent of the sexual revolution in the 1960s syphilis cases began to increase again and continued to increase through the 1970s, with significant spread among men who have sex with men (MSM). Then the human immunodeficiency virus (HIV) and AIDS epidemic began. During the 1980s and early 1990s, AIDS induced changes in sexual behaviors, and syphilis rates in the United States significantly dropped, especially among MSM. However, during this same period, syphilis rates increased among minority heterosexual populations in urban centers. The increase in syphilis rates paralleled the crack cocaine epidemic in these urban populations [12,13]. During this time intense public health measures reduced the number of new cases of syphilis and this trend continued throughout the 1990s. The decline was so significant that by 2000 the incidence was lower than in 1941. This continuous decline in syphilis cases and the concentration of new cases in small urban geographic areas led many to believe that syphilis could be eradicated. The Centers for Disease Control (CDC) developed a National Plan to eradicate syphilis in 1999, which was revised in 2006 [13,14].

From 2001 to 2005 the rates began to increase again, predominantly among MSM. Between 2004 and 2005 the incidence of new cases increased by 11.1%, and in 2004 and 2005, for the first time since the middle 1990s, the incidence began to increase among woman (0.8–0.9 cases per 100,000 population). From the mid-1990s through 2005 the rate of congenital syphilis decreased yearly at a rate of 14.1% [13–15].

From 2013 to 2017 the incidence of primary and secondary syphilis increased by 72.2% (Fig. 1). In 2017 alone it increased by 10.5% (9% in men and 21.2% in women). The increase in women is particularly problematic because it is accompanied by a concomitant increase in congenital syphilis [14,15]. The incidence has also increased significantly in men who have sex with women. The incidence varies by geographic location, with rates in 2017 of 13, 10.2, 8, and 6.2 cases per 100,000 in the west, south, northeast, and midwest regions of the United States, respectively [15] (Fig. 2).

In 2017, the incidence of primary and secondary syphilis increased in all age groups over 15 years. In men, the highest rate of primary and secondary syphilis was in the 25 to 29 year age group (51.9 per 100,000 men), whereas in women the highest rate was in the 20 to 24 year age group (7.8 per 100,000 women) (Fig. 3). From 2016 to 2017, the rates of primary and secondary syphilis infection increased 9.8%, 7.8%, 10.7%, 14.3%, 17.8%, 6.5%, 4.3% 11.8%, and 16.7% for those aged 15 to 19, 20 to 24, 30 to 34, 35 to 39, 45 to 54, 55 to 64, and 65 years or greater, respectively [15,16].

Blacks had the highest rates of primary and secondary syphilis in 2017, with 24.7 cases per 100,000 population–a rate 4.5 times higher than that for whites

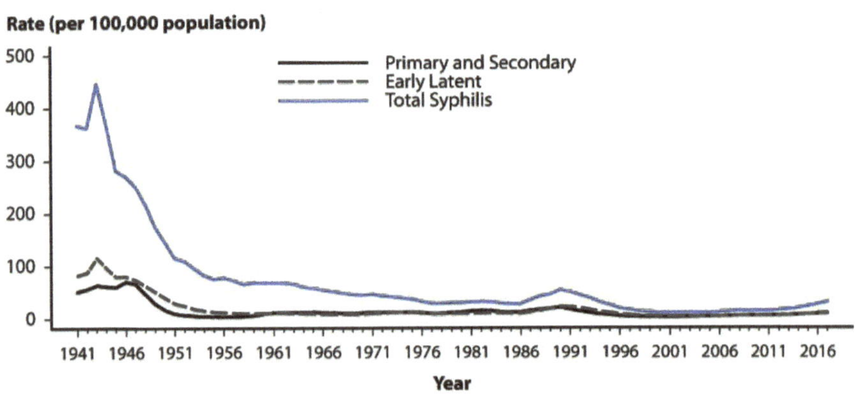

Fig. 1. Syphilis—rates of reported cases by stage of infection, United States, 1941 to 2017. (*From* Centers for Disease Control and Prevention. Sexually transmitted disease surveillance 2017. Atlanta: U.S. Department of Health and Human Services; 2018. https://www.cdc.gov/std/stats17/syphilis.htm.)

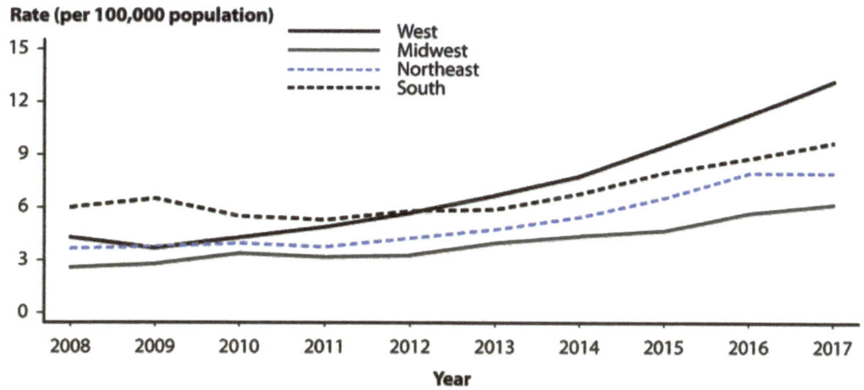

Fig. 2. Primary and secondary syphilis—rates of reported cases by region, United States, 2008 to 2017. (*Data from* Centers for Disease Control and Prevention Sexually Transmitted Disease Surveillance 2017. Atlanta (GA): US Department of Health and Human Services; 2018 https://www.cdc.gov/std/stats.)

(5.4 per 100,000 population). Asians had the lowest rate (4.4 cases per 100,000 population), whereas native Hawaiians and other Pacific Islanders, Hispanics, and American Indian/Native Alaskans had rates of 13.9, 11.8, and 11.1 cases per 100,000 population, respectively [16].

Syphilis continues to have high coinfection rates in persons living with HIV disease. The rates of coinfection are highest in MSM with 45.5% of primary and secondary syphilis cases and lowest in women with 4.5% [16] (Fig. 4).

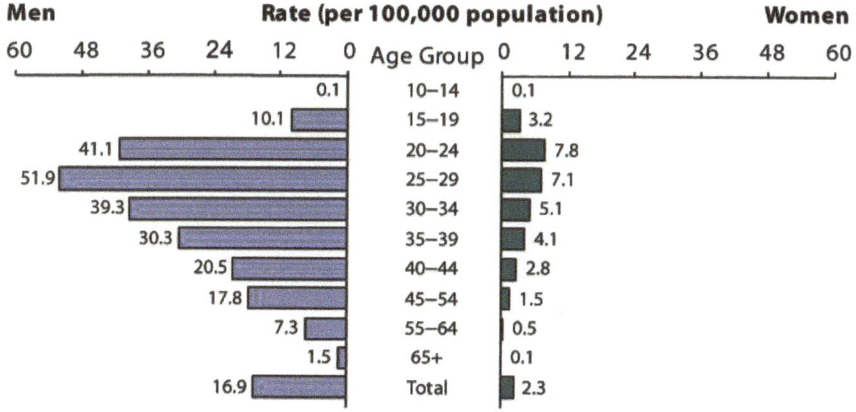

Fig. 3. Primary and secondary syphilis—rates of reported cases by age group and sex, United States, 2017. (*From* Centers for Disease Control and Prevention. Sexually transmitted disease surveillance 2017. Atlanta: U.S. Department of Health and Human Services; 2018. https://www.cdc.gov/std/stats17/syphilis.htm.)

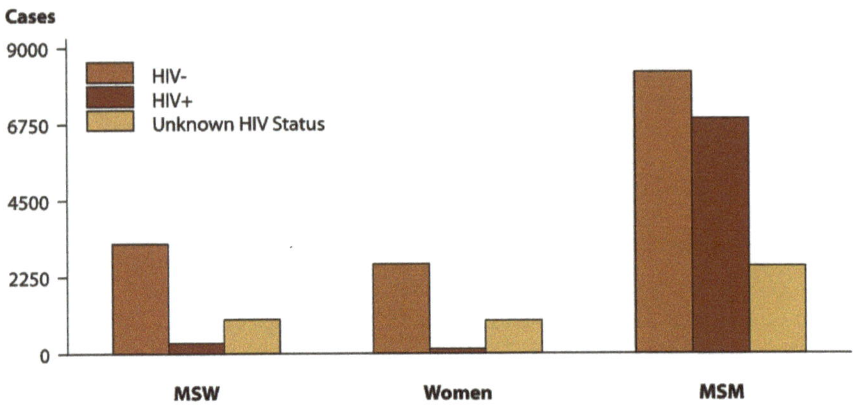

Fig. 4. Primary and secondary syphilis—reported cases by sex, sexual behavior, and HIV, United States, 2017. (*From* Centers for Disease Control and Prevention. Sexually transmitted disease surveillance 2017. Atlanta: U.S. Department of Health and Human Services; 2018. https://www.cdc.gov/std/stats17/syphilis.htm.)

The reasons for the dramatic increase in the incidence of primary and secondary syphilis over the last 5 years continue to be debated. It has been hypothesized that the introduction of HIV preexposure prophylaxis (PrEP) is contributing to the increase among MSM. HIV PrEP is a daily combination pill of the antiretroviral drugs tenofovir and emtricitabine. When taken as directed, PrEP significantly reduces the number of new HIV cases [17]. It is theorized that some MSMs are taking HIV PrEP in place of instead of in addition to the use of condoms, particularly those who engage in receptive anal sex. Volk and colleagues [18] found a 41% decrease in self-reported use of condoms in a cohort of PrEP users. This is an example of "risk compensation." However, other studies have shown no risk compensation in PrEP users [19]. The use of condoms is only partially protective because syphilis only requires direct contact to cause infection, and chancres may be present on many different parts of the body. The increase in primary and secondary syphilis incidence amongst MSMs, including PrEP users, may be partially attributable to increased testing, because continued use of the medication requires an HIV test every 3 months. Frequent interactions with a health care provider bolster opportunities for screening and treatment of other STIs, including syphilis.

Although the burden of disease is disproportionately shared by younger minority male populations, particularly MSMs, the incidence of primary and secondary syphilis cases in the United States is increasing in nearly every demographic, indicating that PrEP use is not the primary reason for the increase. However, in 2017, all races and ethnicities have the highest number of cases of syphilis in the MSM population (Fig. 5).

Rates are increasing in other vulnerable populations. Congenital infections have increased in the United States since 2013, increasing 48.3% to 23.3 cases per 100,000 live births from 2016 to 2017, and resulting in 918 congenital infections

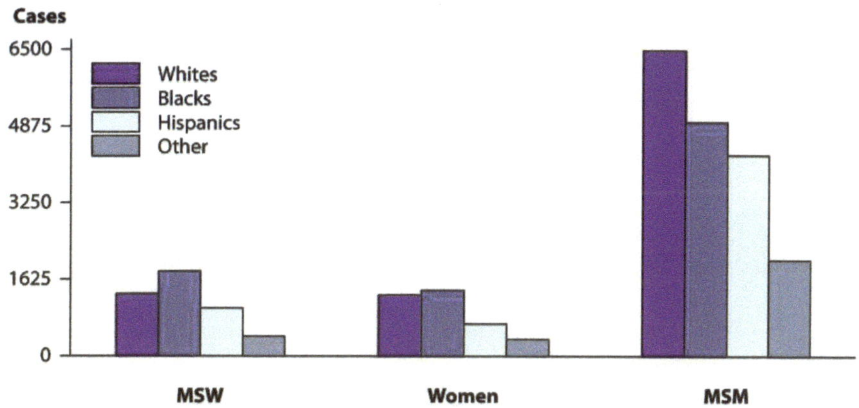

Fig. 5. Primary and Secondary Syphilis — Reported Cases* by Sex, Sexual Behavior, Race, and Hispanic Ethnicity, United States, 2017.

* Of all reported cases of primary and secondary syphilis, 15.0% were among men without data on sex of sex partners, and 0.1% were cases with unknown sex; 5.7% of all cases had missing or unknown race/Hispanic ethnicity. Cases with missing or unknown race/Hispanic ethnicity are included in the "Other" category.

with 64 syphilitic stillbirths and 13 infant deaths. The increase in congenital infections is consistent with the increase in primary and secondary infections in all women (see Fig. 5). The rates of congenital syphilis vary by geographic location, with the highest rate in 2017 being in the West and lowest in the Northeast (37 and 5.7 cases per 100,000 per live births, respectively) [16] (Fig. 6).

The rates of all stages of syphilis have been increasing throughout the twenty-first century, with 2017 having the highest rates since the early 1990s. Early latent syphilis in 2017 increased 17.6%, whereas late latent syphilis increased 17.3%. Neurosyphilis, which can occur at any stage, has remained relatively low with a prevalence of 0.84% between 2009 and 2015. The highest prevalence of neurosyphilis is in those diagnosed with HIV [20].

Although the rates for most STIs have increased since 2013, the increasing rates of primary and secondary syphilis are of particular concern due to the significant morbidity associated with untreated syphilis and the increased risk of congenital syphilis. In 2016 the CDC issued a call to action for health care providers and specific high-risk populations to work together to curb the alarming yearly increase in new syphilis cases [21].

CENTERS FOR DISEASE CONTROL AND PREVENTION (CDC) CALL TO ACTION

Fortunately, *T pallidum* remains sensitive to penicillin. Patients allergic to penicillin have had limited options for treatment, with penicillin desensitization being the recommended course of action. However, the resurgence of syphilis intensifies the need for timely diagnosis and treatment, and alternative

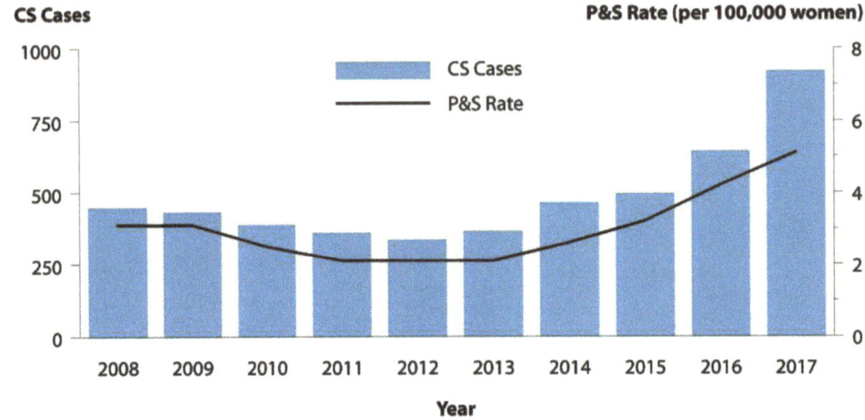

Fig. 6. Prevalence of primary and secondary syphilis and the number of cases of congenital syphilis. CS, congenital syphilis; P&S, primary and secondary syphilis. (*From* Centers for Disease Control and Prevention. Sexually transmitted disease surveillance 2017. Atlanta: U.S. Department of Health and Human Services; 2018. https://www.cdc.gov/std/stats17/syphilis.htm.)

antibiotics are being investigated. Tetracycline and doxycycline have been endorsed as alternative therapies despite a paucity of efficacy data [22]. Doxycycline regimens are preferred due to better compliance with less frequent dosing and fewer gastrointestinal side effects. In more recent studies, doxycycline has been shown to be an effective alternative to penicillin, with 100% effectiveness for early syphilis and 92.4% for all stages at 12 months after treatment [23].

Azithromycin, 2 gm, in a single dose has been used, but *T pallidum* chromosomal mutation associated with azithromycin and other macrolide-resistant drugs and treatment failures have been documented in the United States. Azithromycin should be used with caution and only when treatment with penicillin or doxycycline is not feasible. The CDC states that azithromycin should not be used in MSM, persons with HIV, or pregnant women due to the possibility of an azithromycin-resistant strain of syphilis in these populations. Ceftriaxone can also be used as an alternative therapy to penicillin but should be avoided in patients with severe penicillin allergy. It is essential that all patients treated with alternative therapies have careful clinical and serologic follow-up [24]. However, penicillin is the only treatment used in pregnant women diagnosed with syphilis. Doxycycline is contraindicated for use in pregnancy; therefore, if a pregnant woman is penicillin allergic, penicillin desensitization and treatment with penicillin is recommended [24] (Table 1).

The resurgence in syphilis has also focused attention on improving its diagnosis. Currently, there are 2 main techniques for detecting spirochetes associated with syphilis. Direct detection testing methods include dark-field microscopy, nucleic acid amplification methods, direct fluorescent antibody

Table 1
2015 CDC STI treatment guidelines for syphilis

	Infants (>1 mo age) & children	Adults	Alternative nonpregnant adult treatment
Primary and secondary syphilis	Benzathine penicillin G, 50,000 units/kg IM, up to the adult dose of 2.4 million units in a single dose	Benzathine penicillin G, 2.4 million units IM in a single dose	Doxycycline, 100 mg, twice daily for 14 d, tetracycline, 500 mg, 4 times daily for 14 d. Ceftriaxone, 1–2 gm, daily IM or IV for 10–14 d
Early latent syphilis	Benzathine penicillin G, 50,000 units/kg IM, up to the adult dose of 2.4 million units in a single dose	Benzathine penicillin G, 2.4 million units IM in a single dose	Doxycycline, 100 mg, twice daily for 14 d, tetracycline, 500 mg, 4 times daily for 14 d. Ceftriaxone, 1–2 gm, daily IM or IV for 10–14 d
Late latent syphilis OR latent syphilis of unknown duration	Benzathine penicillin G, 50,000 units/kg IM, up to the adult dose of 2.4 million units, administered as 3 doses at 1-wk interval (total 150,000 units/kg up to the adult total dose of 7.2 million units)	Benzathine penicillin G, 7.2 million units total, administered as 3 doses of 2.4 million units IM each at 1-wk interval	Doxycycline, 100 mg, twice daily or tetracycline, 500 mg, 4 times daily for 28 d.
Tertiary with normal CSF *Examination*		Benzathine penicillin G, 7.2 million units total, administered as 3 doses of 2.4 million units IM each at 1-wk interval	If allergic to penicillin consult an infectious disease expert
Neurosyphilis and ocular syphilis	Aqueous crystalline penicillin G, 200,000–300,000 units/kg/d IV, administered as 50,000 units/kg every 4–6 h for 10 d	Aqueous crystalline penicillin G, 18–24 million units/d, administered as 3–4 million units IV every 4 h or continuous infusion for 10–14 d	Procaine penicillin G 2.4 million units IM once daily PLUS probenecid, 500 mg, orally 4 times a day, both for 10–14, ceftriaxone, 2 gm, daily either by IM or by IV for 10–14 d

(*continued on next page*)

Table 1
(*continued*)

	Infants (>1 mo age) & children	Adults	Alternative nonpregnant adult treatment
Special note on pregnancy	Pregnant women should be treated with the penicillin regimen appropriate for their stage of infection. Pregnant women who report penicillin allergy should be desensitized and treated with penicillin.		
Special note on persons with HIV	Early latent syphilis = Benzathine penicillin G, 2.4 million units IM in a single dose Late latent syphilis = Benzathine penicillin G, at weekly doses of 2.4 million units for 3 wk Efficacy of alternative regimens in person with HIV infection has not been well studied.		
Special note on infants and children	Birth and maternal records need to be reviewed to assess for congenital vs acquired syphilis. Recommend management by a pediatric infectious disease specialist and evaluation for sexual abuse through consultation with child protection services. In late latent syphilis CSF examination need to rule out neurosyphilis.		
Special note on neurosyphilis and ocular syphilis	Above mentioned treatment is shorter than those used for latent syphilis. Therefore, benzathine penicillin 2.4 million units IM once per week for up to 3 wk can be considered after completion of these neurosyphilis treatment regimens to provide comparable total duration of therapy. In pencillin-allergic patient, ceftriaxone, 2 gm, daily either by IM or by IV for 10–14 d can be used as an alternative or consider penicillin desensitization in consultation with a specialist.		

Abbreviations: IM, intramuscular; IV, intravenous.

Data from Centers for Disease Control and Prevention Sexually Transmitted Disease Treatment Guidelines, 2015. In. Atlanta (GA): US Department of Health and Human Services; 2015.

testing, and histopathologic examination of infected tissues. Direct methods are advantageous because they can detect infection in some patients before they have mounted the measurable antibody response that is required for serologic testing methods. However, access to direct methods, especially dark-field microscopy, is limited in many clinical settings. Although demonstration of *T pallidum* is the definitive method of diagnosis, successful testing with dark-field microscopy has limited sensitivity, thus failure to detect *T pallidum* by this method does not rule out syphilis [25].

Direct fluorescent antibody testing for *T pallidum* is easier to perform than dark-field microscopy but is no longer available in the United States. Detection of *T pallidum* DNA through nucleic acid amplification is also commercially available; however, such testing is not yet approved by Food and Drug Administration [26]. Specimens for testing by this method include CSF, whole blood, serum, or swabs from genital lesions. Preliminary studies have shown *T pallidum* PCR testing has a high degree of accuracy and better sensitivity and specificity than dark-field microscopy; however, more studies are needed to confirm this finding [27].

Indirect serologic testing, the other method used for syphilis diagnosis, is based on the detection of antibodies produced in response to infection. These antibodies fall into 2 categories: nontreponemal test for screening and treponemal test for confirmation [25]. Presumptive diagnosis requires the use of both nontreponemal and treponemal serologic testing.

All nontreponemal tests measure IgG and IgM antiphospholipid antibodies formed by the host in response to lipoid material released by damaged host cells early in the infection and to lipid from the cell surface of the treponeme. The most commonly used nontreponemal tests used in the United States are the Venereal Disease Research Laboratory (VDRL) slide test and the rapid plasma reagin test (RPR). Both tests are inexpensive, can be performed rapidly, and provide semiquantitative results through serial 2-fold dilutions. However, for diagnosis of acute infection the testing must be confirmed by one of the specific treponemal tests to exclude a false-positive result [25]. False-negative results can occur in patients with early primary syphilis (before the development of a host antibody response), latent acquired syphilis of long duration, and late congenital syphilis. Occasionally, in cases where high antibody titers are present, nontreponemal testing may show only a weakly positive or false-negative result, known as the prozone phenomenon. Diluting the serum will subsequently result in a positive result [28]. False-positive results for nontreponemal testing can also occur due to advanced age, certain viral infections (eg, Epstein-Barr, hepatitis, varicella, mumps, and measles), lymphoma, tuberculosis, malaria, endocarditis, autoimmune and inflammatory diseases (eg, rheumatoid arthritis, lupus, vasculitis and thyroiditis, ulcerative colitis), pregnancy, abuse of intravenous drugs, laboratory or technical error, and Wharton jelly contamination when umbilical cord blood specimens are used [25].

Both the RPR and VDRL provide semiquantitative results through serial 2-fold dilutions. These titers can be used to both define disease activity and monitor response to therapy. RPR and VDRL titers differ, with RPR titers generally being higher than VRDL titers. Therefore, the same test must be used to monitor follow-up response to therapy. A sustained 4-fold or greater decrease in titer (equivalent to a change of 2 dilutions, eg, 1:32–1:8) demonstrates adequate treatment. A sustained 4-fold increase after treatment suggests reinfection or relapse. Nontreponemal titers usually decrease 4-fold within 6 to 12 months after therapy for primary or secondary syphilis, and if treated during early primary or secondary syphilis they usually become nonreactive within a year after successful therapy. Patients treated for latent or tertiary syphilis may continue to have low stable titers despite effective therapy [25].

Treponemal tests detect antibody to *T pallidum* proteins: commonly used tests are enzyme immunoassays (TP-EIA), chemiluminescence assay (TP-CIA), and fluorescent treponemal antibody absorption test (FTA-ABS). Treponemal tests are technically more difficult to perform and more expensive than nontreponemal tests. Patients may remain reactive for years regardless of treatment, and titers correlate poorly with disease activity. For this reason, these tests are traditionally used to confirm infection following a positive nontreponemal test and should not be used to evaluate response to therapy, relapse, or reinfection in previous treated patients [25].

The "conventional diagnostic approach" for syphilis serologic testing starts with a nontreponemal test such as the RPR or VRDL and if positive a confirmatory test is performed using one of the treponemal tests such as the TP-PA or FTA-ABS. With early syphilis nontreponemal tests may be positive before the treponemal test is positive. To automate the testing process and reduce costs, some laboratories screen with a treponemal test such as TP-PA or TP-EIA first. With this reverse algorithm or "reverse-sequence screening" a positive treponemal test result is confirmed with a quantitative nontreponemal test (RPR or VDRL). If the results are discordant, a second treponemal test targeting a different *T. pallidum* antigen is performed to confirm the original test. If the second treponemal test is negative and the person is at low risk for syphilis, the original treponemal test result likely will be false positive [26].

None of these current testing methods allow for on-the-spot diagnosis, which delays treatment and increases the likelihood of losing the patient to follow-up. These limitations pose an urgent need for modernizing the testing capabilities such as those that are available for rapid HIV detection.

Additional items in the CDC's Call to Action include the development of electronic health records that include sexual history taking, STI screening, and treatment support documentation that can be easily integrated with public health departments; exploration of all options for the development of a syphilis vaccine; and expanded screening, particularly among the most at-risk populations including pregnant women and MSM, particularly those with HIV.

SUMMARY

Since the start of the twenty-first century rates of syphilis have been gradually increasing and now it is affecting a broader range of age groups, races, ethnicities, and geographic regions of the country. The CDC issued a Call to Action in 2017 to health care providers, researchers, and at-risk populations to work together to curb this resurgence. Syphilis is preventable and curable, and the CDC is calling for a twenty-first century approach to supplement control measures in use since the end of WWII. The Call to Action includes the development of improved electronic health records, modernized blood testing for detection and staging of the infection, expanded treatment options for those for whom penicillin is contraindicated and for whom penicillin is not effective in treating complications of syphilis, and development of a syphilis vaccine. Finally, the CDC is calling on all health care workers to expand screening for syphilis especially among the most at-risk populations including pregnant women and MSM, including those with HIV.

References

[1] Neinstein LS, Gordan CM, Katzman D, et al, editors. Adolescent health care: a practical guide. 5th edition. Philadelphia: Wolters Kluwer Health/Lippincott Williams & Wilkins; 2008.
[2] Tampa M, Sarbu I, Matei C, et al. Brief history of syphilis. J Med Life 2014;7(1):4–10.
[3] Hackett CJ. On the origin of the human treponematoses (pinta, yaws, endemic syphilis and venereal syphilis). Bull World Health Organ 1963;29(1):7–41.
[4] Waugh MA. Role played by Italy in the history of syphilis. Br J venereal Dis 1982;58(2): 92–5.
[5] Radolf JD, Tramont EC, Salazar JC. Syphilis (Treponema pallidum). In: Bennett JE, Dolin R, Blaser MJ, editors. Mandell, Douglas and Bennett's Principles and Practice of Infectious Diseases. 8th edition. Philadelphia: Elsevier Saunders; 2015. p. 2684–709.
[6] Sefton A. The Great Pox that was...Syphilis. J Appl Microbiol 2001;91(4):592–6.
[7] O'Shea JG. 'Two minutes with venus, two years with mercury'–mercury as an antisyphilitic chemotherapeutic agent. J R Soc Med 1990;83(6):392–5.
[8] Willeford WG, Bachmann LH. Syphilis ascendant: a brief history and modern trends. Trop Dis Trav Med Vaccin 2016;2:20.
[9] Rosahn PD. Autopsy studies in syphilis. J Veneral Dis Infect 1947;649(Suppl.1):1–67.
[10] Mahoney JF, Arnold RC, Stermer BL, et al. Penicillin treatment of early syphilis II. JAMA 1944;126:63–7.
[11] White RM. Unraveling the Tuskegee study of untreated syphilis. Arch Intern Med 2000;160: 585–98.
[12] Nakashima AK, Rolfs RT, Flock ML, et al. Epidemiology of Syphilis in the United States, 1941–1993. Sex Transm Dis 1996;23(1):16–23.
[13] Aral SO, Fenton KA, Holmes KK. Sexually transmitted diseases in the USA: temporal trends. Sex Transm infections 2007;83(4):257–66.
[14] Centers for disease control and prevention. Sexually Transmitted Disease Surveillance 2005. Atlanta (GA): US Department of Health and Human Services; 2006.
[15] de Voux A, Kidd S, Grey JA. State-specific rates of primary and secondary syphilis among men who have sex with men — United States, 2015. MMWR Morb Mortal Wkly Rep 2017;66:349–54.
[16] Centers for Disease Control and Prevention. Sexually Transmitted Disease Surveillance 2017. Atlanta, GA: U.S. Department of Health and Human Services; 2018.
[17] Grant RM, Lama JR, Anderson PL, et al. Preexposure chemoprophylaxis for HIV prevention in men who have sex with men. N Engl J Med 2010;363(27):2587–99.
[18] Volk J, Marcus J, Phengrasamy T, et al. No new HIV infections with increasing use of HIV preexposure prophylaxis in a clinical practice setting. Clin Infect Dis 2015;61(10): 1601–3.

[19] Marcus J, Glidden D, Mayer K, et al. No evidence of sexual risk compensation in the iPrEx trial of daily oral HIV preexposure prophylaxis. PLoS One 2013;8(12):e81997.
[20] de Voux A, Kidd S, Torrone EA. Reported cases of neurosyphilis among early syphilis cases-United States, 2009 to 2015. Sex Transm Dis 2018;45(1):39–41.
[21] Centers for Disease Control and Prevention. CDC call to action: let's work together to stem the tide of rising Syphilis in the US. Atlanta (GA): US Department of Health and Human Services; 2017.
[22] Ghanem KG, Erbelding EJ, Cheng WW, et al. Doxycycline compared with benzathine penicillin for the treatment of early syphilis. Clin Infect Dis 2006;42(6):e45–9.
[23] Dai T, Qu R, Liu J, et al. Efficacy of doxycycline in the treatment of syphilis. Antimicrob Agents Chemother 2017;61(1) [pii:e01092-01016].
[24] Centers for Disease Control and Prevention. 2015 sexually transmitted diseases treatment guidelines. Atlanta (GA): US Department of Health and Human Services; 2015.
[25] Ratnam S. The laboratory diagnosis of syphilis. Can J Infect Dis Med Microbiol 2005;16(1): 45–51.
[26] Workowski KA, Bolan GA. Sexually transmitted diseases treatment guidelines, 2015. MMWR Recomm Rep 2015;64(Rr-03):1–137.
[27] Gayet-Ageron A, Sednaoui P, Lautenschlager S, et al. Use of treponema pallidum PCR in testing of ulcers for diagnosis of primary syphilis. Emerg Infect Dis 2015;21(1):127–9.
[28] Liu L-L, Lin L-R, Tong M-L, et al. Incidence and risk factors for the prozone phenomenon in serologic testing for syphilis in a large cohort. Clin Infect Dis 2014;59(3):384–9.

Advances in Pediatrics 66 (2019) 245–261

ADVANCES IN PEDIATRICS

Nonoccupational Postexposure Prophylaxis and Preexposure Prophylaxis for Human Immunodeficiency Virus Prevention in Adolescents and Young Adults

Diane M. Straub, MD, MPH[a,*],
Tanya L. Kowalczyk Mullins, MD, MS[b,c]

[a]Division of Adolescent Medicine, University of South Florida, 2 Tampa General Circle, Suite 500, Tampa, FL 33606, USA; [b]Division of Adolescent and Transition Medicine, Cincinnati Children's Hospital Medical Center, 3333 Burnet Avenue, MLC 4000, Cincinnati, OH 45229, USA; [c]Department of Pediatrics, University of Cincinnati College of Medicine, Cincinnati, OH 45267, USA

Keywords

• Human immunodeficiency virus (HIV) • Prevention • Postexposure prophylaxis • Preexposure prophylaxis

Key points

- Nonoccupational postexposure prophylaxis decreases the risk of human immunodeficiency virus infection when initiated 72 hours or less after sexual, injection drug use, or other potential exposure to the virus.
- Preexposure prophylaxis decreases the risk of human immunodeficiency virus infection by more than 90% with high adherence and is now approved for adolescents in the United States.
- The legal rights of minors to access nonoccupational postexposure prophylaxis and preexposure prophylaxis without parental involvement vary by state; clinicians need to be familiar with their local laws.

INTRODUCTION

Of the nearly 40,000 human immunodeficiency virus (HIV) infections diagnosed in the United States in 2016, 21% were in 13- to 25-year-olds [1]. Among adolescents and young adults, 70% of newly diagnosed infections were

Disclosures: Dr T.L.K. Mullins has no relevant financial relationships to disclose.

*Corresponding author. *E-mail address:* dstraub@health.usf.edu

https://doi.org/10.1016/j.yapd.2019.03.007

attributed to men who have sex with men (MSM) or to MSM and injection drug use, and 24% of cases were attributed to heterosexual contact [1]. HIV disproportionately impacts Black/African American and Hispanic/Latino youth, with 55% of infections among 15- to 25-year-olds diagnosed in Black/African Americans and 23% in Hispanic/Latino youth [1]. Sexual risk behaviors are commonly reported among adolescents and young adults (Table 1).

The risk of acquiring HIV differs by route of exposure. Receptive anal intercourse and needle-sharing injection drug use confer the greatest risk of transmission, with a lower–but still substantial–risk associated with penile–vaginal and insertive anal intercourse [2]. Sexual partners of HIV-infected people are at significant risk of HIV: the 1-year cumulative risk of transmission is 52% for MSM practicing anal sex and 6% to 20% for heterosexuals practicing vaginal and/or anal sex [3]. Although consistent condom use reduces risk [3], condomless sex is frequently reported. HIV transmission after sexual assault has been reported [4–6]; transmission risk may be influenced by trauma, anatomic site of exposure, semen HIV viral load (male perpetrator), and cooccurring genital lesions or sexually transmitted infections (STIs) in either the perpetrator or survivor [4].

NONOCCUPATIONAL POSTEXPOSURE PROPHYLAXIS

Nonoccupational postexposure prophylaxis (nPEP) is the use of antiretroviral medication after isolated sexual, injection drug use, or other nonoccupational

Table 1
Reported HIV risk behaviors among adolescents and young adults

Patient population	Risk behavior	Percent
High school students [77]	Ever had sexual intercourse	40
	Had sexual intercourse in past 3 mo	29
	No condom use at last sex	46
	Alcohol, other substance use before last sex	19
	Never tested for HIV	91
HIV-uninfected men who have sex with men (MSM), ages 18–24 y [78]	Condomless anal sex with male partner past 12 mo	73
	Condomless sex with HIV-infected partner at last sex	17
	No HIV testing past 12 mo	21
	Transactional sex past 12 mo	10
	Any PrEP use past 12 mo	22
HIV-uninfected heterosexuals, ages 18–24 y [79]	Condomless vaginal sex past 12 mo	87–93
	No HIV testing past 12 mo	59
	Transactional sex past 12 mo	6
	Any PrEP use past 12 mo	0.1
HIV-uninfected people who inject drugs, ages 18–24 y [80]	Condomless sex with HIV-infected partner	46
	Shared injection equipment used by other(s) past 12 mo	76
	No HIV testing past 12 mo	45
	Transactional sex past 12 mo	19
	Any PrEP use past 12 mo	0.5

HIV exposure to prevent HIV infection. The US Centers for Disease Control and Prevention (CDC)/Department of Health and Human Services released its most recent nPEP recommendations in 2016 [2].

Research supporting nPEP is limited owing to the ethical and feasibility concerns of conducting a large scale, randomized, placebo-controlled clinical trial of nPEP. Thus, information from occupational PEP among health care workers, observational and case studies of nPEP efficacy in humans, nonhuman primate studies, and expert opinion form the basis for the 2016 nPEP guidelines [2]. The efficacy of occupational PEP was first described in a multinational study that demonstrated an 81% decrease in the odds of transmission in health care workers with percutaneous exposure to HIV who received zidovudine prophylaxis [7]. Intrapartum and postpartum prophylaxis prevents perinatal transmission [8,9], and most seroconversions after nPEP are due to ongoing risk behavior and not seroconversions [2]. A pooled analysis of 10 studies regarding nPEP in 8336 sexually assaulted youth revealed no new HIV infections; however, only 8% were offered nPEP and 1.5% completed treatment [2]. Another analysis of 15 studies in youth who completed nPEP revealed that only 1 of 19 seroconversions was due to failure of nPEP [2]. Studies in nonhuman primates also support the efficacy of PEP, its timing of initiation, and the use of tenofovir as part of the nPEP regimen [10]. Of note, comprehensive reviews of nPEP efficacy include older studies, which used single-dose therapy, as compared with newer studies with better tolerated multiple drug regimens, implying improved efficacy over time.

Safety

Much of the literature on adverse reactions to nPEP includes older regimens that are not currently part of the nPEP guidelines. A systematic review including 24 studies, representing 2166 victims of sexual assault using various nPEP regimens, reported that the most common side effects were nausea, vomiting, diarrhea, and fatigue; notably, only 40% of patients adhered to nPEP [11]. More serious side effects (eg, hepatic and renal toxicity) have occasionally been reported. Because of severe hepatotoxicity, nevirapine is now contraindicated for use as nPEP [12]. A study evaluating the combination of raltegravir, tenofovir disoproxil fumarate (TDF), and emtricitabine reported fewer side effects than historical controls. Side effects included mild, self-limited gastrointestinal complaints, headache, fatigue, and myalgias or arthralgias. Additionally, 57% of participants completed the regimen as prescribed, and 27% adhered to the daily medication, although some participants missed the second daily dose of raltegravir [13]. Among 100 MSM using the combination of dolutegravir, TDF, and emtricitabine as nPEP, 90% reported completion of nPEP with 98% self-reported adherence. Side effects reported included fatigue, gastrointestinal complaints, and headache, as well as mild elevation of alanine aminotransferase without hepatitis and a slight decrease in glomerular filtration rate; however, there were no discontinuations owing to toxicity [14]. Newer, more effective, and better tolerated regimens with fewer and less significant side effects–and once daily dosing–are likely to maximize adherence to and effectiveness of nPEP.

Patient awareness of nonoccupational postexposure prophylaxis

The use of nPEP may be limited owing to potential users being unaware of its existence. In New York City, which has comparatively high HIV prevalence and a highly visible HIV prevention initiative, only 59% of high-risk individuals were aware of nPEP (80% among young MSM of color, 63% among transgender women, and 34% among cisgender women of color) [15]. Ongoing nPEP education and outreach should prioritize high-risk groups and focus on reducing stigma and barriers to access.

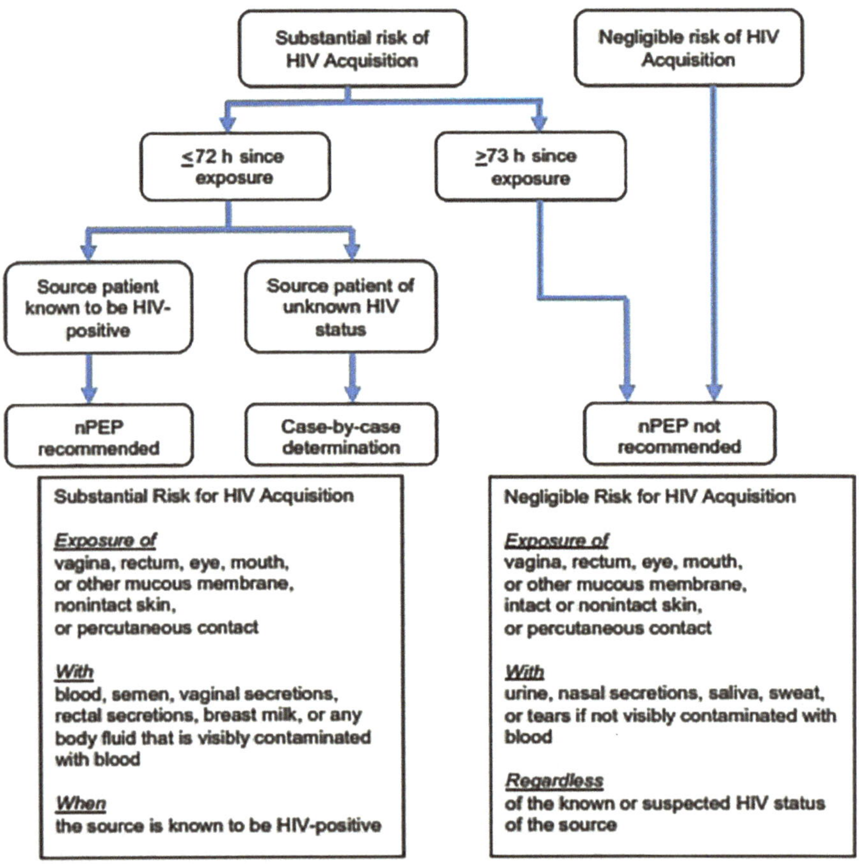

Fig. 1. Algorithm for evaluation and treatment of possible nonoccupational HIV exposure. (*From* Centers for Disease Control and Prevention. Updated guidelines for antiretroviral postexposure prophylaxis after sexual, injection drug use, or other nonoccupational exposure to HIV—United States, 2016. 2016. Available at: https://www.cdc.gov/hiv/pdf/programresources/cdc-hiv-npep-guidelines.pdf. Accessed December 2, 2018.)

Clinical implementation

A summary of the 2016 US CDC nPEP guidelines [2] is as follows.

- Clinicians should evaluate persons rapidly for nPEP when care is sought 72 hours or less after a potential nonoccupational exposure that presents a substantial risk for HIV acquisition. Fig. 1 displays the CDC evaluation and management algorithm, as well as definitions for "substantial risk" and "negligible risk." If the source of the exposure is known to be HIV infected, nPEP is recommended. If the HIV status of the source of exposure is unknown, recommendation for nPEP should be determined on a case-by-case basis. nPEP should not be initiated 73 hours or more after exposure or if there is negligible risk for HIV acquisition.
- At the initial evaluation visit, the clinician should determine the HIV status of the potentially exposed person and the exposure source person (if possible), the timing and characteristics of the exposure for which care is being sought, and the frequency of possible HIV exposures, as well as assessment for other needed treatment or prophylaxis (eg, STIs, pregnancy).
- All persons considered for nPEP should be tested for HIV, preferably using rapid combined antigen/antibody, or antibody blood tests. If rapid tests are unavailable and nPEP is otherwise indicated, it should be started without delay and can be later discontinued if the patient is determined to already be infected or the exposure source is determined to not be infected.
- All persons offered nPEP should be prescribed a 28-day course of a 3-drug antiretroviral regimen.
  - The preferred regimen for otherwise healthy adults and adolescents is TDF 300 mg with emtricitabine 200 mg once daily **plus** raltegravir 400 mg twice daily or dolutegravir 50 mg/d.[a]
  - The alternative regimen for otherwise healthy adults and adolescents is TDF 300 mg with emtricitabine 200 mg once daily **plus** darunavir 800 mg and ritonavir 100 mg/d.
  - For regimens for children, persons with impaired renal function, and pregnant women, see the nPEP guidelines [2].
- All persons evaluated for possible nPEP should also be provided any indicated prevention, treatment, or supportive care for other exposure-associated health risks and conditions (eg, bacterial STIs, traumatic injuries, hepatitis B and C virus infections, or pregnancy).
- All persons who report behaviors or situations that place them at risk for frequently recurring HIV exposures (eg, injection drug use, sex without condoms) or who report receipt of 1 or more courses of nPEP in the past year should be provided risk-reduction counseling and intervention services, including consideration of preexposure prophylaxis (PrEP; discussed elsewhere in this article).
- nPEP should only be provided for infrequent exposures. Patients who have frequent, recurrent exposures should be provided with intensive risk-reduction interventions and consideration of prescription of PrEP. However, if the most recent exposure was within 72 hours of the evaluation, nPEP may be indicated with subsequent transition to PrEP.
- Laboratory testing and the recommended follow-up schedule include HIV, STI, pregnancy, and kidney and liver function testing (Table 2). Ideally, follow-up

should occur at 4 to 6 weeks, 3 months, and 6 months after exposure. Laboratory testing for the exposure source person and for individuals who seroconvert is also outlined [2].

According to the guidelines, nPEP must be initiated within 72 hours of exposure. However, exposures often occur outside of routine office hours when office staff are present to assist with the paperwork that is often required to authorize nPEP. Although manufacturers have patient-assistance programs for those without insurance and copay cards to offset high copays for medications, these programs require knowledge and familiarity on the part of the clinician and the pharmacist, as well as time to complete the necessary forms, such as a letter of medical necessity. Clinicians need to plan ahead to implement office policies to expedite the process of authorizing nPEP to ensure patients can start treatment within the required 72-hour window after exposure. Additionally, nPEP is likely to be more effective the sooner it is started after exposure, so timeliness is critical. One strategy is establishing a relationship with local pharmacies, which can dramatically improve the nPEP process. After-hours and urgent and emergent care centers should identify and develop relationships with 24-hour pharmacies, and encourage them to stock nPEP medications. A pilot program in Florida with an established nationwide retail pharmacy has proven to be an effective collaboration that has improved timely access to nPEP medications (unpublished data, D. Straub, 2018).

---

[a]Since the publication of the nPEP guidelines, additional data suggest safety concerns associated with use of dolutegravir in women at risk for pregnancy. In an ongoing National Institutes of Health-funded observational study in Botswana, a recent preliminary unscheduled data analysis suggested that exposure to dolutegravir-containing regimens at conception may increase the risk of neural tube defects. Four infants with neural tube defects were born to 426 women exposed to dolutegravir at conception, yielding a proportion of 0.9%, as compared with 0.1% in infants of women exposed to other antiretroviral drugs at conception. According to the manufacturer of dolutegravir, a complete package of reproductive toxicology studies showed no evidence of adverse developmental outcomes [16]. Although surveillance is ongoing, as a result of this preliminary data, the CDC recommended in May 2018 that clinicians prescribing nPEP should avoid the use of dolutegravir for nonpregnant women of childbearing potential who are sexually active or have been sexually assaulted and who are not using an effective birth control method, as well as for women early in pregnancy. The preferred regimen for nPEP for these women includes raltegravir, tenofovir, and emtricitabine (as described). Furthermore, all women of childbearing potential starting nPEP should have a pregnancy test performed. If the nPEP regimen for a nonpregnant woman of childbearing potential must include dolutegravir (eg, raltegravir is not available), she should use an effective birth control method until the nPEP regimen is completed. Additionally, dietary folic acid 400 μg is recommended daily [17].

Table 2
Recommended schedule of laboratory evaluations of source and exposed persons for providing nPEP with preferred regimens

Test	Source	Exposed persons			
	Baseline	Baseline	4–6 wk after exposure	3 mo after exposure	6 mo after exposure
		For all persons considered for or prescribed nPEP for any exposure			
HIV Ag/Ab testing[a] (or antibody testing if Ag/Ab test unavailable)	✓	✓	✓	✓	✓[b]
Hepatitis B serology, including: Hepatitis B surface antigen; Hepatitis B surface antibody; Hepatitis B core antibody	✓	✓	—	—	✓[c]
Hepatitis C antibody test	✓	✓	—	—	✓[d]
		For all persons considered for or prescribed nPEP for sexual exposure			
Syphilis serology[e]	✓	✓	✓	—	✓
Gonorrhea[f]	✓	✓	✓[g]	—	—
Chlamydia[f]	✓	✓	✓[g]	—	—
Pregnancy[h]	—	✓	✓	—	—
		For persons prescribed tenofovir DF + emtricitabine + raltegravir or tenofovir DF + emtricitabine + dolutegravir			
Serum creatinine (for calculating estimated creatinine clearance[i])		✓	✓	—	—
Alanine transaminase, aspartate aminotransferase		✓	✓	—	—
	For all persons with HIV infection confirmed at any visit				
HIV viral load	✓	✓[j]			
HIV genotypic resistance	✓	✓[j]			

Abbreviations: Ag/Ab, antigen/antibody combination test; tenofovir DF, tenofovir disoproxil fumarate.

[a]Any positive or indeterminate HIV antibody test should undergo confirmatory testing of HIV infection status.

[b]Only if hepatitis C infection was acquired during the original exposure; delayed HIV seroconversion has been seen in persons who simultaneously acquire HIV and hepatitis C infection.

[c]If exposed person susceptible to hepatitis B at baseline.

[d]If exposed person susceptible to hepatitis C at baseline.

[e]If determined to be infected with syphilis and treated, should undergo serologic syphilis testing 6 mo after treatment.

[f]Testing for chlamydia and gonorrhea should be performed using nucleic acid amplification tests. For patients diagnosed with a chlamydia or gonorrhea infection, retesting 3 months after treatment is recommended (1) for men reporting insertive vaginal, anal, or oral sex, a urine specimen should be tested for chlamydia and gonorrhea, (2) for women reporting receptive vaginal sex, a vaginal (preferred) or endocervical swab or urine specimen should be tested for chlamydia and gonorrhea, (3) for men and women reporting receptive anal sex, a rectal swab specimen should be tested for chlamydia and gonorrhea, and (4) for men and women reporting receptive oral sex, an oropharyngeal swab should be tested for gonorrhea (http://www.cdc.gov/std/tg2015/tg-2015-print.pdf).

[g]If not provided presumptive treatment at baseline, or if symptomatic at follow-up visit.

[h]If a woman of reproductive age, not using effective contraception, and with vaginal exposure to semen.

[i]eCrCl = estimated creatinine clearance calculated by the Cockcroft-Gault formula; eCrClCG = [(140 − age) × ideal body weight] + (serum creatinine × 72) (× 0.85 for females).

[j]At first visit where determined to have HIV infection.

From the Centers for Disease Control and Prevention. Updated guidelines for antiretroviral postexposure prophylaxis after sexual, injection drug use, or other nonoccupational exposure to HIV United States, 2016. 2016. Available at: https://www.cdc.gov/hiv/pdf/programresources/cdc-hiv-npep-guidelines.pdf. Accessed December 2, 2018.

PREEXPOSURE PROPHYLAXIS

PrEP is the use of antiretroviral medications before potential exposure to prevent HIV infection. In the pivotal efficacy trials, use of tenofovir-based PrEP was associated with 44% to 75% decrease in new HIV infections [18–21]. Up to a 92% reduction in infections is achieved with high levels of adherence [20–22]. However, the degree of adherence necessary to achieve high levels of protection depends on the route of exposure: no new HIV infections were documented among MSM taking 4 or more doses of PrEP per week [23], whereas protection in the female genital tract requires daily adherence [24]. In 2012, the US Food and Drug Administration (FDA) approved the first (and currently only) oral medication for PrEP (fixed-dose combination tenofovir disoproxil fumarate-emtricitabine [TDF-FTC; Truvada]) for use in adults. In May 2018, the FDA expanded the indication for TDF-FTC to include adolescents weighing 35 kg or more [25].

Preexposure prophylaxis in adolescents

To date, only 2 published studies describe the results of PrEP trials conducted with adolescents: one study included 18- to 22-year-old MSM [26] and one included 15- to 17-year-old MSM [27]. Both of these US studies were open-label demonstration projects that were not designed to assess efficacy. Among two hundred 18- to 22-year-old MSM, 70% completed the study through week 48. Although most participants reported that taking a daily oral medication was acceptable, adherence waned over time: only 34% of participants were taking 4 or more doses per week at the end of the study [26]. Among the 15- to 17-year-olds, 46 completed the 48-week study, with only 22% reporting taking 4 or more doses per week by the end of the study [27]. In both studies, adherence was 49% to 57% when study visits occurred monthly and then substantially decreased when visits occurred every 3 months [26,27], as currently recommended by the CDC PrEP guidelines [28]. These data, taken together with a metaanalysis demonstrating lower adherence to PrEP in younger users [29], suggest that more frequent follow-up of younger PrEP users may be warranted to bolster adherence.

Safety

Use of tenofovir-based PrEP is associated with dose-dependent decreases in bone density in MSM and transgender women [30,31], heterosexual adults [32], and adult women [33], which has been cited as a barrier to prescribing PrEP to youth [34]. No increase in fractures has been documented in PrEP users [30–33], and bone density recovers after the cessation of PrEP [31,33]. Among 18- to 22-year-old PrEP users, bone density also decreased [35]. Follow-up studies investigating whether bone density among younger PrEP users recovers will be critical to addressing clinician concerns about using PrEP in youth.

Tenofovir-containing PrEP is associated with decreases in renal function among adults [36,37], but these decreases quickly reversed after discontinuation of PrEP [36,37]. Among younger PrEP users, a slight increase in serum creatinine occurred over the first 12 weeks of use, but there was no change in the estimated glomerular filtration rate [35]. Consequently, the CDC PrEP guidelines recommend that patients using PrEP have an estimated creatinine clearance of 60 mL/min or greater [28].

Although HIV viral resistance develops among PrEP users, clinical trial data suggest that it occurs less frequently among those who become HIV infected while using PrEP and more often when PrEP is started in the setting of undetected HIV infection [38–40]. Most new HIV infections that occurred in people taking PrEP were related to poor adherence [41,42], although new infections have been reported among PrEP users with excellent adherence [43]. Among those who become HIV infected while taking PrEP, detection of infection may be delayed [44], but HIV viral load and $CD4^{+}$ T-cell counts are similar to those of people who become infected while taking placebo [45].

Recent implementation studies suggest that some people taking PrEP participate in riskier behaviors. In 1 study, 35% of PrEP users reported less condom use, more condomless sex partners, and more condomless oral sex when compared with nonusers [46]. In another study of MSM who started PrEP, 28% had an increase in STIs from before PrEP to after PrEP [47]. Because a subset of people using PrEP may participate in riskier sexual behaviors, it is critical to routinely screen for STIs in this population as outlined in the PrEP guidelines [28].

Patient uptake and attitudes

The greatest awareness of PrEP is among adult MSM [46,48,49]; however, only 7% to 9% reported taking it [46,48]. Among young transwomen, only 31% were aware of PrEP and 5% reported having taken it [50]. Less than one-quarter of women [51] and 33% of female sex workers reported awareness of PrEP [52]. Similarly, only 18% to 37% of people who inject drugs reported awareness of PrEP [53,54], but only 0.03% to 1.80% had ever taken it [53,54]. Even HIV-infected adults have low awareness of PrEP, although most would encourage PrEP use by HIV-uninfected partners [55]. Among adolescents, 64% of transwomen [56] and 39% of black MSM reported awareness of PrEP [57].

Even though PrEP has been approved by the FDA for use in adults since 2012, few people who are eligible for PrEP have taken it. In 1 study, only 13% of MSM and transwomen who met the criteria for PrEP were taking it; the lowest rate of PrEP use was in 18- to 24-year-olds [58]. The majority of people who have received prescriptions for PrEP to date are 25 to 44 years old and have commercial insurance; 95% are men and 69% are white [59], suggesting that there may be disparities in access and uptake for other age groups (<10% of prescriptions were for 18- to 24-year-olds) [59], women, and other races/ethnicities. Even when prescribed PrEP, many people do not fill the prescription and actually start PrEP [60]. Further, rates of discontinuation are fairly high: only 47% of MSM who initiated PrEP were engaged in PrEP care 13 months later [60].

Potential PrEP users cite barriers including concerns about cost [46], side effects [46], the need for adherence to daily medication [49,61], a lack of perceived risk of HIV infection [49], uncertainty about how to access PrEP [46,61], a lack of awareness of PrEP [46], and a lack of health insurance [46]. PrEP-related stigma is also a significant barrier. Studies describe "PrEP shaming" [61], as well as patient concerns about how PrEP use would be perceived by others [51]. PrEP users report that other people may assume that they participate in risky sex or that they are HIV infected [62]. Even those who may be candidates for PrEP perceived it to be only for those who are "promiscuous". [48] Younger PrEP users, particularly those under age 18 years of age, may face additional barriers to PrEP, including a lack of trust between clinicians and youth, inexperience navigating the health care system, a lack of transportation, cost, and concerns about loss of confidentiality [63].

Clinician attitudes and behaviors

Among clinicians caring for adults, frequently cited barriers to providing PrEP include concerns about patient adherence [64,65], increases in risky behaviors among people taking PrEP [64,65], side effects [64], cost [64,65], lack of clinical time [65], development of HIV resistance [64,65], insufficient infrastructure to provide PrEP [65], failure of PrEP users to keep scheduled follow-up visits [65], and insufficient reimbursement of clinicians for PrEP services [64,65]. Few studies have examined PrEP-related attitudes of clinicians caring for adolescents. Clinicians caring for HIV-infected and -uninfected youth reported concerns including patient adherence, confidentiality, the legal ability to prescribe PrEP confidentially, increases in riskier sexual behaviors, cost/insurance coverage, a lack of organizational resources, and community stigma around HIV [34]. Among physicians from various specialties who provide primary care to adolescents, awareness of PrEP was fairly low, with 37% of physicians reporting some familiarity with PrEP. These primary care physicians identified barriers unique to PrEP use in youth, including the potential impact of PrEP on growth and development, parental opposition to PrEP use, potential breaches of confidentiality, physician concerns about prescribing PrEP to minors, a lack of legal clarity about whether PrEP could be prescribed to youth confidentially, and concerns about whether pharmacists might limit youth access to PrEP. Overall, more physicians reported the intention to recommend PrEP than prescribe it [66], which could impact youth access to PrEP. An online survey of members of the Society for Adolescent Health and Medicine found that 93% had heard of PrEP, 65% were willing to prescribe it to 13- to 17-years-olds, and 78% were willing to prescribe it to 18- to 24-years-olds [67].

Clinical implementation

The only medication currently approved by the US FDA for PrEP is a fixed-dose combination of TDF 300 mg and emtricitabine 200 mg (TDF-FTC) administered once daily. The CDC PrEP guidelines were updated in 2017

[28]. The CDC also published a clinical provider's supplement that provides resources that can be used to provide PrEP care, including counseling resources for clinicians and educational handouts for patients [68]. These documents have not been updated to reflect the recent FDA approval of PrEP for use in adolescents. Several US organizations, including the Society for Adolescent Health and Medicine [69], the American College of Obstetricians and Gynecologists [70], and the International AIDS Society-USA [71], have released statements supporting the use of PrEP among those at risk of HIV infection.

The CDC PrEP guidelines include suggested indications for PrEP (Table 3). Baseline laboratory evaluations should include HIV testing (with an antigen/antibody test [preferred], antibody test, or rapid point-of-care FDA-approved fingerstick blood test), renal function testing (including calculation of estimated

Table 3
Summary of current US PrEP guidance (2017)

	MSM	Heterosexual women and men	Injection drug users
Detecting substantial risk of acquiring HIV infection	HIV-positive sexual partner Recent bacterial STI[a] High number of sex partners History of inconsistent or no condom use Commercial sex work	HIV-positive sexual partner Recent bacterial STI[b] High number of sex partners History of inconsistent or no condom use Commercial sex work In high-prevalence area or network	HIV-positive injecting partner Sharing injection equipment
Clinically eligible	Documented negative HIV test result before prescribing PrEP No signs/symptoms of acute HIV infection Normal renal function; no contraindicated medications Documented hepatitis B virus infection and vaccination status		
Prescription	Daily, continuing, oral doses of TDF/FTC (Truvada), ≤90 d supply		
Other services	Follow-up visits at least every 3 mo to provide the following: HIV test, medication adherence counseling, behavioral risk reduction support, side effect assessment, STI symptom assessment At 3 mo and every 6 mo thereafter, assess renal function Every 6 mo, test for bacterial STIs		
	Do oral/rectal STI testing	For women, assess pregnancy intent Pregnancy test every 3 mo	Access to clean needles/syringes and drug treatment services

[a]Gonorrhea, chlamydia, syphilis for MSM including those who inject drugs.
[b]Gonorrhea, syphilis for heterosexual women and men including those who inject drugs.
From Centers for Disease Control and Prevention. Preexposure prophylaxis for the prevention of HIV infection in the United States—2017 Update: a clinical practice guideline. 2018. Available at: https://www.cdc.gov/hiv/pdf/risk/prep/cdc-hiv-prep-guidelines-2017.pdf. Accessed November 6, 2018.

creatinine clearance using the Cockcroft-Gault formula), hepatitis B serology, and STI testing. An estimated creatinine clearance of less than 60 mL/min is a contraindication to TDF-FTC PrEP. Evaluating hepatitis B status is important because reactivation of hepatitis B and resultant liver toxicity can occur when PrEP is stopped [28]. Hepatitis C testing is recommended for people who have injected drugs. Patients should be counseled that the time required to achieve protective levels of PrEP ranges from 7 days for the rectal compartment to 20 days for blood and the cervicovaginal compartment [28]. The most common side effects include headache and gastrointestinal distress. The CDC recommends that PrEP be limited to a 3-month supply at a time and that patients be evaluated every 3 months for HIV testing, pregnancy testing, PrEP prescription refills, assessment of side effects and adherence, and STI testing. Creatinine clearance should be monitored every 6 months, and the continued need for PrEP should be evaluated every year [28].

Insurance coverage for PrEP and related services varies by carrier. The manufacturer of PrEP (Gilead Sciences, Inc., Foster City, CA) offers a medication assistance program [72]. The web site PleasePrEPMe.org contains links to other potential financial assistance programs [73], and the CDC published a brochure to help patients navigate paying for PrEP [74].

LEGAL ISSUES FOR MINOR-AGED ADOLESCENTS

In all 50 states and the District of Columbia, minors can consent to testing and treatment for STIs without parental consent, and 32 states include HIV as an STI [75]. However, the statutes are less clear regarding HIV prevention. The provision of nPEP could be interpreted as providing treatment, and thus within minor consent rights for those states that include HIV as an STI. For states that do not include HIV as an STI, minor consent for HIV prevention may not be legally permissible. Although the US FDA approved TDF-FTC for PrEP in youth, clinicians considering prescribing PrEP to youth should be familiar with their local legal statutes, because these vary by jurisdiction, and consider using legal expertise to help interpret the statutes where the laws are not clear. A CDC review of legal statutes demonstrated that no states explicitly prohibit minors from accessing PrEP without parental involvement, and 16 states specifically allow minors to access PrEP independently [76]. Additionally, although the age 18 years is considered the age of majority in most states, it varies among different states [76].

Finally, the legal right to consent to confidential health care does not ensure confidential health care, because insurance laws often require explanation of benefits statements be sent to the primary insurance holder. Therefore, a minor's use of insurance benefits for nPEP and PrEP services may be inadvertently communicated to their parent(s). Clinicians attempting to provide HIV prevention services to minors who are seeking confidential care should understand and explain these nuances and potential breaches of confidentiality to their patients.

SUMMARY

The nPEP and PrEP strategies reduce the risk of HIV acquisition. nPEP must be initiated within 72 hours of potential exposure to HIV and current guidelines recommend a 3-drug antiretroviral regimen taken for 28 days. PrEP should be considered for people with an ongoing high risk of HIV infection and current guidelines recommend a daily oral 2 drug antiretroviral regimen. The US CDC maintains updated published guidelines for clinicians who are prescribing nPEP and PrEP. Clinicians should be aware of local legal statutes that may impact the ability to provide confidential nPEP and PrEP services to minor-aged adolescents.

References

[1] Centers for Disease Control and Prevention. HIV surveillance report, 2016; vol 28. 2017. Available at: http://www.cdc.gov/hiv/library/reports/hiv-surveillance.html. Accessed October 30, 2018.

[2] Centers for Disease Control and Prevention. Updated guidelines for antiretroviral Postexposure prophylaxis After sexual, injection drug Use, or other Nonoccupational exposure to HIV—United States, 2016. 2016. Available at: https://www.cdc.gov/hiv/pdf/programresources/cdc-hiv-npep-guidelines.pdf. Accessed December 2, 2018.

[3] Lasry A, Sansom SL, Wolitski RJ, et al. HIV sexual transmission risk among serodiscordant couples: assessing the effects of combining prevention strategies. AIDS 2014;28(10):1521–9.

[4] Centers for Disease Control and Prevention. Sexually transmitted diseases treatment guidelines, 2015. MMWR Recomm Rep 2015;64(No. RR-3):1–137.

[5] Claydon E, Murphy S, Osborne EM, et al. Rape and HIV. Int J STD AIDS 1991;2(3):200–1.

[6] Murphy S, Kitchen V, Harris JR, et al. Rape and subsequent seroconversion to HIV. BMJ 1989;299(6701):718.

[7] Cardo DM, Culver DH, Ciesielski CA, et al. A case-control study of HIV seroconversion in health care workers after percutaneous exposure. N Engl J Med 1997;337(21):1485–90.

[8] Guay LA, Musoke P, Fleming T, et al. Intrapartum and neonatal single-dose nevirapine compared with zidovudine for prevention of mother-to-child transmission of HIV-1 in Kampala, Uganda: HIVNET 012 randomised trial. Lancet 1999;354(9181):795–802.

[9] Moodley D, Moodley J, Coovadia H, et al. A multicenter randomized controlled trial of nevirapine versus a combination of zidovudine and lamivudine to reduce intrapartum and early postpartum mother-to-child transmission of human immunodeficiency virus type 1. J Infect Dis 2003;187(5):725–35.

[10] Irvine C, Egan KJ, Shubber Z, et al. Efficacy of HIV postexposure prophylaxis: systematic review and meta-analysis of nonhuman primate studies. Clin Infect Dis 2015;60(Suppl 3):S165–9.

[11] Chacko L, Ford N, Sbaiti M, et al. Adherence to HIV post-exposure prophylaxis in victims of sexual assault: a systematic review and meta-analysis. Sex Transm Infect 2012;88(5):335–41.

[12] National Institutes of Health. Viramune drug label. 2014. Available at: https://dailymed.nlm.nih.gov/dailymed/drugInfo.cfm?setid=5ec05500-6333-4bd0-ac83-464fad0d5162. Accessed November 12, 2018.

[13] Mayer KH, Mimiaga MJ, Gelman M, et al. Raltegravir, tenofovir DF, and emtricitabine for postexposure prophylaxis to prevent the sexual transmission of HIV: safety, tolerability, and adherence. J Acquir Immune Defic Syndr 2012;59(4):354–9.

[14] McAllister JW, Towns JM, McNulty A, et al. Dolutegravir with tenofovir disoproxil fumarate-emtricitabine as HIV postexposure prophylaxis in gay and bisexual men. AIDS 2017;31(9):1291–5.

[15] Koblin BA, Usher D, Nandi V, et al. Post-exposure prophylaxis awareness, knowledge, access and use among three populations in New York City, 2016-17. AIDS Behav 2018;22(8):2718–32.
[16] World Health Organization. Potential safety issue affecting women living with HIV using dolutegravir at the time of conception. 2018. Available at: http://www.who.int/medicines/publications/drugalerts/Statement_on_DTG_18May_2018final.pdf. Accessed July 16, 2018.
[17] Centers for Disease Control and Prevention. Interim statement regarding potential Fetal Harm from exposure to dolutegravir - Implications for HIV post-exposure prophylaxis (PEP). 2018. Available at: https://www.cdc.gov/hiv/pdf/basics/cdc-hiv-dolutegravir-alert.pdf. Accessed November 12, 2018.
[18] Baeten JM, Donnell D, Ndase P, et al. Antiretroviral prophylaxis for HIV prevention in heterosexual men and women. N Engl J Med 2012;367(5):399–410.
[19] Choopanya K, Martin M, Suntharasamai P, et al. Antiretroviral prophylaxis for HIV infection in injecting drug users in Bangkok, Thailand (the Bangkok Tenofovir Study): a randomised, double-blind, placebo-controlled phase 3 trial. Lancet 2013;381(9883):2083–90.
[20] Grant RM, Lama JR, Anderson PL, et al. Preexposure chemoprophylaxis for HIV prevention in men who have sex with men. N Engl J Med 2010;363(27):2587–99.
[21] Thigpen MC, Kebaabetswe PM, Paxton LA, et al. Antiretroviral preexposure prophylaxis for heterosexual HIV transmission in Botswana. N Engl J Med 2012;367(5):423–34.
[22] Donnell D, Baeten JM, Bumpus NN, et al. HIV protective efficacy and correlates of tenofovir blood concentrations in a clinical trial of PrEP for HIV prevention. J Acquir Immune Defic Syndr 2014;66(3):340–8.
[23] Grant RM, Anderson PL, McMahan V, et al. Uptake of pre-exposure prophylaxis, sexual practices, and HIV incidence in men and transgender women who have sex with men: a cohort study. Lancet Infect Dis 2014;14(9):820–9.
[24] Cottrell ML, Yang KH, Prince HM, et al. A translational pharmacology approach to predicting outcomes of preexposure prophylaxis against HIV in men and women using tenofovir disoproxil fumarate with or without emtricitabine. J Infect Dis 2016;214(1):55–64.
[25] Gilead Sciences Inc. Package labeling: TRUVADA® (emtricitabine/tenofovir disoproxil fumarate) tablets. 2018. Available at: https://www.accessdata.fda.gov/drugsatfda_docs/label/2018/021752s055lbl.pdf. Accessed November 6, 2018.
[26] Hosek SG, Rudy B, Landovitz R, et al. An HIV preexposure prophylaxis demonstration project and safety study for young MSM. J Acquir Immune Defic Syndr 2017;74(1):21–9.
[27] Hosek SG, Landovitz RJ, Kapogiannis B, et al. Safety and feasibility of antiretroviral preexposure prophylaxis for adolescent men who have sex with men aged 15 to 17 years in the United States. JAMA Pediatr 2017;171:1063–71.
[28] Centers for Disease Control and Prevention. Preexposure prophylaxis for the prevention of HIV infection in the United States—2017 Update: a clinical practice guideline. 2018. Available at: https://www.cdc.gov/hiv/pdf/risk/prep/cdc-hiv-prep-guidelines-2017.pdf. Accessed November 6, 2018.
[29] Yun K, Xu JJ, Zhang J, et al. Female and younger subjects have lower adherence in PrEP trials: a meta-analysis with implications for the uptake of PrEP service to prevent HIV. Sex Transm Infect 2018;94(3):163–8.
[30] Liu AY, Vittinghoff E, Sellmeyer DE, et al. Bone mineral density in HIV-negative men participating in a tenofovir pre-exposure prophylaxis randomized clinical trial in San Francisco. PLoS One 2011;6(8):e23688.
[31] Mulligan K, Glidden DV, Anderson PL, et al. Effects of emtricitabine/tenofovir on bone mineral density in HIV-negative persons in a randomized, double-blind, placebo-controlled trial. Clin Infect Dis 2015;61(4):572–80.
[32] Kasonde M, Niska RW, Rose C, et al. Bone mineral density changes among HIV-uninfected young adults in a randomised trial of pre-exposure prophylaxis with tenofovir-emtricitabine or placebo in Botswana. PLoS One 2014;9(3):e90111.

[33] Mirembe BG, Kelly CW, Mgodi N, et al. Bone mineral density changes among young, healthy African women receiving oral tenofovir for HIV preexposure prophylaxis. J Acquir Immune Defic Syndr 2016;71(3):287–94.
[34] Mullins TL, Zimet G, Lally M, et al. Adolescent human immunodeficiency virus care providers' attitudes toward the use of oral pre-exposure prophylaxis in youth. AIDS Patient Care STDS 2016;30(7):339–48.
[35] Havens PL, Stephensen CB, Van Loan MD, et al. Decline in bone mass with tenofovir disoproxil fumarate/emtricitabine is associated with hormonal changes in the absence of renal impairment when used by HIV-uninfected adolescent boys and young men for HIV preexposure prophylaxis. Clin Infect Dis 2017;64(3):317–25.
[36] Gandhi M, Glidden DV, Mayer K, et al. Association of age, baseline kidney function, and medication exposure with declines in creatinine clearance on pre-exposure prophylaxis: an observational cohort study. Lancet HIV 2016;3(11):e521–8.
[37] Mugwanya KK, Wyatt C, Celum C, et al. Reversibility of glomerular renal function decline in HIV-uninfected men and women discontinuing emtricitabine-tenofovir disoproxil fumarate pre-exposure prophylaxis. J Acquir Immune Defic Syndr 2016;71(4):374–80.
[38] Lehman DA, Baeten JM, McCoy CO, et al. Risk of drug resistance among persons acquiring HIV within a randomized clinical trial of single- or dual-agent preexposure prophylaxis. J Infect Dis 2015;211(8):1211–8.
[39] Liegler T, Abdel-Mohsen M, Bentley LG, et al. HIV-1 drug resistance in the iPrEx preexposure prophylaxis trial. J Infect Dis 2014;210(8):1217–27.
[40] Mugwanya KK, Baeten JM. Safety of oral tenofovir disoproxil fumarate-based pre-exposure prophylaxis for HIV prevention. Expert Opin Drug Saf 2016;15(2):265–73.
[41] Delaugerre C, Rodriguez C, Capitant C, et al. Drug resistance among patients who acquired HIV infection in a preexposure prophylaxis trial. AIDS 2018;32(16):2353–61.
[42] Sivay MV, Li M, Piwowar-Manning E, et al. Characterization of HIV seroconverters in a TDF/FTC PrEP study: HPTN 067/ADAPT. J Acquir Immune Defic Syndr 2017;75(3):271–9.
[43] Thaden JT, Gandhi M, Okochi H, et al. Seroconversion on preexposure prophylaxis: a case report with segmental hair analysis for timed adherence determination. AIDS 2018;32(9): F1–4.
[44] Donnell D, Ramos E, Celum C, et al. The effect of oral preexposure prophylaxis on the progression of HIV-1 seroconversion. AIDS 2017;31(14):2007–16.
[45] Grant RM, Liegler T, Defechereux P, et al. Drug resistance and plasma viral RNA level after ineffective use of oral pre-exposure prophylaxis in women. AIDS 2015;29(3):331–7.
[46] Strauss BB, Greene GJ, Phillips G, et al. Exploring patterns of awareness and use of HIV pre-exposure prophylaxis among young men who have sex with men. AIDS Behav 2017;21(5): 1288–98.
[47] Beymer MR, DeVost MA, Weiss RE, et al. Does HIV pre-exposure prophylaxis use lead to a higher incidence of sexually transmitted infections? A case-crossover study of men who have sex with men in Los Angeles, California. Sex Transm Infect 2018;94(6):457–62.
[48] Eaton LA, Kalichman SC, Price D, et al. Stigma and conspiracy beliefs related to pre-exposure prophylaxis (PrEP) and interest in using PrEP among black and white men and transgender women who have sex with men. AIDS Behav 2017;21(5):1236–46.
[49] Holloway IW, Tan D, Gildner JL, et al. Facilitators and barriers to pre-exposure prophylaxis willingness among young men who have sex with men who use geosocial networking applications in California. AIDS Patient Care STDS 2017;31(12):517–27.
[50] Kuhns LM, Reisner SL, Mimiaga MJ, et al. Correlates of PrEP indication in a multi-site cohort of young HIV-uninfected transgender women. AIDS Behav 2016;20(7):1470–7.
[51] Calabrese SK, Dovidio JF, Tekeste M, et al. HIV pre-exposure prophylaxis stigma as a multidimensional barrier to uptake among women who attend Planned Parenthood. J Acquir Immune Defic Syndr 2018;79(1):46–53.

[52] Peitzmeier SM, Tomko C, Wingo E, et al. Acceptability of microbicidal vaginal rings and oral pre-exposure prophylaxis for HIV prevention among female sex workers in a high-prevalence US city. AIDS Care 2017;29(11):1453–7.
[53] Bazzi AR, Biancarelli DL, Childs E, et al. Limited knowledge and mixed interest in pre-exposure prophylaxis for HIV prevention among people who inject drugs. AIDS Patient Care STDS 2018;32(12):529–37.
[54] Shrestha R, Karki P, Altice FL, et al. Correlates of willingness to initiate pre-exposure prophylaxis and anticipation of practicing safer drug- and sex-related behaviors among high-risk drug users on methadone treatment. Drug Alcohol Depend 2017;173:107–16.
[55] Farthing H, Rodriguez A, Armstrong M, et al. Discomfort discussing HIV/AIDS and lack of awareness are barriers to partner-to-partner pre-exposure prophylaxis education. Int J STD AIDS 2018;30(2):147–53.
[56] Wood SM, Lee S, Barg FK, et al. Young transgender women's attitudes toward HIV pre-exposure prophylaxis. J Adolesc Health 2017;60(5):549–55.
[57] Arrington-Sanders R, Morgan A, Oidtman J, et al. A medical care missed opportunity: pre-exposure prophylaxis and young black men who have sex with men. J Adolesc Health 2016;59(6):725–8.
[58] Shover CL, Javanbakht M, Shoptaw S, et al. HIV preexposure prophylaxis initiation at a large community clinic: differences between eligibility, awareness, and uptake. Am J Public Health 2018;108(10):1408–17.
[59] Huang YA, Zhu W, Smith DK, et al. HIV preexposure prophylaxis, by race and ethnicity - United States, 2014-2016. MMWR Morb Mortal Wkly Rep 2018;67(41): 1147–50.
[60] Hojilla JC, Vlahov D, Crouch PC, et al. HIV pre-exposure prophylaxis (PrEP) uptake and retention among men who have sex with men in a community-based sexual health clinic. AIDS Behav 2018;22(4):1096–9.
[61] Hubach RD, Currin JM, Sanders CA, et al. Barriers to access and adoption of pre-exposure prophylaxis for the prevention of HIV among men who have sex with men (MSM) in a relatively rural state. AIDS Educ Prev 2017;29(4):315–29.
[62] Dubov A, Galbo P Jr, Altice FL, et al. Stigma and shame experiences by MSM who take PrEP for HIV prevention: a qualitative study. Am J Mens Health 2018;12(6):1843–54.
[63] Doll M, Fortenberry JD, Roseland D, et al. Linking HIV-negative youth to prevention services in 12 U.S. cities: barriers and facilitators to implementing the HIV prevention continuum. J Adolesc Health 2018;62(4):424–33.
[64] Bacon O, Gonzalez R, Andrew E, et al. Brief report: informing strategies to build PrEP capacity among San Francisco Bay Area clinicians. J Acquir Immune Defic Syndr 2017;74(2):175–9.
[65] Petroll AE, Walsh JL, Owczarzak JL, et al. PrEP awareness, familiarity, comfort, and prescribing experience among US primary care providers and HIV specialists. AIDS Behav 2017;21(5):1256–67.
[66] Mullins TLK, Idoine CR, Zimet GD, et al. Primary care physician attitudes and intentions toward use of HIV pre-exposure prophylaxis in adolescents n one metropolitan region. J Adolesc Health 2019;64(5):581–8.
[67] Hart-Cooper GD, Allen I, Irwin CE Jr, et al. Adolescent health providers' willingness to prescribe pre-exposure prophylaxis (PrEP) to youth at risk of HIV infection in the United States. J Adolesc Health 2018;63(2):242–4.
[68] Centers for Disease Control and Prevention. Preexposure prophylaxis for the prevention of HIV infection in the United States - 2017: clinical providers' supplement. 2018. Available at: http://www.cdc.gov/hiv/pdf/PrEPProviderSupplement2017.pdf. Accessed November 6, 2018.
[69] Society for Adolescent Health and Medicine. HIV pre-exposure prophylaxis medication for adolescents and young adults: a position paper of the Society for Adolescent Health and Medicine. J Adolesc Health 2018;63(4):513–6.

[70] Committee on Gynecologic Practice. ACOG Committee Opinion no 595: preexposure prophylaxis for the prevention of human immunodeficiency virus. Obstet Gynecol 2014;123(5):1133–6.
[71] Gunthard HF, Saag MS, Benson CA, et al. Antiretroviral drugs for treatment and prevention of HIV infection in adults: 2016 Recommendations of the International Antiviral Society-USA Panel. JAMA 2016;316(2):191–210.
[72] Gilead Sciences Inc. How can you get help paying for TRUVADA for PrEP®?. 2018. Available at: https://www.truvada.com/how-to-get-truvada-for-prep/truvada-cost. Accessed November 26, 2018.
[73] PleasePrEPMe. PleasePrEPMe. 2018. Available at: www.pleaseprepme.org. Accessed February 6, 2018.
[74] Centers for Disease Control and Prevention. Paying for PrEP. 2015. Available at: https://www.cdc.gov/hiv/pdf/risk/prep/cdc-hiv-paying-for-prep.pdf. Accessed November 26, 2018.
[75] Guttmacher Institute. Minors' access to STI services. 2018. Available at: https://www.guttmacher.org/state-policy/explore/minors-access-sti-services. Accessed February 1, 2018.
[76] Centers for Disease Control and Prevention. Minors' consent laws for HIV and STI services. 2018. Available at: https://www.cdc.gov/hiv/policies/law/states/minors.html. Accessed November 26, 2018.
[77] Centers for Disease Control and Prevention. 2017 Youth risk behavior survey data. 2017. Available at: https://www.cdc.gov/yrbs. Accessed October 30, 2018.
[78] Centers for Disease Control and Prevention. HIV Infection Risk, Prevention, and Testing Behaviors Among Men Who Have Sex With Men National HIV Behavioral Surveillance 23 U.S. Cities, 2017. HIV Surveillance Report Special Report 22. 2019; Available online at: https://www.cdc.gov/hiv/pdf/library/reports/surveillance/cdc-hiv-surveillance-special-report-number-22.pdf. Accessed April 30, 2019.
[79] Centers for Disease Control and Prevention. HIV Infection, Risk, Prevention, and Testing Behaviors Among Heterosexuals at Increased Risk for HIV Infection National HIV Behavioral Surveillance 17 U.S. Cities, 2016. HIV Surveillance Report Special Report 19. https://www.cdc.gov/hiv/pdf/library/reports/surveillance/cdc-hiv-surveillance-report-number-19.pdf. Accessed April 30, 2019.
[80] Centers for Disease Control and Prevention. HIV infection, risk, prevention, and testing behaviors among persons who inject drugs – National HIV Behavioral Surveillance: injection drug use, 20 US Cities, 2015. HIV surveillance special report 18. 2018. Available at: http://www.cdc.gov/hiv/library/reports/hiv-surveillance.html. Accessed October 30, 2018.

Advances in Pediatrics 66 (2019) 263–280

ADVANCES IN PEDIATRICS

Clostridium difficile Infection in Children

Ana M. Alvarez, MD, FPIDS[a,b],
Mobeen H. Rathore, MD, CPE, FPIDS[a,b,*]

[a]Pediatric Infectious Diseases and Immunology, University of Florida Center for HIV/AIDS Research, Education and Service (UF CARES), 910 North Jefferson Street, Jacksonville, FL 32209, USA; [b]Wolfson Children's Hospital, 800 Prudential Drive, Jacksonville, FL 32207, USA

Keywords

• *Clostridium difficile* • Infection • Children • Antibiotics

Key points

- The incidence of *Clostridium difficile* infection (CDI) in children has increased remarkably in the past decade. Unlike cases in adults, most pediatric cases are community associated.
- Certain precautions when ordering CDI testing are recommended because of the inability of the currently available tests to differentiate disease from asymptomatic colonization.
- The management of CDI is complicated by an increasing incidence of severe disease and a high rate of recurrences.
- New therapies and strategies for the treatment and prevention of CDI seem promising, but more studies in children are needed.
- Strong infection prevention and control programs, including antibiotic stewardship, are essential to control *C difficile* transmission.

INTRODUCTION

Clostridium difficile infection (CDI) is the leading cause of health care–associated diarrhea in the United States [1], and it is one of the most common health care–associated infections, surpassing methicillin-resistant *Staphylococcus aureus* (MRSA) in some areas of the country [2]. Once thought of as only a

Disclosure: The authors have no relevant disclosures.

*Corresponding author. Pediatric Infectious Diseases and Immunology, University of Florida Center for HIV/AIDS Research, Education and Service (UF CARES), 910 North Jefferson Street, Jacksonville, FL 32209, USA. *E-mail address:* mobeen.rathore@jax.ufl.edu

https://doi.org/10.1016/j.yapd.2019.03.010

hospital-acquired infection mostly affecting adults, CDI has emerged as an important community-associated infection in adults and children over the last decade [3]. In 2013, the Centers for Disease Control and Prevention (CDC) categorized *C difficile* as one of 3 urgent threats among 18 drug-resistant threats in the United States, requiring urgent public health attention [4]. This article summarizes epidemiologic trends and updated recommendations for the diagnosis, treatment, and prevention of CDI in children. It also discusses emerging treatment and prevention strategies.

PATHOGENESIS

C difficile is an anaerobic, spore-forming, gram-positive bacillus. The spores are dormant in the environment, including health care facilities. They can also be found in low levels in the food supply [5]. They are resistant to acid, heat, antibiotics, and most disinfectants. The spores germinate after they reach the intestine, where *C difficile* can overgrow if there are alterations of the intestinal microbiota (intestinal dysbiosis). Not all strains of *C difficile* are pathogenic. In the intestine, the pathogenic strains are able to produce toxins A and B, which are responsible for the clinical manifestations by disrupting the cytoskeletal structure of the epithelial cells [6]. Toxin B is the most important virulent factor and it is more potent than toxin A in causing mucosal damage. Strains not producing toxin A can be as virulent as strains producing both toxins [7]. Infections outside the intestine are rare. Other factors affecting the pathogenesis include colonization with nontoxigenic strains, production of antibodies against toxins, and variable expression of toxin receptors in the intestine [5].

The transmission of *C difficile* spores can be the result of person-to-person spread through the fecal-oral route or direct exposure to contaminated surfaces, including hands. Transmission from asymptomatic carriers and health care personnel is well known [8]. The incubation period from colonization to infection has not been clearly established but it has been estimated to vary from 2 days to more than a week [2].

Risk factors

Several risk factors have been associated with CDI. However, antibiotic exposure is the most important for both community-associated and health care–associated CDI (HA-CDI) [8,9]. Disease usually occurs 5 to 10 days after starting antibiotics but has been described on the first day of treatment and up to 10 weeks after antibiotic cessation [10]. Certain antibiotic classes, such as cephalosporins, fluoroquinolones, and lincosamides, have been more frequently associated with CDI, but any antibiotic can be responsible for CDI. *C difficile* infection can also occur without antibiotic exposure [9]; antibiotic exposure was not identified as a risk factor in more than 40% of children with CDI [9]. Other identified risk factors in children include acid suppression medications (ie, proton pump inhibitors [PPIs] and histamine-2 receptor antagonists) [11] and gastrointestinal feeding devices [12].

Use of PPIs or narcotics, leukocytosis greater than 15×10^9/L, increased serum creatinine level greater than 1.5-fold from baseline, and older age have been identified as risk factors for severe disease in adults [13]. Risk factors for severe disease reported in children include exposure to multiple classes of antibiotics in the 30 days before infection [14] and the presence of a gastrostomy tube [15].

EPIDEMIOLOGY

Since 2002, there has been a remarkable increase in the rates of CDI, as well as in the severity of the illness. The increase in incidence rates has also been observed in children [16,17]. For example, CDI incidence increased from 2.6 to 32.6 per 100,000 population from 1991 through 2009 in children residing in Minnesota. Most of the cases were acquired in the community [8]. The overall CDI incidence increase has been attributed at least in part to the emergence of a hypervirulent strain of *C difficile* known as the North American pulse-field gel electrophoresis type 1 ribotype 027 (NAP1), identified in the mid-2000s [2]. However, in the pediatric population this NAP1 strain is only present in 10% to 20% of cases, which suggests that there are other factors driving the increased incidence and severity of CDI in children [14,18].

Another phenomenon observed in the mid-2000s was the increased incidence of CDI cases in the community, in people without the classic high-risk factors [19]. For surveillance purposes, CDI case definitions have been standardized as shown in Box 1 [2].

Based on CDC surveillance data from 2009 to 2011, out of 984 cases of community-associated CDI (CA-CDI), 82% were associated with exposure to ambulatory health care facilities and 36% were not exposed to antibiotics within 12 weeks of diagnosis. However, 31% of cases without antibiotic exposure had received PPIs [3].

In the largest active population-based surveillance of pediatric CDI in the United States, 71% were CA-CDI. There were no significant differences regarding demographics, exposures, and clinical characteristics among different age groups. However, the group with the highest burden was children 1 to 3 years old, suggesting true disease and not asymptomatic colonization in this group. Children less than 12 months of age were excluded [20].

Box 1: Epidemiologic definitions

Health care facility-onset CDI: cases occurring more than 3 days after admission to the facility (ie, on or after day 4 of hospitalization)

Community-onset, health care facility-associated CDI: cases occurring within 28 days after discharge from a health care facility (ie, postdischarge cases)

Community-associated CDI: cases occurring in patients with no inpatient stay in the previous 12 weeks.

Data from McDonald LC, Gerding DN, Johnson S, et al. Clinical practice guidelines for Clostridium difficile infection in adults and children: 2017 update by the Infectious Diseases Society of America (IDSA) and Society for Healthcare Epidemiology of America (SHEA). Clin Infect Dis 2018;66:e1–48.

A few studies have found differences among children with CA-CDI compared with children with HA-CDI, such as lower rates of exposure to antibiotics, immunosuppressants, acid suppressants, and narcotics [21,22], and fewer comorbid conditions, fewer prior surgical procedures, and a trend toward more complicated courses and a higher proportion of recurrences in children with CA-CDI [22].

In general, special populations at increased risk of CDI include patients with inflammatory bowel disease (IBD), patients with chronic renal disease, solid organ transplant recipients, and hematopoietic stem cell transplant (HSCT) recipients. In addition, these patients have higher CDI-associated morbidity and mortality as well as increased risk of recurrences [2]. In children in particular, the conditions associated with increased risk for CDI include cancer [23,24], transplant [25], IBD [26], cystic fibrosis [27], Hirschsprung disease (HD), and structural or postoperative intestinal disorders [28].

The incidence of CDI in children with cancer has been reported as more than 15 times greater than in children without cancer. Their increased susceptibility to CDI is caused by factors such as increased health care contact, immunosuppression caused by chemotherapy, and repeated and/or prolonged exposure to broad-spectrum antibiotics [24]. Variations in the risk of HA-CDI among different antipseudomonas β-lactam antibiotics has been reported in children with leukemia [29]. Specifically, cefepime and ceftazidime were independently associated with CDI. In the same study, the investigators found that even 1 additional day of exposure to antipseudomonas β-lactam antibiotics in the last 30 days increased the risk for CDI [29]. A prospective study of *C difficile* colonization in this population reported that approximately one-third of their pediatric oncology patients were colonized on admission, and more than half of their patients with history of CDI remained persistently or intermittently colonized during a follow-up period of up to 20 weeks after diagnosis and treatment. Many of their patients were colonized with different strains, which suggests either carrying multiple strains or acquisition of new strains. They also showed a high acquisition rate in newly diagnosed oncology patients [23]. The acquisition can occur during hospitalization or ambulatory visits, or in the community. These patients probably represent a large reservoir for HA-CDI [24].

Data on the risk of CDI in pediatric transplant recipients are lacking. However, based on data in the adult population, it is predicted that these patients have very high risk for CDI. Several risk factors for the development of CDI in adult transplant patients have been reported retrospectively. These risk factors include acute graft-versus-host disease, chemotherapy before conditioning for HSCT, broad-spectrum antibiotic use, colonization with vancomycin-resistant enterococci, cord blood as the source for stem cells, and total body irradiation of at least 12 Gy [25].

The prevalence of CDI in pediatric patients with IBD seems to vary significantly from one center to another, ranging from 3.5% to 69% [30]. These children do not seem to share the same risk factors for CDI as the general population or other pediatric subgroups. For example, antibiotic exposure does not seem to play a role. However, most experts believe that IBD plays an important role, in addition to the frequent use of immunosuppressive therapies and health care–based services [26]. In a recent prospective, multicenter study of the occurrence and course of CDI among 211 European children with IBD, the investigators found an overall 1-year occurrence of 11.5%, and an asymptomatic colonization rate of 28.5%. CDI was associated with a more severe IBD course (ie, more active disease, higher number of hospitalizations, and more intensification of immunosuppressive or biologic therapy). Antibiotics, immunosuppressive therapy, and PPIs were not predisposing factors [26].

Children with HD are particularly susceptible to CDI because of colonic stasis and altered intestinal microbiota. The role of CDI in Hirschsprung-associated enterocolitis (HAEC), a condition that frequently complicates the HD course, has been investigated with conflicting conclusions. Many investigators have found high rates of *C difficile* isolation in patients with HD and HAEC. In addition, severe pseudomembranous colitis in patients with HD has been reported with and without *C difficile* isolation. However, a causal association has not been established, partly because of the high rate of asymptomatic colonization in young children [28].

CLINICAL PRESENTATION

The clinical spectrum of CDI is wide, from asymptomatic colonization to severe, sometimes fatal disease.

Colonization

Colonization with *C difficile* seems to occur soon after birth. However, the reported colonization rates in neonates have a wide variation from 2.5% to 90%. It seems to be more common in premature babies than in full-term babies. These rates increase with age to peak at 1 year [31], probably because of low resistance to colonization caused by immature intestinal flora. Formula-fed infants have higher colonization rates of *C difficile* than breast-fed infants [32]. Disease can occur in this age group, but it is rare, possibly because of the lack of intestinal toxin receptors in infants [31].

Colonization is transient and can be caused by different strains in the same patient [2]. After the first year of life, colonization rates decrease with increasing age and in children more than 2 years of age the rates are similar to adults' rates (1%–3%) [32]. However, rates of colonization in hospitalized children seem to be higher, with one center reporting colonization in up to 24% using polymerase chain reaction among pediatric patients aged 1 to 18 years. The prevalence did not vary markedly with age [33]. Pediatric oncology patients in particular seem to have higher rates of colonization, up to 33% [23].

Disease

By far, the most common clinical manifestations of *C difficile* involve the gastrointestinal tract. However, extracolonic manifestations have been reported.

Gastrointestinal manifestations: an acute diarrheal illness is the classic presentation, which can be mild to severe. The clinical features include profuse watery diarrhea with more than 6 stools per day, fever, and abdominal cramping or pain. Vomiting is not common but can present in one-third of the patients. Approximately one-quarter of the patients have bloody stools, but grossly bloody stools are seen in less than 15% of patients [21]. Children with severe CDI can present with severe abdominal pain and distension, hemodynamic instability, hypoalbuminemia, increased age-adjusted creatinine level, leukocytosis, and lactic acidosis. Some of these patients do not present with diarrhea because of prolonged paralytic ileus [10,21].

Complications associated with CDI include pseudomembranous colitis, pneumatosis intestinalis, toxic megacolon, intussusception, rectal prolapse, gastrointestinal perforation, sepsis, and death. In population-based studies, 8% to 9% of children with CDI experienced severe disease, and 0.7% to 3% had CDI-associated complications [14,21]. However, these numbers were higher in a cohort of hospitalized children with CDI, with 59% of them having severe disease and 17% to 31% having CDI-associated complications, depending on the definition used [34].

Extracolonic manifestations include bacteremia, skin and soft tissue infections, osteomyelitis, and reactive arthritis [35]. These manifestations are rare, especially in children.

A recurrent CDI case is defined as an episode of symptom onset and positive assay result following an episode with positive assay result in the previous 2 to 8 weeks for epidemiologic purposes [2]. Recurrences typically occur 1 to 3 weeks after the initial episode. The recurrence rates are similar in children and adults (20%–30%). A few studies have identified certain risk factors predisposing children to have recurrent CDI: malignancy, antibiotic exposure, recent surgery, presence of tracheostomy tube, receipt of concomitant antibiotics during the first episode, and CA-CDI [36–38]. The risk of further recurrences increases with each successive recurrence [2]. In addition, the mortality risk is 33% higher in patients with recurrent CDI compared with those without recurrence [39].

DIAGNOSIS

Challenges in the diagnosis of CDI in children are underscored by the difficulty in distinguishing colonization from symptomatic infection. Available laboratory tests, including molecular assays, do not help to make that distinction, which highlights the importance of a thorough clinical evaluation, including looking for other causes of diarrhea and careful assessment of response to therapy. However, validated clinical criteria are lacking.

Testing all children with diarrhea for CDI may lead to misdiagnosis and inappropriate and unnecessary treatment, therefore it is not recommended [40,41]. Indications for testing should incorporate factors such as clinical presentation, age, exposure to antibiotics or gastric acid suppressants, and the predisposing conditions described earlier (eg, having a gastrointestinal feeding device, malignancy, transplantation, IBD).

Based on clinical presentation, CDI testing is indicated for patients with new-onset diarrhea (3 or more unformed stools in 24 hours) with no other clearly attributable cause (eg, IBD exacerbation, laxatives, intensive chemotherapy, enteral tube feeding) [2,10]. In particular, diarrheal illnesses are frequent and more commonly caused by viral agents in children. It is difficult to distinguish CDI from the other viral causes of diarrhea in children. However, symptoms like fever, nausea, and vomiting are more prominent with viral infections than with CDI.

Recommended restrictions/precautions when ordering CDI testing in children include [2,10]:

- Discourage testing infants less than 12 months of age
- In toddlers 1 to 2 years of age with diarrhea, limit testing to those in whom other infectious or noninfectious causes of diarrhea have been excluded
- In children 3 years of age or older, limit testing to those with prolonged or worsening diarrhea who also have relevant exposures (eg, antibiotic exposure, health care system contact) and/or CDI risk factors

The diagnosis of CDI is most commonly based on laboratory methods to detect *C difficile* toxins or toxin gene s in stools of patients with diarrhea. Unless ileus or toxic megacolon is suspected, laboratory tests for *C difficile* should not be ordered on formed stools. In many institutions the laboratory rejects stool samples that are not liquid or soft (ie, take the shape of the container). This measure can improve the specificity of the tests [2].

Available diagnostic tests include nucleic acid amplification tests (NAATs) to detect genes responsible for the production of toxins A and B, enzyme immunoassay (EIA) to detect free toxins A and B, enzyme immunoassay for glutamate dehydrogenase, toxigenic culture, and the cell culture cytotoxic assay to detect the toxins. These last 2 tests are rarely used for routine testing because they require technical expertise and are labor intensive [2].

The Infectious Diseases Society of America (IDSA) and the Society for Healthcare Epidemiology of America (SHEA) have recently published clinical practice guidelines for CDI [2]. With regard to the most appropriate tests for CDI, they recommend the use of tests that are more specific, such as EIA toxin assays as part of a multitest algorithm rather than NAAT alone for institutions with no clinical data who accept all unformed samples for testing. In contrast, they recommend NAAT alone or a multitest algorithm for institutions that have preagreed criteria for accepting the samples [2].

Tests of cure are not recommended because greater than 60% of patients remain positive even after successful treatment and shedding of *C difficile* in the stools can persist for several months [2,10].

TREATMENT AND PREVENTION

The first consideration when deciding the management of patients with CDI should be the discontinuation of ongoing antibiotic therapy as soon as possible. The continuation of such therapy is associated with suboptimal clinical response and increased risk of recurrence [38,42]. If antibiotics for a concomitant infection need to be continued, it is advisable to use antibiotics with the narrowest spectrum possible for that infection. Consideration to shorten the duration of antibiotic therapy is also recommended [2].

The use of antimotility drugs (eg, loperamide) has been associated with poor outcomes, and it is generally discouraged [10]. However, it might be safe to use them once specific antibiotic treatment of CDI has been started [2].

Empiric therapy for CDI should be started when the results of testing will be delayed for more than 48 hours and/or when patients show signs of severe or fulminant infection. Otherwise, it is recommended to wait for positive laboratory results before starting treatment [2].

Asymptomatic colonization should not be treated [2,10].

The first-line antibiotics for CDI include vancomycin and metronidazole. Vancomycin, administered orally, is the only US Food and Drug Administration (FDA)–approved agent for the treatment of CDI in children. Because it is not absorbed through the gastrointestinal tract, it achieves high fecal concentrations without the risk of adverse effects with systemic administration. The oral formulation is expensive; however, the intravenous (IV) formulation of vancomycin is less expensive and it can used for oral administration. Vancomycin administered intravenously is not effective for CDI because it does not reach the gastrointestinal tract [10]. The use of oral vancomycin is fraught with concerns about perturbation of the intestinal microbiota and risk of increasing intestinal colonization with vancomycin-resistant enterococci. However, this has been shown to occur with metronidazole as well [43].

Metronidazole, administered orally, is absorbed quickly. It is then excreted through the biliary system and secreted across inflamed intestinal mucosa, achieving high fecal levels. Those levels decline as the mucosal inflammation decreases. Because of systemic absorption, side effects are more common and include nausea, vomiting, abdominal cramps, and metallic taste. Serious complications, such as peripheral neuropathy and encephalopathy, are less common. These complications seem to occur more often in adults, but pediatric cases have been reported [44,45].

Rifaximin is a rifamycin derivative approved for treatment of travelers' diarrhea in individuals 12 years of age or older. Because it is minimally absorbed, well tolerated, and active against *C difficile*, its role for treatment of CDI has been investigated with promising results. In a small, prospective, single-blind, single-center study comparing the efficacy and recurrence rate of metronidazole with rifaximin in children between 12 and 18 years of age with IBD and mild to moderate CDI, the investigators found no significant difference between the two regimens. This finding suggests that rifaximin could be a good choice for these patients, especially if they do not tolerate metronidazole [46]. Other studies of rifaximin for treatment of recurrent CDI have shown a modest decrease in the rate of recurrent diarrhea when used immediately after a standard anti-CDI course [47,48]. The major concern with its use is the issue of resistance: the rate of resistance among *C difficile* isolates [49] and the risk of inducing resistance to all rifamycins among intestinal flora [50].

Nitazoxanide is an antiparasitic agent with good activity against anaerobic bacteria, including *C difficile* [51]. A few small studies have shown nitazoxanide's efficacy to be comparable with vancomycin and metronidazole in the treatment of CDI [52], and a good response to it in patients who failed treatment with metronidazole [53].

Fidaxomicin has not been FDA approved for use in children with CDI. In spite of this, 16% of pediatric infectious diseases specialists who responded to a survey about their practices related to CDI reported using it for severe or recurrent CDI [54]. In a phase 2a open-label study in children with CDI, fidaxomicin for 10 days had promising results, with good tolerability and excellent clinical response rate (92%). However, the recurrence rate was higher than in some adult studies (31.4% vs 12.7%–15.4%) [55]. Phase 3 clinical trials in children are ongoing.

There is limited information available about the antibiotic susceptibility of *C difficile* isolates obtained from children. A single-center study found that most of the pediatric isolates were susceptible to first-line and second-line antibiotics (100% susceptible to vancomycin and metronidazole and 98% susceptible to rifaximin), and had favorable minimum inhibitory concentrations to fidaxomicin. This susceptibility pattern did not differ between the initial and subsequent isolates from children with recurrent CDI [55]. Adult populations tend to have more resistant strains [49,56,57].

The definitive treatment of CDI depends on the age of the patient; whether it is the first episode, first recurrence, or subsequent recurrences; and the severity of the illness.

For example, in adults, there is substantial evidence that vancomycin is superior to metronidazole for CDI. In contrast, fidaxomicin seems to be better than vancomycin [58]. This superiority has been proved particularly in patients in whom concomitant antibiotics for other infections cannot be discontinued [42]. Therefore, for adults with a first or recurrent episode of CDI, either vancomycin or fidaxomicin is recommended rather than metronidazole. Metronidazole is only considered acceptable for an initial CDI episode if it is nonsevere and if the access to vancomycin or fidaxomicin is limited [2].

In children, comparative data for different regimens are lacking. There are limited data suggestive of inferiority of metronidazole compared with vancomycin with regard to failure rates [34]. Metronidazole seems to work well for the first episode of CDI in children, and it is the preferred regimen of most pediatric infectious diseases specialists in North America for a mild first episode of CDI in children without comorbidities [54]. In addition, because complications and mortality in children with CDI are rare, it is difficult to compare the outcomes with different regimens. The new clinical practice guidelines from IDSA and SHEA recommend either metronidazole or vancomycin for the initial or first recurrent CDI episode in children, as long as it is nonsevere. For a severe first episode and for second or greater recurrence, vancomycin should be used [2]. Metronidazole should not be used for subsequent recurrences because of the risk for neurotoxicity [10,44]. The best treatment of children with second or greater episodes of recurrent CDI has not been studied well. Recommendations are extrapolated from limited data in adults [59], and include the use of tapered or pulse regimens of vancomycin alone or followed by rifaximin or nitazoxanide [10]. Table 1 provides a summary of the treatment recommendations for the first episode of CDI and Table 2 shows recommended regimens for recurrent CDI in children.

Newer antibiotics being developed to treat *C difficile* include surotomycin (a lipopeptide), cadazolid (a novel oxazolidinone-fluoroquinolone hybrid), and ridinilazole (a novel, narrow-spectrum, nonabsorbable antibiotic) [60].

The approach of using vancomycin or metronidazole for primary or secondary prophylaxis has gained attention in recent years and has been tried anecdotally. Literature on this is limited to a few retrospective studies using vancomycin in high-risk adults, showing promising results [61–63], and 1 prospective study using metronidazole [64]. The ideal dose and duration have not been determined, and there are no data in children. At this time, there are not sufficient robust data to support this approach.

Given the limitations of standard antibiotic therapy against recurrent CDI, and based on the understanding of the role of intestinal dysbiosis in the pathogenesis of CDI, several biotherapeutic approaches have been developed for

Table 1
Recommended regimens for the treatment of first episode of *Clostridium difficile* infection in children

Severity	Antimicrobial agent	Dose and duration
Mild to moderate	Metronidazole[a] Or	30 mg/kg/d PO every 6 h (preferred) Or IV every 6 h for 10 d (maximum 500 mg/dose)
	Vancomycin	40 mg/kg/d, PO, every 6 h for 10 d (maximum 125 mg/dose)
Severe[b]	Vancomycin	40 mg/kg/d, PO, every 6 h for 10 d (maximum 125 mg/dose)
Severe and complicated[c]	Vancomycin[d] Plus metronidazole	Same doses as above for 10 d

Abbreviation: PO, by mouth.

[a]Consider switching to vancomycin if failure to respond in 5 to 7 days [10].

[b]Severe: should be considered in the presence of severe abdominal pain and distension, hemodynamic instability, hypoalbuminemia, worsening renal function, leukocytosis, and lactic acidosis [10,14,21].

[c]Complicated: intensive care unit admission, hypotension or shock, pseudomembranous colitis, pneumatosis intestinalis, toxic megacolon, intussusception, rectal prolapse, gastrointestinal perforation, surgical intervention because of CDI and/or sepsis [10,14,21].

[d]If complicated with ileus or toxic colitis and/or significant abdominal distension, add vancomycin, 500 mg/100 mL normal saline enema, as needed every 8 hours until improvement [10].

Adapted from McDonald LC, Gerding DN, Johnson S, et al. Clinical practice guidelines for Clostridium difficile infection in adults and children: 2017 update by the Infectious Diseases Society of America (IDSA) and Society for Healthcare Epidemiology of America (SHEA). Clin Infect Dis 2018; 66:e1–48; and American Academy of Pediatrics. Clostridium difficile. In: Kimberlin DW, Brady MT, Jackson MA, Long SS, eds. Red Book: 2018 Report of the Committee on Infectious Diseases. American Academy of Pediatrics; 2018;288–92.

Table 2
Recommended regimens for the treatment of recurrent *Clostridium difficile* infection in children

For first recurrent episode of CDI		
Severity	**Antimicrobial agent**	**Dose and duration**
Mild to moderate	Metronidazole Or	30 mg/kg/d PO every 6 h (preferred), OR IV every 6 h for 10 d (maximum 500 mg/dose)
	Vancomycin	40 mg/kg/d, PO, every 6 h for 10 d (maximum 125 mg/dose)
Severe	Vancomycin	40 mg/kg/d, PO, every 6 h for 10 d (maximum 125 mg/dose)
For second or greater episode of recurrent CDI		
Initial dose of vancomycin	**Tapered dose of vancomycin**	**Additional agent**
10 mg/kg/dose (maximum 125 mg) PO 4 times a day for 7 d	Then same dose, 3 times a day for 7 d Then twice a day for 7 d Then once a day for 7 d Then once every other day for 7 d Then every 72 h for 7 d	None
10 mg/kg/dose (max. 125 mg) PO 4 times a day for 14 d	Then same dose, twice a day for 7–14 d Then once daily for 7–14 d Then every 2–3 d for 2–8 wk	None
10 mg/kg/dose (max. 125 mg) PO 4 times a day for 14 d	None	Then rifaximin[a] PO 400 mg 3 times a day for 14 d Or Nitazoxanide PO twice a day for 10 d: 100 mg: 1–3 y of age 200 mg: 4–11 y of age 500 mg: ≥12 y of age

[a]Rifaximin is not FDA approved in children less than 12 years of age, but it is poorly water soluble and minimally absorbed. It should be avoided if the patient recently has received rifaximin for CDI or another indication [2,10].

Adapted from McDonald LC, Gerding DN, Johnson S, et al. Clinical practice guidelines for Clostridium difficile infection in adults and children: 2017 update by the Infectious Diseases Society of America (IDSA) and Society for Healthcare Epidemiology of America (SHEA). Clin Infect Dis 2018; 66:e1–48; and American Academy of Pediatrics. Clostridium difficile. In: Kimberlin DW, Brady MT, Jackson MA, Long SS, eds. Red Book: 2018 Report of the Committee on Infectious Diseases. American Academy of Pediatrics; 2018;288–92.

the treatment and prevention of CDI. Clinical trials are ongoing for some of them and some are being used for salvage therapy with varying degrees of success. They include fecal microbiota transplant (FMT), oral administration of nontoxigenic *C difficile* spores, and probiotics [65].

FMT consists of the administration of fecal content from a healthy donor into the gastrointestinal tract of a patient with CDI, with the goal of providing a preformed healthy balanced intestinal flora to patients with recurrent CDI in order to achieve a cure [66]. Beneficial effects include restoration of the recipient's gastrointestinal microbiota, which then inhibits *C difficile* colonization, and eliciting an immunologic response that facilitates the eradication of *C difficile* [67]. It has proved to be effective in adults with recurrent CDI with high success rates. In a systematic review, the rate of resolution of symptoms without recurrences was 75% in 2 randomized controlled trials (RCTs), and 85% in 21 case-series studies [68]. The routes of delivery include nasoenteric tubes, colonoscopy, enemas, and oral capsules with concentrated fecal microbes. However, it has not been shown that the route affects the efficacy of FMT. Adverse events are uncommon, and include gastrointestinal symptoms (eg, nausea, vomiting, flatulence, bloating, abdominal and/or rectal discomfort), headaches, and transient fever [67–69]. There are no published RCTs in children and the experience, although limited, is increasing.

A recent review summarizes the current pediatric data on FMT [69]. As of 2017, the investigators had found 45 reported cases of the use of FMT in children aged 1.1 to 19 years with recurrent CDI. After the intervention, there was symptomatic improvement in 89% of the children. There was a relapse in only 4% of the children. However, the follow-up period varied from 2 months to 4 years. Of note, 29% of these children had IBD. No serious adverse events (SAEs) or infectious complications were reported, and mild adverse events (eg, transient abdominal pain and mucoid stools) related to FMT occurred in 6% [69]. One of the concerns with FMT is the risk for acquired infections, especially when used in immunocompromised hosts. In a multicenter retrospective review of FMT in immunocompromised patients (75 adults and 5 children), the investigators found a cure rate of 78% (62 out of 80) after a single FMT, and an overall cure (defined as resolution of CDI after 1 or more FMTs) of 89%. After a follow-up period of 12 weeks, they found no infections related to the procedure. However, 15% of the patients experienced SAEs that included 10 hospitalizations and 2 deaths (1 was related to aspiration during the sedation for the FMT, the second death was unrelated) [70]. Adequate screening of donors minimizes infectious complications.

Even with limited pediatric data, 23 of 125 (18%) pediatric infectious diseases specialists who reported using alternative therapies for recurrent or severe CDI would recommend using FMT, especially for the third or later recurrence [54]. Perceived advantages of FMT include less risk of drug allergy; fewer exposures to antibiotics, which decreases development of antimicrobial resistance; higher cure rates in adults; and potential lower cost (considering avoiding multiple course of antibiotics and hospitalizations for recurrences) [65,66]. Based on evidence from studies done in the adult population and limited pediatric data, it seems reasonable to consider FMT for children with multiple recurrences, following standard treatment courses [2]. Potential benefits should be weighed against known and theoretic risks.

Nontoxigenic *C difficile* (NTCD) therapy focuses on the ability of this strain to outcompete and replace the toxigenic strain. A phase 2 randomized, double-blind, placebo-controlled trial showed significant difference in CDI recurrence rate compared with the placebo group (11% vs 30%; $P = .006$). Reduced recurrence rate correlated with NTCD colonization. However, colonization was transient (100% of patients lost colonization by 22 weeks) [65,71].

The efficacy and safety of probiotics in the prevention of CDI in adults and children undergoing antibiotic therapy have been studied in randomized trials. Based on a recent systematic review, the evidence suggests with moderate certainty that probiotics are effective in reducing the risk of CDI in these patients. The calculated reduction was 60% and the results were similar in adults and in children, inpatients and outpatients, and with different products and doses. However, the reduction was significantly higher (70%) in patients at higher risk for CDI. In the same review, probiotics also seemed to be safe [72].

Immunologic therapies for CDI include passive infusion of antibodies and active immunization. Serum antitoxin antibody levels are higher in patients with asymptomatic *C difficile* colonization than in patients with CDI, suggesting a protective effect [65]. The potential benefits of IV immunoglobulin have led to anecdotal use and retrospective evaluation, showing promising results. However, controlled clinical trials have not been done. In contrast, monoclonal antibodies against toxin A (actoxumab, Merck & Co., Inc) and toxin B (bezlotoxumab [Zinplava], Merck & Co., Inc.) have been developed and studied in clinical trials. In 2 phase III RCTs, patients receiving bezlotoxumab alone or combined with actoxumab had lower CDI recurrences than placebo (15.7% and 14.9% vs 25.7%, respectively; $P = .0003$). Actoxumab alone did not decrease the recurrence rate compared with placebo. The combination of both monoclonal antibodies did not offer an advantage compared with bezlotoxumab alone, suggesting that antibodies against toxin B could play a more important role in the prevention of recurrences [65,73]. Bezlotoxumab was FDA approved in October 2016 for the prevention of recurrent CDI in patients 18 years of age or older.

Vaccines targeted against *C difficile* toxins have the potential to provide longer-term protection compared with the monoclonal antibodies, and 3 candidate vaccines, targeting both toxins, have been developed and are undergoing RCTs. In phase II trials, all of them showed high immunogenicity and satisfactory safety. The Sanofi Pasteur toxoid vaccine is currently undergoing a phase III trial [60].

INFECTION PREVENTION AND CONTROL

Prevention of transmission of *C difficile* is challenging because the spores are resistant to commonly used alcohol-based hand sanitizers and cleaning agents, they can persist on environmental surfaces for months, and they can be transmitted from person to person through direct contact, via contaminated environmental surfaces and through the contaminated hands of other people, including health care personnel. Guidelines for infection prevention and control were published recently within the clinical practice guidelines from IDSA and SHEA [2] and are summarized as follows:

1. Whenever possible, patients with suspected or confirmed CDI should be isolated in a private room. If this is not possible, patients infected or colonized with the same organisms (eg, MRSA, VRE) can be cohorted.
2. Health care personnel must wear gloves and gowns on entry to a room of a patient with CDI, and while caring for that patient.
3. Health care personnel should perform hand hygiene before and after contact with a patient with CDI, and after removal of gloves. Soap and water or alcohol-based product can be used in routine or endemic settings. However, soap and water is preferred in outbreaks or hyperendemic settings, because it is more efficacious in removing spores from the hands.
4. Use disposable patient equipment when possible. When reusable equipment is used, it should be cleaned and disinfected thoroughly. A sporicidal agent (eg, hypochlorite) is preferred.
5. Consider terminal room cleaning or daily cleaning with a sporicidal agent in hyperendemic or outbreaks settings, or when there are repeated CDI cases in the same room. There is not consistent evidence that this measure reduces CDI in nonoutbreak situations.
6. Quality of environmental cleaning should be monitored.

Another important aspect of infection prevention and control for CDI is the reduction of patients' susceptibility to CDI. Because antibiotic exposure is the most important risk factor for HA-CDI, avoiding or minimizing this exposure is essential. To this end, it is recommended to minimize the frequency and duration of high-risk antibiotics (eg, fluoroquinolones, clindamycin and cephalosporins) to reduce the risk for CDI and to implement of an antibiotic stewardship program [2]. The effect of antibiotic stewardship programs (ASPs) on the incidence of CDI and infections with antibiotic-resistant bacteria was analyzed in a systematic review. The investigators found that ASPs reduced the incidence of CDI by 32% [74].

Infection prevention and control efforts should include not only hospital settings but also outpatient settings, especially in patient populations at increased risk of CDI because of the shift of care of these patients to ambulatory settings.

SUMMARY

It is important for pediatricians to recognize the increasing incidence of CDI in children, not only in the health care settings but also in the community. There are many risk factors for CDI in children, but the exposure to antibiotics is still the most important risk factor. The challenges clinicians face include a 20% to 30% rate of recurrent CDI and the occurrence of rare but severe and complicated disease. Standard therapies are not always effective. New treatment and prevention strategies are promising, but more studies involving children are urgently needed. The role of infection prevention and control, as well as antibiotic stewardship, is of utmost importance.

References

[1] Lessa FC, Mu Y, Bamberg WM, et al. Burden of *Clostridium difficile* infection in the United States. N Engl J Med 2015;372:825–34.
[2] McDonald LC, Gerding DN, Johnson S, et al. Clinical practice guidelines for *Clostridium difficile* infection in adults and children: 2017 update by the Infectious Diseases Society of America (IDSA) and Society for Healthcare Epidemiology of America (SHEA). Clin Infect Dis 2018;66:e1–48.
[3] Chitnis AS, Holzbauer SM, Belflower RM, et al. Epidemiology of community-associated *Clostridium difficile* infection, 2009 through 2011. JAMA Intern Med 2013;173:1359–67.
[4] Centers for Disease Control and Prevention. Antibiotic resistance threats in the United States Report 2013. Available at: https://www.cdc.gov/drugresistance/threat-report-2013/pdf/ar-threats-2013-508.pdf. Accessed August 10, 2018.
[5] Leffler DA, Lamont JT. *Clostridium difficile* infection. N Engl J Med 2015;372:1539–48.
[6] Voth DE, Ballard JD. *Clostridium difficile* toxins: mechanism of action and role in disease. Clin Microbiol Rev 2005;18:247–63.
[7] Lyras D, O'Connor JR, Howarth PM, et al. Toxin B is essential for virulence of *Clostridium difficile*. Nature 2009;458:1176–9.
[8] Caroff DA, Yokoe DS, Klompas M. Evolving insights into the epidemiology and control of *Clostridium difficile* in hospitals. Clin Infect Dis 2017;65:1232–8.
[9] Adams DJ, Eberly MD, Rajnik M, et al. Risk factors for community-associated *Clostridium difficile* infection in children. J Pediatr 2017;186:105–9.
[10] American Academy of Pediatrics. Clostridium difficile. In: Kimberlin DW, Brady MT, Jackson MA, et al, editors. Red book: 2018 Report of the Committee on Infectious Diseases. 31st edition. Itaska (IL): American Academy of Pediatrics; 2018. p. 288–92.
[11] Nylund CM, Eide M, Gorman GH. Association of *Clostridium difficile* infections with acid suppression medications in children. J Pediatr 2014;165:979–84.
[12] Sandora TJ, Fung M, Flaherty K, et al. Epidemiology and risk factors for *Clostridium difficile* infection in children. Pediatr Infect Dis J 2011;30:580–4.
[13] Shivashankar R, Khanna S, Kammer PP, et al. Clinical factors associated with development of severe *Clostridium difficile* infection. Clin Gastroenterol Hepatol 2013;11:1466–71.
[14] Kim J, Shaklee JF, Smathers S, et al. Risk factors and outcomes associated with severe *Clostridium difficile* infection in children. Pediatr Infect Dis J 2012;31:134–8.
[15] Kuiper G, van Prehn J, Ang W, et al. *Clostridium difficile* infections in young infants: case presentations and literature review. IDCases 2017;10:7–11.
[16] Nylund CM, Goudie A, Garza JM, et al. *Clostridium difficile* infection in hospitalized children in the United States. Arch Pediatr Adolesc Med 2011;165:451–7.
[17] Zilberberg MD, Tillotson GS, McDonald C. *Clostridium difficile* infections among hospitalized children, United States, 1997-2006. Emerg Infect Dis 2010;16:604–9.
[18] Toltzis P, Kim J, Dul M, et al. Presence of the epidemic North American pulsed field type 1 *Clostridium difficile* strain in hospitalized children. J Pediatr 2009;154:607–8.
[19] Centers for Disease Control and Prevention. Severe *Clostridium difficile*-associated disease in populations previously at low risk – four states, 2005. MMWR Morb Mortal Wkly Rep 2005;54:1201–5.
[20] Wendt JM, Cohen JA, Mu Y, et al. *Clostridium difficile* infection among children across diverse US geographic locations. Pediatrics 2014;133:651–8.
[21] Crews JD, Koo HL, Jiang ZD, et al. A hospital-based study of the clinical characteristics of *Clostridium difficile* infection in children. Pediatr Infect Dis J 2014;33:924–8.
[22] Tschudin-Sutter S, Tamma PD, Naegeli AN, et al. Distinguishing community-associated from hospital-associated *Clostridium difficile* infections in children: implications for public health surveillance. Clin Infect Dis 2013;57:1665–72.
[23] Dominguez SR, Dolan SA, West K, et al. High colonization rate and prolonged shedding of *Clostridium difficile* in pediatric oncology patients. Clin Infect Dis 2014;59:401–3.

[24] Kim J. *Clostridium difficile* in pediatric oncology patients: more questions than answers. Clin Infect Dis 2014;59:404–5.
[25] Nicholson MR, Osggod CL, Acra SA, et al. *Clostridium difficile* infection in the pediatric transplant patient. Pediatr Transplant 2015;19:792–8.
[26] Martinelli M, Strisciuglio C, Veres G, et al. *Clostridium difficile* and pediatric inflammatory disease: a prospective, comparative, multicenter, ESPGHAN study. Inflamm Bowel Dis 2014;20:2219–25.
[27] Theunissen C, Knoop C, Nonhoff C, et al. *Clostridium difficile* colitis in cystic fibrosis patients with and without lung transplantation. Transpl Infect Dis 2008;10:240–4.
[28] McLaughlin D, Friedmacher F, Puri P. The impact of *Clostridium difficile* on paediatric surgical practice: a systematic review. Pediatr Surg Int 2014;30:853–9.
[29] Fisher BT, Sammons JS, Li Y, et al. Variation in risk of hospital-onset *Clostridium difficile* infection across beta-lactam antibiotics in children with new-onset acute lymphoblastic leukemia. J Pediatric Infect Dis Soc 2014;2:329–35.
[30] Pant C, Anderson MP, Deshpande A, et al. Health care burden of *Clostridium difficile* infection in hospitalized children with inflammatory bowel disease. Inflamm Bowel Dis 2013;19: 1080–5.
[31] Enoch DA, Butler MJ, Pai S, et al. *Clostridium difficile* in children: colonization and disease. J Infect 2011;63:105–13.
[32] Tamma PD, Sandora TJ. *Clostridium difficile* infection in children: current state and unanswered questions. J Pediatric Infect Dis Soc 2012;1:230–43.
[33] Leibowitz J, Soma VL, Rosen L, et al. Similar proportions of stool specimens from hospitalized children with and without diarrhea test positive for *Clostridium difficile*. Pediatr Infect Dis J 2015;34:261–6.
[34] Khana S, Baddour LM, Huskins WC, et al. The epidemiology of *Clostridium difficile* infection in children: a population-based study. Clin Infect Dis 2013;56:1401–6.
[35] Horton DB, Strom BL, Putt ME, et al. Epidemiology of *Clostridium difficile* infection-associated reactive arthritis in children: an underdiagnosed, potentially morbid condition. JAMA Pediatr 2016;170:e160217.
[36] Nicholson MR, Thomsen IP, Slaughter JC, et al. Novel risk factors for recurrent *Clostridium difficile* infection in children. J Pediatr Gastroenterol Nutr 2015;60:18–22.
[37] Kociolek LK, Palac HL, Patel SJ, et al. Risk factors for recurrent *Clostridium difficile* infection in children: a nested case-control study. J Pediatr 2015;167:384–9.
[38] Tschudin-Sutter S, Tamma PD, Milstone AM, et al. Predictors of first recurrence of *Clostridium difficile* infections in children. Pediatr Infect Dis J 2014;33:414–6.
[39] Olsen MA, Yan Y, Reske KA, et al. Recurrent *Clostridium difficile* infection is associated with increased mortality. Clin Microbiol Infect 2015;21:164–70.
[40] Kociolek LK, Patel SJ, Zheng X, et al. Clinical and microbiologic assessment of cases of pediatric community-associated *Clostridium difficile* infection reveals opportunities for improved testing decisions. Pediatr Infect Dis J 2016;35:157–61.
[41] Kociolek LK, Bovee M, Carter D, et al. Impact of a healthcare provider educational intervention on frequency of *Clostridium difficile* polymerase chain reaction testing in children: a segmented regression analysis. J Pediatric Infect Dis Soc 2017;6:142–8.
[42] Mullane KM, Miller MA, Weiss K, et al. Efficacy of fidaxomicin versus vancomycin as therapy for *Clostridium difficile* infection in individuals taking concomitant antibiotics for other concurrent infections. Clin Infect Dis 2011;53:440–7.
[43] Al-Nassir WN, Sethi AK, Li Y, et al. Both oral metronidazole and oral vancomycin promote persistent overgrowth of vancomycin-resistant enterococci during treatment of *Clostridium difficile*-associated disease. Antimicrob Agents Chemother 2008;52:2403–6.
[44] Kuriyama A, Jackson JL, Doi A, et al. Metronidazole-induced central nervous system toxicity: a systematic review. Clin Neuropharmacol 2011;34:241–7.
[45] Gaye A, Sanghavi A. Metronidazole-induced encephalopathy in a pediatric patient. J Allergy Clin Immunol 2007;119:S38.

[46] Gawronka A, Banasiuk M, Lachowicz MS, et al. Metronidazole or rifaximin for treatment of *Clostridium difficile* in pediatric patients with inflammatory bowel disease: a randomized clinical trial. Inflamm Bowel Dis 2017;23(12):2209–14.
[47] Matila E, Arkkila P, Mattila PS, et al. Rifaximin in the treatment of recurrent *Clostridium difficile* infection. Aliment Pharmacol Ther 2013;37:122–8.
[48] Garey KW, Ghantoji SS, Shah DN, et al. A randomized, double-blind, placebo-controlled pilot study to assess the ability of rifaximin to prevent recurrent diarrhoea in patients with *Clostridium difficile* infection. J Antimicrob Chemother 2011;66:2850–5.
[49] Reigadas E, Muñoz-Pacheco P, Vasquez-Cuesta S, et al. Rifaximin-resistant *Clostridium difficile* strains isolated from symptomatic patients. Anaerobe 2017;48:269–72.
[50] Farrell DJ. Rifaximin in the treatment of irritable bowel syndrome: is there a high risk for development of antimicrobial resistance? J Clin Gastroenterol 2013;47:205–11.
[51] Freeman J, Baines SD, Todhunter SL, et al. Nitazoxanide is active against *Clostridium difficile* strains with reduced susceptibility to metronidazole. J Antimicrob Chemother 2011;66: 1407–8.
[52] Musher DM, Logan N, Bressler AM, et al. Nitazoxanide versus vancomycin in *Clostridium difficile* infection: a randomized, double-blind study. Clin Infect Dis 2009;48:e41–6.
[53] Musher DM, Logan N, Mehendiratta V, et al. *Clostridium difficile* colitis that fails conventional metronidazole therapy: response to nitozoxanide. J Antimicrob Chemother 2007;59:705–10.
[54] Sammons JS, Gerber JS, Tamma PD, et al. Diagnosis and management of *Clostridium difficile* infection by pediatric infectious diseases physicians. J Pediatric Infect Dis Soc 2014;3: 43–8.
[55] O'Gorman MA, Michaels MG, Kaplan SL, et al. Safety and pharmacokinetic study of fidaxomicin in children with *Clostridium difficile*-associated diarrhea: a phase 2a multicenter clinical trial. J Pediatric Infect Dis Soc 2018;7:210–8.
[56] Kociolek LK, Gerding DN, Osmolski JR, et al. Differences in molecular epidemiology and antibiotic susceptibility of *Clostridium difficile* isolates in pediatric and adult patients. Antimicrob Agents Chemother 2016;60:4896.
[57] Curry SR, Marsh JW, Shutt KA, et al. High frequency of rifampin resistance identified in in epidemic *Clostridium difficile* clone from a large teaching hospital. Clin Infect Dis 2009;48: 425–9.
[58] Nelson RL, Suda KJ, Evans CT. Antibiotic treatment for *Clostridium difficile*-associated diarrhea in adults. Cochrane Database Syst Rev 2017;(3):CD004610.
[59] McFarland LV, Elmer GW, Surawicz CM. Breaking the cycle: treatment strategies for 163 cases of recurrent *Clostridium difficile* disease. Am J Gastroenterol 2002;97:1769–75.
[60] Martin J, Wilcox M. New and emerging therapies for *Clostridium difficile* infection. Curr Opin Infect Dis 2016;29:546–54.
[61] Van Hise NW, Bryant AM, Hennessey EK, et al. Efficacy of oral vancomycin in preventing recurrent *Clostridium difficile* infection in patients treated with systemic antimicrobial agents. Clin Infect Dis 2016;63:651–3.
[62] Carignan A, Poulin S, Martin P, et al. Efficacy of secondary prophylaxis with vancomycin for preventing recurrent *Clostridium difficile* infections. Am J Gastroenterol 2016;111: 1834–40.
[63] Papic N, Maric LS, Vince A. Efficacy of oral vancomycin in primary prevention of *Clostridium difficile* infection in elderly patients treated with systemic antibiotic therapy. Infect Dis (Lond) 2018;50:483–6.
[64] Tobar-Marcillo M, Guerrero-Duran M, Avecillas-Segovia A, et al. Metronidazole in the prevention of antibiotic-associated diarrhoea and *Clostridium difficile* infection in high-risk hospitalized patients. Gastroenterol Hepatol 2018;41:362–8.
[65] Kociolek LK, Gerding DN. Breakthroughs in the treatment and prevention of *Clostridium difficile* infection. Nat Rev Gastroenterol Hepatol 2016;13:150–60.

[66] Khan MY, Dirweesh A, Khurshid T, et al. Comparing fecal microbiota transplantation to standard-of-care treatment for recurrent *Clostridium difficile* infection: a systematic review and meta-analysis. Eur J Gastroenterol Hepatol 2018; https://doi.org/10.1097/MEG.0000000000001243.
[67] Walia R, Kunde S, Mahajan L. Fecal microbiota transplantation in the treatment of refractory *Clostridium difficile* infection in children: an update. Curr Opin Pediatr 2014;26:573–8.
[68] Drekonja D, Reich J, Gezahegn S, et al. Fecal microbiota transplantation for *Clostridium difficile* infection: a systematic review. Ann Intern Med 2015;162:630–8.
[69] Chen B, Avinashi V, Dobson S. Fecal microbiota transplantation for recurrent *Clostridium difficile* infection in children. J Infect 2017;74:S120–7.
[70] Kelly CR, Ihunnah C, Fischer M, et al. Fecal microbiota transplant for treatment of *Clostridium difficile* infection in immunocompromised patients. Am J Gastroenterol 2014;109:1065–71.
[71] Mills JP, Rao K, Young VB. Probiotics for prevention of *Clostridium difficile* infection. Curr Opin Gastroenterol 2018;34:3–10.
[72] Goldenberg JZ, Yap C, Lytvyn L, et al. Probiotics for the prevention of *Clostridium difficile* diarrhea in adults and children [review]. Cochrane Database Syst Rev 2017;(12):CD006095.
[73] Wilcox MH, Gerding DN, Poxton IR, et al. Bezlotoxumab for prevention of recurrent *Clostridium difficile* infection. N Engl J Med 2017;376:305–17.
[74] Baur D, Gladstone BP, Burkert F, et al. Effect of antibiotic stewardship on the incidence of infection and colonization with antibiotic-resistant bacteria and *Clostridium difficile* infection: a systematic review and meta-analysis. Lancet Infect Dis 2017;17:990–1001.

FSC
www.fsc.org
MIX
Papier | Fördert
gute Waldnutzung
FSC® C083411

Kolibri 360 GmbH
Ferdinand-Jühlke-Straße 7
99095 Erfurt, Deutschland
produktsicherheit@kolibri360.de